Essentials of
Biopharmaceutics
and
Pharmacokinetics

for BPharm, MPharm and Research Scholars

Second Edition

Essentials of
Biopharmaceutics
and
Pharmacokinetics

for BPharm, MPharm and Research Scholars

Second Edition

Ashutosh Kar

Professor Emeritus
Lingaya's University, Faridabad, India

Formerly
Professor, Department of Pharmaceutical Sciences
Apeejay Stya University, Gurugram, India

Professor, School of Pharmacy, Addis Ababa University
Addis Ababa, Ethiopia

Dean, Chairman and Professor, Faculty of Pharmaceutical Sciences
Guru Jambheshwar University, Hisar, India

Professor, School of Pharmacy, Al Arab Medical University
Benghazi, Libya

Professor and Head, Department of Pharmaceutical Chemistry
Faculty of Pharmaceutical Sciences, University of Nigeria
Nsukka, Nigeria

Professor and Head, Department of Pharmaceutical Science
College of Pharmacy, Delhi University
New Delhi, India

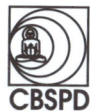

CBSPD

CBS Publishers & Distributors Pvt Ltd

New Delhi • Bengaluru • Chennai • Kochi • Kolkata • Lucknow • Mumbai
Hyderabad • Jharkhand • Nagpur • Patna • Pune • Uttarakhand

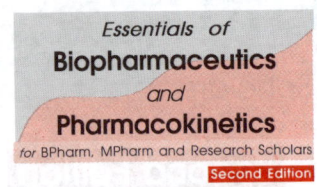

ISBN: 978-93-88327-53-4

Second Edition: 2019

Reprint: 2022

First Edition: 2011

Published by Satish Kumar Jain and produced by Varun Jain for

CBS Publishers & Distributors Pvt Ltd

4819/XI Prahlad Street, 24 Ansari Road, Daryaganj, New Delhi 110 002, India.
Ph: 23289259, 23266861, 23266867   Website: www.cbspd.com
Fax: 011-23243014   e-mail: delhi@cbspd.com; cbspubs@airtelmail.in.

Corporate Office: 204 FIE, Industrial Area, Patparganj, Delhi 110 092
Ph: 011-4934 4934   Fax: 011-4934 4935   e-mail: publishing@cbspd.com; publicity@cbspd.com

Branches

- **Bengaluru:** Seema House 2975, 17th Cross, K.R. Road, Banasankari 2nd Stage, Bengaluru 560 070, Karnataka, India
  Ph: +91-80-26771678/79   Fax: +91-80-26771680   e-mail: bangalore@cbspd.com
- **Chennai:** 7, Subbaraya Street, Shenoy Nagar, Chennai 600 030, Tamil Nadu, India
  Ph: +91-44-26680620, 26681266   Fax: +91-44-42032115   e-mail: chennai@cbspd.com
- **Kochi:** 42/1325, 1326, Power House Road, Opp KSEB, Power House, Ernakulam 682 018, Kochi, Kerala, India
  Ph: +91-484-4059061-67   Fax: +91-484-4059065   e-mail: kochi@cbspd.com
- **Kolkata:** 6/B, Ground Floor, Rameswar Shaw Road, Kolkata 700 014, West Bengal, India
  Ph: +91-33-25633055/56   e-mail: kolkata@cbspd.com
- **Lucknow:** Basement, Khushnuma Complex, 7-Meerabai Marg (Behind Jawahar Bhawan) Lucknow 226001, India
  Ph: +91-522-4000032   e-mail: tiwarilucknow@cbspd.com
- **Mumbai:** PWD Shed, Gala no. 25/26, Ramchandra Bhatt Marg, Next to JJ Hospital Gate no. 2, Opp. Union Bank of India, Noorbaug, Mumbai-400009, Maharashtra, India
  Ph: +91-22-66661880, 66661889   e-mail: mumbai@cbspd.com

Representatives

- **Hyderabad**   0-9885175004
- **Patna**   0-9334159340
- **Jharkhand**   0-9811541605
- **Pune**   0-9623451994
- **Nagpur**   0-9421945513
- **Uttarakhand**   0-9716462459

Printed at: Neekunj Print Process, Haryana, India

to
my beloved parents, sisters and brother
others and my wife
who helped me build-up my life

our sons, daughters-in-law and grand children
who thrilled my life with joy and cheers

my esteemed teachers and taughts
(in India, Nigeria, Libya and Ethiopia)

the august authors; home and abroad
whomsoever the book owes

the people who meticulously toil, to make fruitful the soil
forever and now

Almighty God's eternal blessings,
I respectfully bow, bow and bow

"To teach is to learn twice"

Joseph Jouberi

"Belive in yourself!
Have faith in your abilities!
Without a humble but reasonable confidence in your own powers you
cannot be successful or happy."

Norman Vincent Peale

"Education is a progressive discovery of our own ignorance"

Will Durant

Preface to the Second Edition

Biopharmaceutics and pharmacokinetics are indeed two well-recognized quantitative disciplines. The major aim and objective is meticulously focused to the readers, so as to provide them with an in-depth basic knowledge and understanding of the cardinal fundamental principles of two integrant subjects, namely: Biopharmaceutics and pharmacokinetics. In fact, the overall broad-based generalized intentions are geared significantly to the benefit of its end-users so as to enable them in the specialized applications to the development of both drug product (dosage form) and drug therapy with utmost precision, skill, and accuracy.

The second edition of *Essentials of Biopharmaceutics and Pharmacokinetics* has been thoroughly revised, expanded and updated to the entire benefits of its august readers. Importantly, the popular textual content remains viable and versatile in teaching students the much needed relevant basic concepts, ideas and documented evidences that may be intelligently applied to the thorough understanding and appreciating the complex issues that are intimately associated with the ever increasing and expanding processes (intricate) pertaining and efficacious drug therapy episodes.

The text has been duly classified into five major sections.

Section 1 Biopharmaceutics and Pharmacokinetics: What do they mean?

Section 2 Biopharmaceutics

Section 3 Pharmacokinetics

Section 4 Clinical Pharmacokinetics

Section 5 Bioavailability and Bioequivalence

The present compendium also includes appendices at the end comprising eight subject related most valuable and indispensable information so that the textbook may also serve the purpose of a handy reference book perceptively.

Certain improvements in this edition include predominantly the restructuring of chapters and contents to focus and reflect the latest PCI curriculum in pharmaceutical sciences being implemented from the academic session 2017, in all Indian universities. Special intrinsic care has been duly taken to revise and also to incorporate the latest concepts in the domain of biopharmaceutics and pharmacokinetics. All the figures in each chapter have been redrawn, duly modified, and given in a coloured scheme so that students must get an added-advantage of the neat and well-elaborated diagrams wherever inserted in the text.

I earnestly confides and believes that this text does integrate the underlying fundamental scientific principles and dictums along with clinical pharmacy practice, and also encourage the brilliant students in the field of drug product development with great zeal and gusto. Besides, this revised and expanded edition will vehemently provide a positive help and cater to the basic requirement of all aspirant UG/PG pharmacy students of all Indian universities and also professional courses abroad.

I like to place on record the tremendous help, keen interest, and excellent cooperation by shri Satish Kumar Jain, Hon'ble MD, CBS Publishers & Distributors, New Delhi, for bringing out this book in a record time frame.

Ashutosh Kar

Preface to the First Edition

*E*ssentials of Biopharmaceutics and Pharmacokinetics correlates the intricacies involved in the interdisciplinary interaction of two qualitative subjects. The text has been designed in a manner so as to help its readers comprehend the subject with the insight of a researcher. The primary objective of this textbook is to provide the reader an in depth knowledge of the principles of biopharmaceutics and pharmacokinetics, which could be extended wisely to the product development as well as the drug therapies. The teachers indeed would find the subject matter quite user-friendly and the students shall be able to grasp the basic concepts of complex topics like critical drug delivery modalities and effective safe drug therapy.

The pharmacy degree (BPharm) students in all Indian universities shall be duly benefitted from this textbook because the course content in it has been carefully developed as per the latest prescribed syllabi for BPharm. This book shall further enrich the knowledge of R&D scientists in the pharmaceutics in particular.

The entire course content has been categorized into five sections.

Section 1 Biopharmaceutics and Pharmacokinetics: What do they mean?

Section 2 Biopharmaceutics

Section 3 Pharmacokinetics

Section 4 Clinical Pharmacokinetics

Section 5 Bioavailability and Bioequivalence

Each section in the book deals with a brief introduction, definition, classification, exemplification, laws, graphics, diagrammatic representations, illustrations and highlights, and concludes with selected biography and review questions.

Besides maintaining a logical chain of continuity in all five sections in a lucid manner, an attempt has been made to include very interesting examples that will create enough interest in the fields of biopharmaceutics and pharmacokinetics.

I solemnly believes that this book will provide a positive help and an urgent need to all aspirant UG/PG pharmacy students across various Indian universities. Any suggestions for improvement of the book are invited.

I would like to place on record the excellent help and cooperation by the entire publishing team of Elsevier in bringing out this book in a record time frame.

Ashutosh Kar

Contents

5. Bioavailability and Bioequivalence   (298–361)

Chapter

1

INTRODUCTION TO BIOPHARMACEUTICS AND PHARMACOKINETICS

1.1. INTRODUCTION

Since 1960s till date, most **Pharmaceuticals** right from the *generic* **Analgeric Tablet** being used extensively in the *Community Pharmacy* to the *state-of-the-art* **Immunotherapy** being practiced in *super-specialized* **Hospitals**, invariably subjected to a vigorous research and development (R&D) episode prior to the ultimate approval by the **United States-Food and Drug Administration [US-FDA].**

Importantly, the meticulous systematic well-defined *in-vivo* overall *performance, safety*, and *efficaciousness* of the **Drug Products** (or **Dosage Forms**) are ascertained and established due to: " the various *Physiochemical Characteristics* of the so-called **Active Pharmaceutical Ingredient (API) or Drug Substance, and also the precise and exact route of administration (*viz.,* IV, IM, SC, CSF) are regarded to be the most reliable and critical determinants perceptively."**

In addition, the characteristic features of the '**drug substance**' and its respective '**dosage form**' are being engineered with utmost care and precision and tested to yield a fairly '**stable drug product**' that:

" **on being administered to the respective patients does afford the so-called desired** *Therapeutic Response* **perceptively".**

 NOTE Hence, both *Pharmaceuticals Scientist* and *Pharmacist* should thoroughly understand and comprehend these inherent '*Complex Relationships*' in the use and development of Pharmaceuticals for the benefit of the patients.

Critical Importance of Drug Substance and Drug Formulation

In order to fully understand and illustrate the critical importance of **Drug Substance** and **Drug Formulation** upon these most *vital, prevalent*, and *important* aspects, such as:

- **Absorption Pattern of Drug**, and
- **Distribution Profile of Drug** *in-vivo*,

one would certainly take cognizance of the so-called:

" **sequence of events that essentially precede elicitation of a** *drug's therapeutic effect* **precisely".**

Following are the *four* **sequential stages** that need to ascertain the **Drug's Therapeutic efficacy** predominantly:

➢ *First* the **Drug** in its *Dosage Form* (or **Drug Product**) is administered in the patient *via* **oral, IV, SC, transdermal route of administration.**

➢ *Secondly* the **Drug** gets subsequently released right from the *Dosage Form* (or **Drug Product**) precisely in a **predictable and charactericable modality.**

➢ *Thirdly* certain fraction of the **Drug** gets duly **absorbed from the site of administration** – critically into:

• **Surrounding tissues**, or

• **Various parts of the body*.**

➢ *Fourthly* the **Drug** gains an access to the **site-of-action.** Thus, in a situation when the **drug concentration at the site-of-action** does exceed categorically, at:

"**Minimum Effective Concentration (MEC)**",

one may observe a positive **pharmacologic response**.

Remarks: Importantly, it is quite necessary to ascertain the *actual dosing regimen* (*viz.*, **Dose, Dosage Form, Dosing Interval**) very meticulously in the **Clinical Trials** so as to obtain the accurate and precise **drug concentration at the very site-of-action.**

 NOTE   **Amazingly, the ensuring** *sequence-of-events* **gets affected profoundly, at times seem to be** *orchestrated* **by the respective design of the Dosage Form, Drug itself, or even both.**

This chapter deals specifically with *two* **extremely important aspects,** namely *Biopharmaceutics* and **Pharmacokinetics**. These would be treated individually and briefly in the sections that follow.

Definition and Scope: **Biopharmaceutics** refers to the study of relationship existing *physical, chemical and biological characteristic features* of matter in relation to **drugs, drug products, drug availability and actions.**

1.2. HISTORICAL PERSPECTIVE OF BIOPHARMACEUTICS

Historically, the **Pharmaceutical Scientists** made a genuine effort towards the *systematic evaluation* of the *relative availability* of 'Drug' to the human or animal body in vivo after due administration of the respective **Dosage Form** (or **Drug Product**) and ultimately comprising the following *three* aspects:

• **Particular pharmacologic activity profile,**
• **Clinical responses**, and
• **Possible toxic activity feature.**

Example

Isoproterenol-α, β-adrenergic agonist used as a **Bronchodilator** represents a typical example that shows different pharmacologic activity with different routes of administration, such as:

---

*   That is, quite similar to the '**Oral Dosage Forms**'.

Isoproterenol

Intravenous (IV) administration causes an enhancement in the heart rate. Oral administration shows practically little effect on heart rate.

Interestingly, the **Degree of Bioavailability** also varies appreciably from one particular drug product (**manufactured by 'A'**) to another product (**manufactured by 'B'**) containing the same 'Drug' even though the route of administration remains the same. Nevertheless, the actual observed difference in the **Bioavailability** of the drug substance may be shown by carefully examining the difference in the **specific therapeutic effectiveness of the drug products or the dosage forms.**

It may, however, be concluded that the following *three* **important aspects,** namely:

- **precise nature of the drug molecule**.
- **actual route of administration of the dosage form**, and
- **critical formulation of the drug product may accurately establish and determine whether the 'administered secondary pahramaceutical product' is deemed to be**

  (a) **effective therapeutically,**
  (b) **toxic in nature,** and
  (c) **devoid of any apparent pharmacologic effect.**

As to date, **Biopharmaceutics** has virtually emerged as the most versatile and well-developed scientific discipline that actually looks at closely the prevailing inter-relationship among the following *three* **critical aspects,** such as:

- **drug's physicochemical features,**
- **drug product (dosage form) in which medicament is administered**, and
- **route of drug administration [*i.e.*, intramuscular (IM), intravascular (IV), subcutaneous (SC)] exerting its effect upon the ensuing rate as well as degree of systemic drug absorption.**

In other words, **Biopharmaceutics** predominantly gets influenced by *four* **cardinal circumstances,** which essentially contributes towards:

- **actual stability of the drug within the dosage form,**
- **actual release pattern of the drug from the dosage form,**
- **actual rate of dissolution or release profile of the drugs at the site of absorption (*in vivo*),** and
- **actual absorption of the drug systematically.**

Fig:1.1. illustrates, the detailed **Block-Diagram** of the so-called '*General Scheme*' that elaborates comprehensively the **dynamic** relationship prevailing explicitly amongst the **Drug-Dosage Form- Pharmacological- and/or Clinical Pharmacokinetic-Response** predominantly.

Remarks: The everexpanding discipline of **Biopharmaceutics** critically focuses upon the following *two* **aspects** generously:

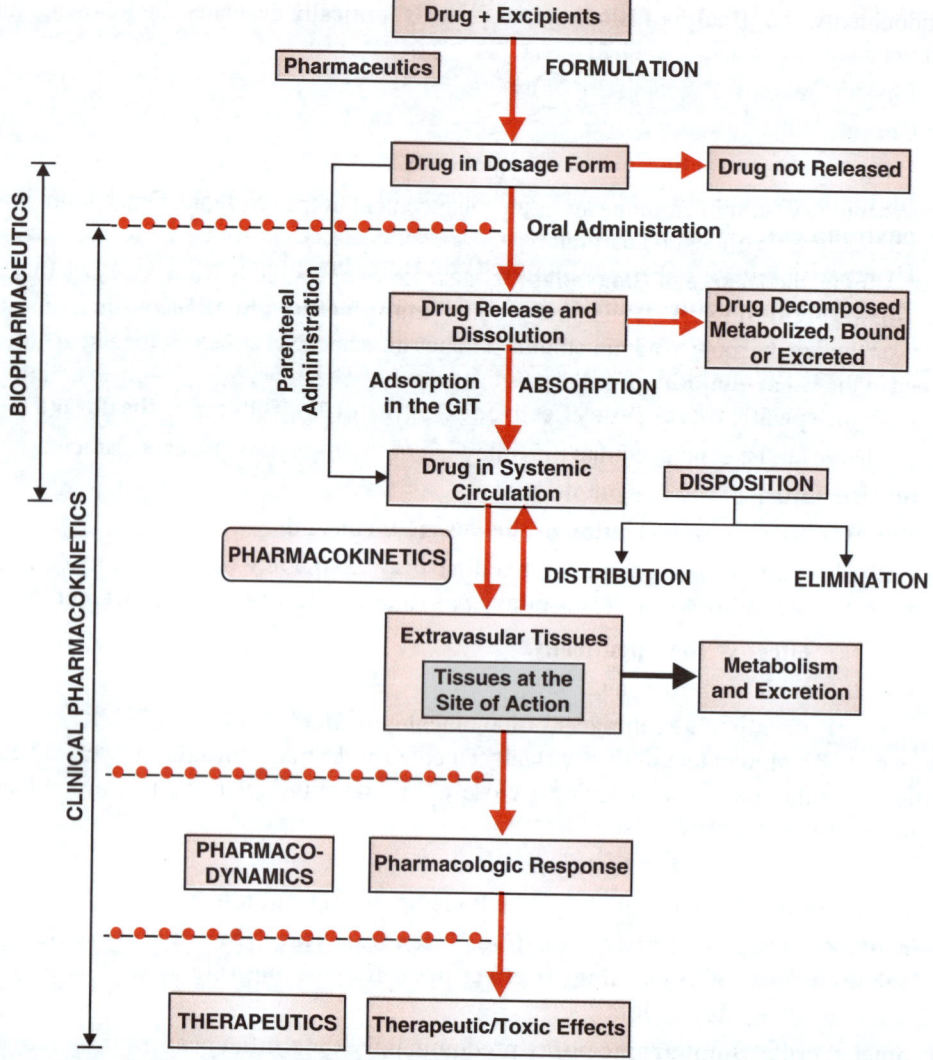

Fig. 1.1: Diagrammatic Representation of a 'General Scheme' Demonstrating Evidently the Dynamic Relationship Existing Among Drug Dosage Form Pharmacologic or Clinical Pharmacokinetic Response.

- **Fundamental Scientific Principles;** and
- **Detailed *in-vivo* Investigative Studies**.

Thus, we may have the following glaring scientific revelations:

In vitro investigative studies : Essentially comprise an array of pharmacologic test apparatus, *e.g.*, **analgesiometer activity cage, rota-rod apparatus, conditioned-avoidance response apparatus**; and

In vivo investigative studies : Essentially includes rather complex evaluations engaging **healthy human subjects** or even **healthy laboratory** animals (*with known strains*).

Undoubtedly, the '**Realm of Biopharmaceuticals**' critically evaluates the following much-needed valuable information as/stated under:

- **Physical–chemical properties of drugs,**
- **Commercial production of drugs,**
- **Large scale production of the dosage forms based solely upon the actual observed biologic response of the active constituent (drug) in a typical physiological environment,**
- **Drugs with a preplanned (anticipated) therapeutic applications,** and
- **Establish the specific 'route of administration' of the drug product.**

1.3. EXTRAVASCULAR ADMINISTRATION OF A DRUG

A **drug** on being administered to a subject by an **Extravascular Route** (*i.e.*, **outside the vessel**) should by all means be transferred right from the **Dosage Form** (*viz.* **tablet, capsule, injection**) to the '**Circulating Blood**' so as to remain **Bioavailable**. It is, therefore, suggested emphatically that **Bioavailability** involves as a necessary consequence the following *two* **vital and important aspects,** namely:

- **Exact and precise quantum of drug entering the blood stream,** and
- **Rate at which drug gains entry to blood stream**

Biopharmaceutics, therefore, may be defined as '**the critical study of such factors that eventually influence the bioavailability**[*] **and the subsequent utilization of this accumulated knowledge in order to optimize the ultimate clinical success of the Drug Products**'.

Earlier, it was believed that the actual prevailing **Therapeutic Response of a Drug** is predominantly by virtue of its **Intrinsic Pharmacologic Activity.**[*] Nevertheless, as to date, it is reasonably understood and overwhelmingly conceptualized that the '**dose-response relationship**' duly accomplished after the administration of a drug *via* different routes, such as: **oral, SC** and **parenteral**, do not show the same response. In addition, there are certain obvious noticeable variations in the critical anticipated response when the 'same drug' is being administered either at **different dosage forms** or **identical dosage forms** (*produced by several manufacturers*), which exclusively depend, in turn, on a host of **cardinal governing factors,** namely:

- **Physiochemical parameters of the drug,**
- **Presence of several excipients in the dosage form,**
- **Method of formulation adopted,** and
- **Actual route of administration of a drug.**

Bearing in mind the importance and impact of the above-cited **intricacies, technicalities,** and **therapeutic evaluations of a Dosage Form** necessitated the development and evolution of an altogether new and separate '**discipline**' termed as **Biopharmaceutics** so as to take care of all important criteria/factors, which ultimately exert a gainful and visible response upon the **therapeutic effectiveness of a drug.**

---

[*] **Bioavailability**: It refers to the rate and extent of absorption of a drug from a dosage form into the inner compartments of the body.

[**] **Intrinsic Pharmacologic Activity**: It refers to the pharmacologic activity with respect to these degree of response initiated as a result of a drug-receptor interaction.

1.4. SCOPE OF BIOPHARMACEUTICS

In the recent past, the scope of **Biopharmaceutics** has attained a glorious new height. Impotantly, almost all **Pharmaceuticals** ranging from the simple **Generic Analgesic Dosage Forms** [*viz.* **Acetaminophen Tablets (USA), Paracetamol Tablets (Asia)** and its branded counterparts: **Tylenol (McNeil consumer), Valadol (Squibb), Tapar (Parke-Davis)**] that are being sold either as **'Over-the-Consumer (OTC) Drugs'** or in the **Community Pharmacy'** across the globe in comparison to the highly sophisticated state-of-the-art medicaments invariably used for **immunotherapy** in modern specialized hospitals [*viz.*, **Mithracin (Pfizer-Roaring, Dome)-Antineoplastic Agent, Harmony] [Abbott]- antipsychotics**] are being subjected to both meticulous development and extensive research before getting the due approval from the **US-FDA***:

Besides, there are quite a few **critical determinants** pertaining to the *in vivo* **performance, efficiency and safety of the Dosage Form or Drug Product** or **Secondary Pharmaceutical Product** that are entirely dependent upon such crucial factors as given below:

- **Active Pharmaceutical Ingredient(s) (APIs) in relation to their inherent physiochemical properties,**
- **Dosage Form (*i.e.*, Formulated Product) itself,** and
- **Route of administration of medicament.**

Biopharmaceutics Classification Systems (BCS)- Interestingly, as an integral segment of :

- **Safety** and
- **Efficacy**

The overall assessment of a **Generic Drug Product**, the recognized *Regulatory Bodies* do critically need an elaborated and comprehensive **Bioavailability (BA) Study** (see also *section 1.10*) together with a **Bioequivalence (BE) study** *vis-à-vis* the research-based **Innovator Product** perceptively, whose actual **Safety** as well as **Efficacy aspects** would have been adequately ascertained *via* the so-called stipulated expensive *Clinical Trials* [*i.e.*, an absolute mandatory conditionalities laid down by **US-FDA** for approved marketing the respective **Dosage Forms** globally].

Besides, such investigative studies do need an *in-vivo* **comparisons** of the resulting **Plasma-Drug Concentration** in the *healthy human subjects* perceptively between:

- **Actual Test and** - **Reference Products**

Consequently, the **BCS** was eventually introduced and promulgated along with certain specified guidelines from the **US-FDA** ultimaltely.

NOTE | The Regulatory Objective of the BCS is to render the *Drug Development and Review Phenomenon* by recommending a clear strategy for replacing certain BE studies with *Surrogate in-vitro* Dissolution Tests.

The progress in the domain of **Pharmaceuticals Technology** has made it possible to preplan about the characteristic features of both the **Drug** (*e.g.*, through **Prodrugs**) and the **Secondary Pharmaceutical Product** via carefully engineered means, thereby producing a fairly stable drug

---

*   **US-FDA:** United States Food and Drug Administration.

product, which on being administered to a patient gives rise to appropriate and desired therapeutic response significantly.

In short, it may be added that both the **Pharmacist** and the **Pharmaceutical Scientist** may have to play a big, pivotal and responsible job with utmost concerned efforts to understand thoroughly these intricate, transcrucial and complex relationships so as to apprehend the appropriate *usage* and *meaningful* development of Pharmaceuticals of the **Future.**

1.5. VARIANTS IN BIOPHARMACEUTICS

Biopharmaceutics refers to the science that:

"**Examines critically the inherent relationship of the so-called** *Physicochemical characteristic features* **of the Drug substance, the** *Dosage Form* **in which the drug is being administered, and finally the route of administration upon the rate and the** *degree of systemic absorption of the Drug*".

The enormous scientific revelations and literature survey that the discipline **Biopharmaceutics** essentially involves are the following *four* **cardial** aspects perceptively, such as:

    (a) **Stability of the** *Drug* **within the** *Drug Product* **(or Dosage Form);**

    (b) **Release pattern of the** *Drug* **from the** *Drug Product*;

    (c) **Rate of Dissolution/Release profile of the** *Drug* **at the** *absorption site;* and

    (d) **Critical** *Systemic Absorption* **of the** *Drug.*

Fig:1.2 depicts a *general scheme* between the **Drug Substances** and the **Drug Product** *vis-a-vis* the resulting **Pharmacologic Effect.**

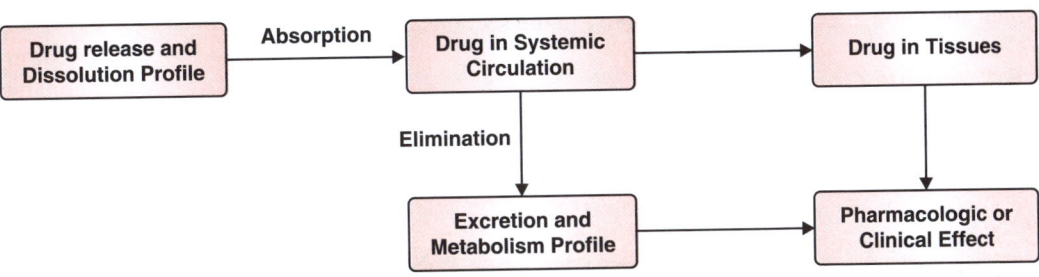

Fig. 1.2: Representation of the Scheme Depicting Dynamic Relationship between the Drug and the Drug Product *vis-a-vis* the Pharmacologic Effect.

Having mustered a fairly sufficient understanding of the **Basics of Biopharmaceutics**, it is indeed a prime requirement to have a closer look at the various **Variants in Biopharmaceutics**, such as:

- **Pharmacokinetics**,
- **Clinical Pharmacokinetics**,
- **Pharmacodynamics**,
- **Toxicokinetics and Clinical Toxicology,** and
- **Bioavailability**.

which shall now be discussed briefly in this introductory chapter so as to familiarize the readers with these above-mentioned terminologies. The objective is to recognize the inherent importance of these factors in the *design, formulation,* and *large-scale production of drug products* across the globe to help ultimately the mankind to lead a **'better quality of life'**.

1.6. PHARMACOKINETICS

Pharmacokinetics refers to –'**the study of how compounds (or *chemical entities*) are absorbed, distributed, metabolized, and eliminated (ADME) by the body. (*i.e.*, the study of how the body acts upon the drug)'**.

Alternatively, **Pharmacokinetics** relates to '**the study of the quantitative relationships pertaining to the rates of drug absorption, distribution, and elimination processes *i.e.*, the data used to establish the specific dosage amount and frequency for the desired therapeutic response'**.

In true sense, the volume of data so generated may be used both intelligently and judiciously to:

> ➤ **obtain and ascertain the precise and exact '*dosage regimen'*,** and
> ➤ **establish perceptively the frequency of a drug to accomplish the so-called desired and intended therapeutic response predominantly.**

Pharmacokinetics may be further studied, explored, and expatiated under the following *three* **heads**, namely:

- *Modus Operandi,*
- **Salient Features of Pharmacokinetics**, and
- **Experimental Aspects of Pharmacokinetics,**

which shall now be discussed individually in the sections that follows:

1.6.1. *Modus Operandi*

The **Extravascular Administration of Drugs** may be achieved in a variety of mean and ways, such as:

- **Buccal,**
- **Intramuscular (IM),**
- **Intravenous (IV),**
- **Intraocular (IO),**
- **Intraoperative,**
- **Intraparietal,**
- **Intraperitoneal,**
- **Intrarenal,**
- **Intraspinal,**
- **Intrathecal,**
  Intravesical,
  Intraventricular,
  Rectal,
  Subcutaneous (SC), and
  Topical,

and the results thus obtained when plotted between the **Observed Plasma Concentration and Time (in hours),** distinctly show an initial increase followed by a subsequent decrease, as illustrated in Figure 1.3. However, the **observed drug plasma concentration evidently passes** *via* **a maximum value** C_{max} at time T_{max}.

It is, however, pertinent to state here that the administered **'Drug'** should be released right from the **Dosage Form** (*viz*. **Tablet, Capsule, Injection**) *via* several **Physiological Barriers** (*viz*. **Biological Membranes, Body Fluid**) in order to gain its legitimate entry into the circulating blood, as depicted explicitly in Fig. 1.4.

In fact, an elaborated study of the aforesaid phenomenon should usually comprise the following *two* aspects, namely:

- **Total quantum of drugs absorbed** *in-vivo,* and
- **Rate of absorption of drug.**

1.6.2. *Salient Features of Pharmacokinetics*

These essentially include the following *five* important aspects, namely:

1. **Experimental segment of pharmacokinetics includes** *three* **cardinal points:**
   - **Critical development of newer biological sampling techniques,**
   - **Latest analytical techniques [*e.g.*, liquid chromatography–mass spectrometry, gas chromatography and mass spectrometry, high performance liquid chromatography (HPLC), reversed-phase HPLC, differential scanning calorimetry]: for the assay of drugs and metabolites*,** and
   - **Various procedures, which categorically facilitate data collection and manipulation.**

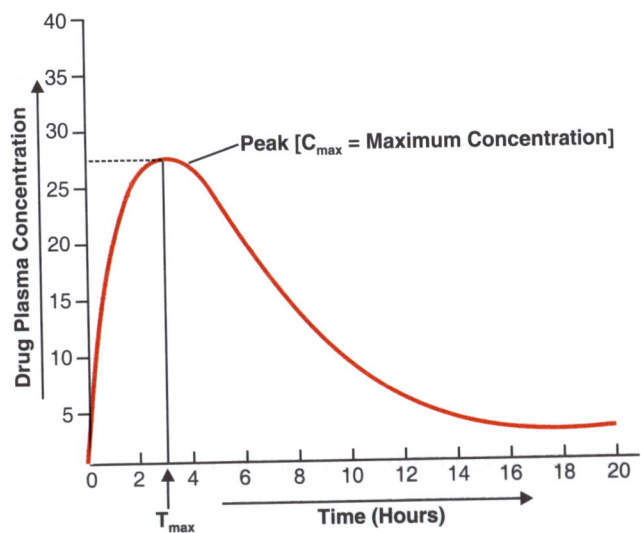

Fig. 1.3: A Plot between Drug Plasma Concentration vs. Time (hours) Following Administration of Drug *via* Extravascular Route.

---

* Kar A: **Pharmaceutical Drug Analysis,** 3rd ed., New Age International, Pvt Ltd, New Delhi, 2016.

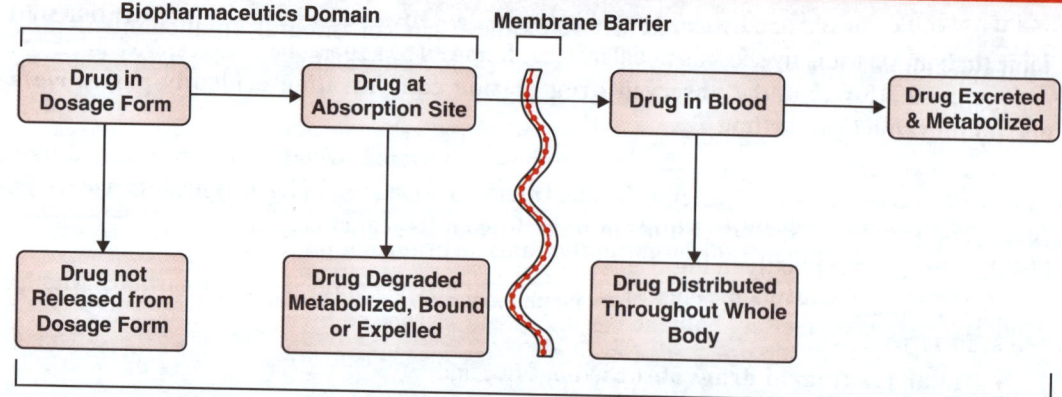

Fig. 1.4: Drug in Dosage form Shown in Pharmaceutics Domain and in Pharmacokinetics Domain.

2. Theoretical segment of **Pharmacokinetics** embraces critically the meticulous and development of an array of **Sophisticated Pharmacokinetics Models** which may be responsible for the precise prediction of drug deposition soon after drug administration *via* a known route.

3. **Biostatistics: Biostatistics** refers to 'the application of statistical processes and methods to the analysis of biological data'. It essentially forms an integral part of the **Pharmacokinetics Studies** to determine **vital aspects,** namely:

   • **Pharmacokinetics Parameter,**

   • **Data Interpretation,**

   • **Predict the Actual Designing of 'Optimal Dosing Regimen' for Individuals or Groups of Patients,** and

   • Applicable to Various Pharmacokinetics Models to Determine both

      (a) **Data Error and**

      (b) **Structural Model Deviations.**

4. **Computational and Mathematical Techniques** based on the *theoretical aspects* pertaining to a host of **Pharmacokinetics Methods.**

5. Exercising and implementing of **'Classical Pharmacokinetics'**, which critically deals with the study of **Absolute Theoretical Models** that solely forms the centre of activity with respect to the following *two* **features**, such as:

   • **Model Development,** and

   • **Parameterization.**

1.6.3. *Experimental Aspects of Pharmacokinetics*

The **experimental aspects of Pharmacokinetics** essentially involves the following *three* **vital and important** features, such as:

• **Specific Development of Biologic Sampling Methods,**

• **Analytical Techniques for the Measurement of Drugs and Metabolites,** and

• **Typical Procedures that Essentially Facilitate Data Collection and Manipulation.**

Besides, the **application of statistics** does form an integral component of most **Pharmacokinetic Investigative Studies.** However, the **Statistical Procedures** are being used solely for:

- **Pharmacokinetics Parameter Estimation**, and
- **Data Interpretation**,

so as to accomplish finally the very **purpose of designing and predicting the so-called optimized dosing regimens for either individuals or groups of patients.**

Advantages of Statistical Methods: These are exclusively applied to the **Pharmacokinetics Models** to estimate precisely both the ensuring **Data Error** and **Structural Model Deviations** perceptively. Also the intelligent usage of **mathematical and computational procedures** do critically form the so-called **Theoretical Basis of a Host of Pharmacokinetics Methodologies.**

1.7. CLINICAL PHARMACOKINETICS

Clinical Pharmacokinetics refers to 'the application of Pharmacokinetics principles for the Rational Design of an individualized dosage regimen'.

However, the *two* **major objectives** are as given below:

> Maintenance of maximum drug concentration at the receptor-site in order to accomplish the desired therapeutic response for a pre-determined period, and

> Manipulation of any Advance Drug Response (ADR) or Toxic Effects of the Drug being tested.

Another school of thought relates the application of **Pharmacokinetics** to the safe and effective therapeutic management of an individual patient exclusively.

Interestingly, the necessity related to a '**Drug Therapy**' more or less designates, an unpredictable, hit-and-miss, absolute gamble; nevertheless, the gainful optimization of the ensuing '**Benefit-to-Risk**' ratio is the ultimate reward. In fact, the factual statement entirely based upon the so-called population averages crucially refer to as one's acclaimed knowledge on drug action(s).

In actual practice, while expressing critically the '**Normal Dosage Regime**n' of a **drug product,** the so-called anticipated results are invariably projected as a '**Statistical Most Probable Best Guess**' that may be termed as follows:

- **Usual dosage of a drug** and
- **Actions and adverse drug reactions.**

As-to-date, medical practitioners or clinicians do have a tendency to recognize that each and every individual subject is altogether '**different**'; and, therefore, the usual '**Practice of Medicine**' predominantly tries to;

- **Predict and avoid 'Non average Complications',** or
- **Readjust therapeutic approach solely based on the specific observations pre-emptively.**

The influx of **Newer Drug Products** in the past couple of decades have urgently necessitated the particular active and vigilant consideration(s) being more important than the prevailing characteristics features pertaining to the ensuing **drug-patient interaction that may eventually enhance the** possibility and likelihood of attaining a rather more definite **favourable benefit-to-risk ratio perceptively.**

The survey of literature reveals that there are several excellent examples of drug substance that obviously illustrates and expatiate the fundamental clinical usage of the **Principles of Pharmacokinetics** in accomplishing a positive improvement in the prospects related to the **magnificent success in drug therapy.**

Thus, one may come across *individualized* **'Pharmacokinetics Variations'**, which may categorically come into play in such *in vitro* processes, namely **ADME**. Consequently, the aforesaid biological phenomena are duly influenced, affected and guided by disease conditions, age, drugs and the like.

Clinical Pharmacokinetics in true sense makes use of the **well-defined, recognized and accepted methodologies so as to counteract or negate these influences by intelligently and skillfully affording individualization of drug therapy.** It has been duly observed and established that two major situations invariably come into being on account of either **intra-individual variation or inter-individual variation, for instance:**

- **Subtherapeutic response of a drug product, wherein the concentration of the drug stands below the minimum effective concentration (MEC), or**
- **Toxic response of drug product, wherein the concentration of the drug remains above the minimum toxic concentration (MTC),**

which would perhaps predominantly need an immediate adjustment to the prevailing dosing regimen. Thus, **Clinical Pharmacokinetics** predominantly involves the broad application of various **Pharmacokinetic Methodologies** in the domain of **drug therapy**. It will be worthwhile to impress at this point in time that '**Clinical Pharmacokinetics**' critically embraces a purely multidisciplinary approach with respect to the individually optimized dosing strategies that are exclusively based upon the patient's actual disease condition *vis-a-vis* patient-specific related careful thoughts.

In the light of the aforesaid statement of facts and observations, one may safely come to a meaningful conclusion. That the valuable and informative inputs derived from the extensive and intensive studies pertaining to the **Clinical Pharmacokinetics of drug products in various disease conditions do require input from medical research as well as pharmaceutical research.**

Based on the **National Vital Statistics Report (2003)*** of the **rate of death**** from 10 most glaring causes of death in the United States, which has been duly provided in Table 1.1.

1.7.1. *Therapeutic Drug Monitoring (TDM) and Pharmacokinetics*

Quite recently, the tentacles of **Pharmacokinetics** have been duly explored, evaluated and utilized effectively in most versatile and urgently needed **Therapeutic Drug Monitoring (TDM)**. Importantly, TDM is generally applicable to extremely **potent drug substances,** *viz.* **Aminoglycosides: Streptidine, Spectinamine** and **Anticonvulsants: Sulthiame, Valproic Acid**, usually having a narrow therapeutic range in order to accomplish the following **two main objectives:**

- **To optimize efficacy of drug product,** and
- **To check and prevent any possible adverse toxicity.**

Therefore, in order to carry out **TDM** in a methodical manner, it is absolutely necessary to place the patient under constant vigil for monitoring in *two* **accepted means**, namely:

---

* National Vital Statistics Report (USA): **52** (3), 2003.

** Age-adjusted death rates by male-female ratio.

- **Plasma-Drug concentration levels** (*e.g.*, Theophylline, Hydrocortisone), and
- **Particular Pharmacodynamic end point,** *viz.* prothrombin-clotting time (*e.g.*, Warfarin, Heparin)

Table 1.1. Observed Ratio of Age-adjusted Death Rates Obtained by Male-Female Ratio Derived from 10 Leading Causes of Death in the United States (2003)

S. No.	Disease Conditions	Rank	Male-Female Ratio
1	Heart disease	1	1.5
2	Malignant neoplasms	2	1.5
3	Cerebrovascular disease	3	4
4	Chronic liver respiration disease	4	1.4
5	Accidents and others	5	2.2
6	Diabetes mellitus	6	1.2
7	Pneumonia and influenza	7	1.4
8	Alzheimer	8	0.8
9	Nephritis, nephritic syndrome	9	1.5
10	Septicaemia	10	1.2

NOTE The clinical Pharmacokinetics service attached to modern hospitals does provide requisite urgent pharmacokinetics and drug-analysis services that are more or less indispensable for 'safe-drug monitoring'.

1.8. PHARMACODYNAMICS

Pharmacodynamics relates to 'the study of the physiological effects and mechanisms of action of a chemical entity (compound), and how this varies with either concentration/ dosage or the study of how the drug acts upon the body'.

Alternatively, **Pharmacodynamics refers to** 'the study of absorption, distribution, metabolism, and excretion (ADME) drug *i.e.*, explaining the mechanism of action and its biochemical and physiological effects perceptively'.

Pharmacodynamics turns to the information of the in-depth study of **ADME of a drug with specific reference to its:**

- **Mechanism of action,**
- **Biochemical reaction,** and
- **Physiological effect.**

In other words, **Pharmacodynamics** designates 'the study of drugs and their subsequent actions upon the living organism'.

Pharmacodynamics invariably described the character of the specific concentration of a drug at the very site of action *vis-à-vis* its ensuing relationship to the magnitude of observed physiological effects.

In a rather much simpler version, **Pharmacodynamics** deals with what the drug actually does to the body very much in contrast to **'Pharmacokinetics',** which is essentially a study of what the body does to the drug.

Another school of thought defines **Pharmacodynamics** as 'refurbishing and surrogating the ensuing relationship between the concentration of the drug at the 'Receptor Site' (*i.e.,* site of action) and the corresponding pharmacologic response, *i.e.,* the various biochemical and physiological effects, which ultimately are responsible for the interaction of a 'drug molecule with the receptor'.**

In this manner, the interaction of a drug molecule with a receptor initiate a remarkable sequence of molecular event that may give rise to either a **pharmacological response or a toxic response**.

The skillful and judicious design of the so-called **Pharmacokinetics-Pharmacodynamic Model,** in fact, offers an excellent bridge of relationship between *two* **important entities**:

- **Plasma-drug level,** and
- **Drug concentration at the receptor site,**

thereby establishing and ascertained the intensity as well as time course of the drug under investigation.

1.9. TOXICOKINETICS AND CLINICAL TOXICOLOGY

Toxicokinetics refers to the critical and specific application of pharmacokinetic principles to the so-called:

"Design, Conduct, and Interpretations of drug safety evaluation studies in a comprehensive manner".*

The above findings were used in validating the dose-related exposure to animals subsequently. Importantly, the resulting **Toxicokinetic Data** does help in a big way in the critical interpretations of the ensuing **toxicological findings** in the animals. Thus, the results were carefully extrapolated *vis-a-vis* the resulting data to humans perceptively.

Obviously, the **Toxicokinetic Investigative Studies** are invariably carried out in healthy laboratory animals in the course of the so-called **Proclinical Drug Development** episodes, which may even be extended beyond to maintain the continuity profile after 'drug' has been subjected to the **test in the Clinical Trials.****

Clinical Toxicology relates **to 'the study of the Adverse Drug Effects (ADE) and the respective toxic substances (*poisonous*) in the body'**.

Observations: They essentially comprise

1. The '**Pharmacokinetics**' of a drug usually in an **over-medicated** (*intoxicated*) patient may

---

* Leal M *et al*: **Use of Toxiokinetic Principles in Drug Development: Bridging Preclinal and Clinical Studies**, In: Yakobi A *et al* (Eds.): *Integration of Pharmacokinetics, Pharmacodynamics, and Toxicokinetics in Rational Drug Development*, Plenum Press, New York, pp: 55-67, 1993.

** Clinical Trial: It refers to a carefully designed and executed investigation of the 'drug' being adminstered to human subjects. The main goal is to define the clinical efficiency and pharmacological effects (e.g., toxicity, side-effects, incompatibilities or interactions). US-FDA requires strict testing of all new drugs before their approval for use as therapeutic agents.

be very different *vis-a-vis* the **Pharmacokinetic**s of the *same drug* being given in relatively **lower-therapeutic dose levels.**

2. However, at **very high-doses** the observed drug concentration present in the human body may saturate the enzymes that are involved perceptively in:

- **Absorption**
- **Biotransformation** and
- **Active Renal Excretions Mechanisms,**
  - thereby altering the ensuing **Pharmacokinetic profiles from linear to non-linear Pharmacokinetics ultimately.**

1.10. BIOAVAILABILITY

Bioavailability refers to '**the precise proportion of a medicine (drug product or dosage form) reaching the systemic circulation soon after a specific-predetermined-route of administration'.**

First-Pass Metabolism-It relates to the most prevalent and significant factor in the determination of **Bioavailability** profile of a **Drug Product (Medicine).** Furthermore, it critically ascertains the so-called **presystemic metabolism** taking place either at the intestine or the liver perceptively.

Examples: A few classical examples essentially comprise:

- An array of **lipid-soluble medicines** *viz.*, β**-Blockers***[**metaprolol**®], a few *Tricyclic Antidepressant Drugs,* and an altogether different *opiate* Analgesics are affected quite severely.
- Besides, the food may also affect the **bioavailability** *via* several proven and established means and ways, such as:
  - **Modification of Gastric Emptying Process,** and
  - **Hence slowing Medicine Absorption Profile.**

> **NOTE** **Ingested Calcium may specifically combine with Medicines (drug substances)** *viz., Tetracyclines* **further reduce the absorption of Ca^{2+} systematically.**

US-FDA defines '**Bioavailability**' as '**the rate and extent to which the drug substances gets absorbed and becomes available at the site of action'.**

Based on the extensive and intensive survey of literature reveals that there are *four* **distinct and important Functional Terminologies for Bioavailability,** namely:

- **Absolute Bioavailability,**
- **Relative Bioavailability,**
- **Quantifying Absolute Availability,** and
- **Quantifying Relative Availability,**

which shall now be discussed individually in the sections that follows:

---

* β**-Blockers:** It is also known as: **Beta-Adrenoreceptor Blocking Drugs** or **Beta Blockers (Metapcolol**®]-that eventually inhibit the effects caused by the stimulation of β$_1$- and β$_2$-**adrenergic neurons.**

1.10.1. *Absolute Bioavailability*

Bioavailability refers to 'a comparison of the extent of a drug being absorbed *in vivo via* altogether different means, using IV administration as a standard procedure.* That is without considering the rate of absorption. Nevertheless, the 'absolute bioavailability' is namely guided by such vital and important characteristics features, such as:

- **Active substance (*i.e.*, drug), and**
- **Absorption receptor site.**

1.10.2. *Relative Bioavailability*

In true sense, the critical importance for the evaluation of the **Secondary Pharmaceutical Products** (or) **Dosage Forms** actually looked at from a **formulator's point of view** in an event when a newer pharmaceutical formulation is being crafted and designed. In actual practice, one may eventually come across *two* **possible options,** namely:

- *First*, that exclusively deals with the so-called **Comparative Bioavailability** when the rate and degree of absorption are duly subjected to comparison by a '**generic equipment**' *vis-a-vis* an '**Innovative-Researched Product**'. As a result, one would favourably expect that the ensuing **Pharmacokinetic Parameters** must agree very intimately for the aforesaid *two* formulations (*viz.* generic/researched product). Thus, the *two* altogether different drug products are regarded overwhelmingly to be **Bioequivalent.**
- *Second,* that critically demands to alter and modify the existing **Pharmacokinetic profile** of the so-called **Patent Formulation,** *e.g.*, **modified drug-release dosage form(s).** obiviously, in such an instance one may make use of the **Pharmacokinetic profile** of the '**Patent Formulation**' as an ideal means of comparison to access and record the extent of absorption.

Interestingly, the most relevant and important definitions of their relationships are intelligently pieced together and depicted in Figure 1.5

In short, it may be added that while '**Clinical Pharmacokinetics**' studies are found to be useful in determining the safety and efficacy of **Dosage Forms** (or **Drug Product**), and the **Bioavailability studies** are meant to define the overall ensuing effect of changes taking place in the **physiochemical characteristics** of.

- **Drug Substance, and**
- **Effect of Drug Product (or Dosage form),**

upon the **Pharmacokinetics of the Drug.**

1.10.3. *Qualifying Absolute Availability*

The **Absolute Availability of a Drug** represents precisely the **Systemic Availability** of a **Drug** after an **extravascular administration** (*viz.* oral, rectal, SC, transdermal) *vis-a-vis* **IV dosing alternatively.**

In general, the **Absolute Availability of a Drug** is measured by comparing meticulously two vital aspects, namely:

- **Respective Area Under Curves (AUCs) after oral, rectal, SC, transdermal administrations, and**
- **Corresponding IV administration.**

---

* That is without considering the rate of absorption.

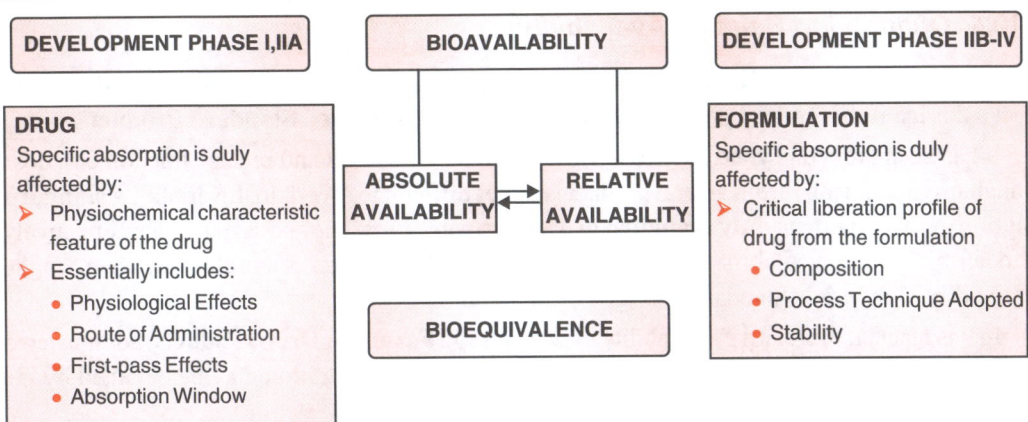

Fig. 1.5: Bioavailability and Related Terminologies.

However, the measurement of **Absolute Availability** may be carried out so far as both 'V_d*' and k ** remain grossly independent of the route of administration.

Importantly, one may obtain the **Absolute Availability,** after due oral administration by making use of the ensuing '**Plasma Concentration Data**' as given below:

$$\text{Absolute availability F} = \frac{(\text{AUC})_{PO}/\text{Dose}_{PO}}{(\text{AUC})_{IV}/\text{Dose}_{IV}} \tag{a}$$

Besides, the **Absolute Availability** may also be represented as a fraction or as a percent by multiplying **F×100.** On the basis of the **Urinary Drug Excretion Data,** one may express the **Absolute Availability** as stated below:

$$\text{Absolute availability} = \frac{(\text{DU})^{\infty}_{PO}/\text{Dose}_{PO}}{(\text{DU})^{\infty}_{IV}/\text{Dose}_{IV}} \tag{b}$$

Important points: Following are four **important points** pertaining to **Absolute Availability.**

1. It is equal to 'F' *i.e.,* **the critical fraction of the dose or the bioavailable dose**.
2. It is variably expressed as a percent, *i.e.,* **F = 1 or 100%**
3. Intravascularly administered drugs get absorbed almost completely, for instance, IV Bolus.*** Injection, wherein **F = 1**, because almost complete absorption occurs.
4. Extravascularly administered drugs, *e.g.,* **oral route (PO)**, the observed absolute bioavailability 'F' perhaps may not exceed beyond **100% (*i.e.,* F > 1).**

Equations **(a)** and **(b)** given above actually determine the **Absolute Bioavailability 'F'**, where **PO** designated an oral route, and other **Extravascular Route(s)** of drug administration, such as:

- **SC route,**
- **Intraperitoneal route,** and
- **Rectal route.**

---

* V_d: Volume of distribution.

** k: Overall drug elimination rate constant [$k = k_e + k_m$], where k_e = excretion rate constant [first order] k_m = metabolism rate constant [first order].

***   It refers to the **volume of drug given rapidly by IV route 1.**

1.10.4. *Quantifying Relative Availability*

Importantly, the **Relative Availability** (or apparent) refers to the availability of a drug right from a dosage form (or drug product) *vis-a-vis* another '**Recognized Standard Product**'.

It has been proved beyond any reasonable doubt that the exact and precise fraction of a dose available systematically from an oral product is rather difficult to ascertain. Invariably, a **standard solution of the pure drug duly evaluated in a 'Crossover Study'** may be accomplished effectively by determining the availability of drug in the **Dosage Form** (*i.e.,* **Formulation**) *vis-a-vis* the availability of drug in a Standard Dosage Formulation'.

In this manner, the relative availability of two **Dosage Forms** (or **Drug Products**) administered at the identical dosage level and by the identical route of administration may be obtained by the help of the following expression:

$$\text{Relative availability} = \frac{(AUC)_A}{(AUC)_B} \qquad \text{(c)}$$

where, **A** = drug in a dosage form and

       B = recognized reference standard.

The resulting fraction when multiplied by 100 gives rise to the corresponding **Relative Availability.**

In a situation, when different dosage levels are duly administered, a necessary correction as applicable for the exact '**size of the dose**' needs to be incorporated as shown in the following equation:

$$\text{Relative availability} = \frac{(AUC)_A/\text{Dose}_A}{(AUC)_B/\text{Dose}_B} \qquad \text{(d)}$$

Alternatively, one may even make use of the '**Urinary Excretion Data**' in order to measure the relative availability, so far as one maintains to collect the '**Total Quantum of Intact Drug**' excreted in the urine. Thus, it is possible to determine the per cent **Relative Availability** by making use of the **Urinary Excretion Data** as given in the following expression:

$$\text{Percent relative availability} = \frac{(Du)_A^{\infty}}{(Au)_B^{\infty}} \times 100 \qquad \text{(e)}$$

where, **(Du)** = **Total amount of drug excreted in the urine.**

1.11. BIOEQUIVALENCE

Bioequivalence relates to a specific instance when *two* medicines (**Drug Products or Dosage Form**) are said to be **bioequivalent** when they contain the same amount of an identical active chemical entity (compound); and when their **bioavailability** remains the same on being administered in equal doses under similar parameters.

Bioequivalent (Biological Equivalent) relates to '**those equivalents that when administered in the same quantum do provide the same biological or physiological availability profile –as measured precisely by blood-levels and urine-levels**'.

Bioequivalence designates a relative term that essentially denotes that the drug present in two or more *identical dosage forms* (or **drug product**), critically reaches the ensuing systemic circulation usually:

- **At the same relative rate,** and
- **At the same relative degree.***

Obviously, the critical appearance and observations of the statistically significant differences in the *two* or *three* or even more dosage form do indicate the **Bioequivalence.**

1.11.1. *Bioequivalence: The Canadian Regularly Perspective*

Canada enjoys the reputation of being one of the pioneers in the critical application of the 'Concept of Bioequivalence', by virtue of the imposition of **compulsory and mandatory 'Licensing Legislation',** which with effect from **1969 to 1988** (almost a span of two decades) not only promulgated but also facilitated the gainful entry of the '**Generic Drug Product****'.

- **Westlake (1973)***** postulated an artitrary standard of almost 80% extant of bioavailability with respect to a reference product, The **Exprt Advisory Committee on Bioavailability** was duly established in 1974, which eventually carried out and examined several approaches for the in-house stydies due to the urgent and crucial lack of the much-needed statistical procedures for both **Bioavailability** and **Bioequivalence.**

Examples

Phenylbutazone Equivalence Study: **McGilveray *et al*. (1978)** specifically studied the **Plasma Concentration Derived Data**, for instance:

- **Area under the concentration-time curve (AUC),** and
- **Maximum observed concentration (C_{max}).**

which were adequately examined after

  (a) **Transformation to corresponding log value, and**
  (b) **Confidence intervals (CI) up to 95%.**

Table: 1.2 records the different categories of complicated drug substances in the critical and precise assessment of the **Bioequivalence Values** perceptively.

The **Canadian Approach** and **Suggestion to Bioequivalence** predominantly helps in the judicious and logical classification of **Orally Administered Drugs** into *two* **main categories,** namely:

---

* That is, their ensuing plasma concentration-time profiles shall be more or less quite identical without any appreciable observed '**statistical differences**'.

** **Generic Drug Product**s: It essentially refers to a chemically equivalent copy of a brand-name drug whose patent has expired legally.

*** Westlake (1973): Use of Statistical Methods in Evaluation of *in vivo* Performance of Dosage Forms, *J Pharm Sci.*, **62**: 1579-1589, 1973.

- **Uncomplicated Class**, and
- **Complicated Class.**

Table 1.2. Complicated Drug *vis-a-vis* Their Variants for Bioequivalence Evaluation Studies

S. No.	Complicated Variants
1	Sustained (or modified) drug release secondary pharmaceutical products
2	Drugs having either variable or complicated pharmacokinetics profiles, namely: (a) Nonlinear kinetics (*viz.* those having an appreciable first-pass effect say > 40%) (b) Variable kinetics on account of different 'genetic phenotypes'* (c) Stereochemical effects, *viz.* inversion of configuration in vivo and (d) Prolonged plasma half-life (t_{12})
3	Drugs for which the exact 'time of onset of the effect' as well as the precise 'rate of absorption' are equally of prime importance
4	Highly toxic drugs as well as those with a narrow therapeutic range
5	Unabsorbable drug substances and whose therapeutic remains active locally in the GI tract.
6	Typical drugs having no clear cut known measurable technique either sensitive enough or dependable enough to estimate blood concentration up to at least terminal plasma half-lives
7	Combination dosage forms (or drug products)
8	Most biological products, *e.g.*, typhoid vaccine, γ-globulin

Very much in time and in line with the nature and degree of commonly encountered **Bioequivalence problems**.** Various researchers making dedicated contributions across the globe on crucial bioequivalence problems thought it worthwhile to ponder over such cardinal aspects thoughtfully as:

- **Strictly adhere to 'one basic protocol'** *viz.* **single-dose crossover,** and
- **A critical predetermined universally acceptable decision protocol** *viz.* **CI 90% pertaining to the 'relative mean parameter' necessarily falling within the range of 80-120% or 80-125% may not be suitable, practical and feasible for most drug variants,** *e.g.*, **α-lactoms, metronidazole, chloroquine and sulpha drug.**

Interestingly, from a close look of the contents given in Table 1.2, we may find the various types of drugs (or even their respective drug products) that are regarded to be explicitly and overwhelmingly complicated in terms of their critical '**Bioequivalence Assessment**'.

1.11.2. *Uncomplicated Drugs*

The **Uncomplicated Drugs** invariably refer to the various '**Oral Drug Product**' duly marketed as the common conventional formulations, which do not find their place under single or several complicated categories (Table 1.2).

---

* **Genetic Phenotype:** the expression of the genes (pertaining to reproduction) duly presented in an individual.

** **Expert Advisory Committee on Bioavailability:** Report on bioavailability of oral dosage formulations of drug used for systemic effects. Drugs with uncomplicated characteristics, drug Directorate, Health Protection Branch, Health and Family Welfare Canada, 1990.

1.11.3. *Guidelines for Equivalence Studies*

It is, however, pertinent to state here that while making for formulating the guidelines for **Bioequivalence Studies** for the actual conduct and careful analysis, the following array of pivotal factors must be considered, such as:

- **Physiochemical characteristic features,**
- **Pharmacokinetics profile of the drug,**
- **Vital and important clinical aspect,** and
- **A host of methodological aspects,**

for both classification of aforesaid drugs (*viz.* **Complicated ones and Uncomplicated ones as well**).

1.11.4. *Plasma-Drug Concentration Versus Time Curve*

The **Plasma-Drug Concentration** *versus* time curve is usually obtained by determining precisely the **Drug Concentration in Plasma Samples** meticulously drawn at predetermined/ programmed time interval (in hours) soon after a **Drug Product** is duly administered to a patient.

1.11.5. *Modus Operandi*

The various steps that are essentially involved in the preparation of plasma-drug concentration versus time curve are enumerated as follows:

1. The actual concentration obtained after a single oral dose of a drug product being analyzed in each plasma sample is duly plotted on a rectangular coordinate graph paper by taking:
   - **Plasma-drug concentration along *Y*-axis,** and
   - **Time interval* (in hours) along *X*-axis, to obtain a typical curve, as illustrated in Figure 1.5.**
2. Figure 1.6 distinctly elaborates the various observed **Pharmacokinetic** and **Pharmacodynamic** parameters.

Explanations

These essentially comprise:

The various vital and important aspects of the **Plasma-Drug Concentration *Vs* Time Curve** are explained duly as under:

1. Administered drug does have a remarkable tendency to reach the general (systemic) circulation, thereby giving rise to the attainable drug concentration in plasma to a maximum level.
2. Invariably, one may observe critically that the absorption of a drug is found to be more fast and rapid *vis-a-vis* its elimination phenomenon.

---

    *   **Time Interval**: It refers to the corresponding 'time' at which the 'plasma sample' was collected duly from the patient after the administration of the drug product.

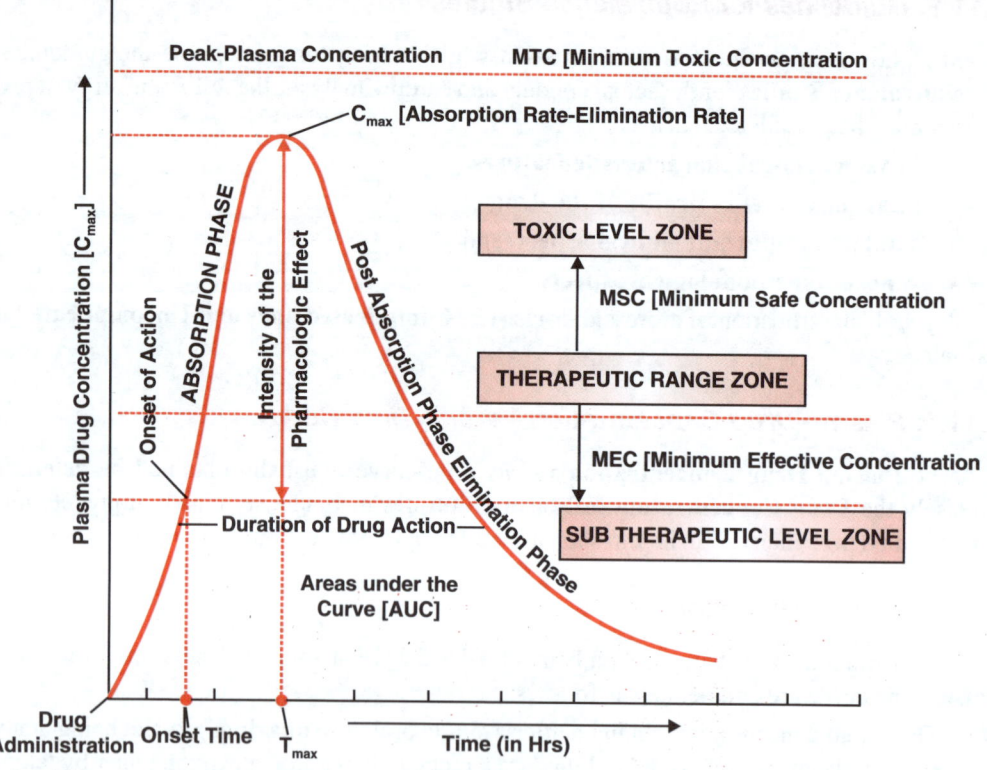

Fig. 1.6: Diagrammatic Representation of a Typical Plasma-Drug Concentration *vs* Time Curve Showing Explicitly Pharmacokinetics Pharmacodynamic Parameters accomplish after Oral Administration of a Single Dose.

3. Importantly, the drug soon after its absorption right into the systemic circulation gets eventually distributed to most of the tissues in the body and ultimately, undergoes elimination simultaneously.

4. Interestingly, the process of 'elimination' may be gainfully accomplished by
   - excretion,
   - biotransformation or
   - a combination of both processes.

5. There are *three* **distinct cut-off points along the Y-axis**, representing **Plasma-Drug Concentration (C_{max})** in Figure 1.5, namely:

   MTC: Minimum toxic concentration,

   MSC: Maximum safe concentration, and

   MEC: Minimum effective concentration.

   MEC: Such drugs that act specifically upon the **Autonomus Nervous System**, namely:
   - **Norepinephrine-acting on the sympathetic system,** and
   - **Acetylcholine-acting on the parasympathetic system.**

It is absolutely necessary and useful to know the actual concentration of 'drug substance' which would just afford a bare **minimum level of pharmacologic effect.** At this point in time, let us assume that the prevailing concentration of the drug substance duly presented in the plasma remains to be in perfect equilibrium status with the tissue; the ensuing **MEC** duly designates the minimum concentration of drug required actually at the receptor to exhibit the anticipated pharmacologic effect.

MTC: Likewise, **MTC** designates the prevailing drug concentration required to cause just a bare minimum extent of toxic effect.

6. The intensity of the **pharmacologic effect (as shown in the apex segment of Fig.1.5) is observed to be proportional to the number of drug receptor occupied predominantly.** Nevertheless, this specific pharmacologic action is distinctly reflected in the observation that the higher plasma-drug concentrations do exhibit a greater pharmacologic response up to a maximum degree.

7. The **duration of drug action (as shown in the lower segment of AUC in Fig. 1.5) is shown by the difference between the onset time and the time needed for the drug to decline back to MEC.**

8. **AUC***: In fact, the wisdom and skill of a **Pharmacokinetics** may also elaborate and describe the respective **Plasma-Drug Level Concentration** Vs **Time Curve** of the following *three* **Pharmacokinetics terms,** namely:
   - **Peak plasma level,**
   - **Time for peak plasma level,** and
   - **AUC**

9. **AUC:** It is virtually guided by *three* **cardinal factors,** such as:
   - **Absorption phase,**
   - **Postabsorption phase,** and
   - **Elimination phase.**

10. **Average rate of drug absorption:** It is represented by the **Time of Peak Plasma Level *vis-à-vis* Time of Maximum Drug Concentration recorded in the plasma.**

11. **Peak Plasma Concentration**: The **Peak plasma Concentration** or **Maximum Drug Concentration** is intimately dependent upon the following *three* **cardinal factors,** such as:
   - **Directly related to the dose**
   - **Rate constant for absorption,** and
   - **Elimination constant of the drug.**

A Few extra terms you must know!

Dosage Regimen: It is the method that should be used to administer the appropriate quantity of the drug.

Drug Disposition: Distribution and elimination play a role in the therapeutic activity of a drug and are together referred to as drug disposition.

---

* **AUC:** It is related to the actual quantum of drug being absorbed systemically.

Drug Distribution: The relative motion of drug between different compartments of the body (*e.g.*, blood and extravascular tissue) is known as drug distribution.

Elimination: This is the process in which of drug activity is terminated (through biotransformation) and drug metabolites are removed from the body (excretion).

ADME: Absorption, distribution, metabolism and excretion.

KADME: Kinetics of ADME or pharmacokinetics.

\multicolumn{3}{c}{**SUGGESTED READINGS**}		

Gibaldi M	:	**Biopharmaceutics and Clinical Pharmacokinetics** 4th ed., Pharma Book Syndicate, Hyderabad, 2006.
Lutz R and Dedrick: R	:	**Physiological Pharmacokinetics: Reference to Human Risk Assesment,** In: Li AP (Ed): *Toxicity Testing: New Applications and Applications in Human Risk Assessment,* Raven, New York, pp: 129-149, 1985.
Rowl and N and Tozor T	:	**Clinical Pharmacokinetics: Concepts and Applications**, 3rd ed., Lea & Febiger, Philadelphia, PA, (USA), 1995.
Shargel L *et al.*	:	**Applied Pharmaceutics & Pharmacokinetics,** 5th ed., McGraw Hill, New Delhi, 2005.
Tipnis HP	:	**Bioavailability and Bioequivalence**, New Age International Publishers, New Delhi, 1996.
Welling P and Tse E	:	**Pharmacokinetics**, Applied Therapeutics, Marcel Dekker, New York, 1993.
Winters ME	:	**Basic Clinical Pharmacokinetics,** Applied Therapeutics, Vancouver, WA, 1994.

Chapter

2

BIOPHARMACEUTICS

2.1. INTRODUCTION

In a broader view of the relative importance of underlying facts the **Pharmacokinetics** essentially comprises the so-called:

"intrinsic study of almost all the controlling rate processes". However, it is invariably termed as: '**ADE-Kinetics**' due to its respective **Absorption-Distribution-Elimination kinetic profile,** - which may be illustrated in Fig: 2.1.

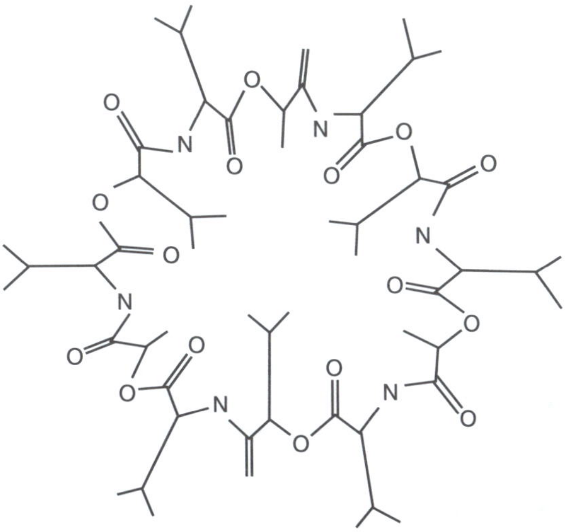

Fig. 2.1: Representation of the ADE-Kinetics of a Drug *In-Vivo* Showing Explicitly Biopharmaceuties and Disposition.

Based on the aforesaid statement of facts "it may be inferred that **Biopharmacokinetics** exclusively deals with the vital and important **Absorption Phenomenon of a Drug** *In-Vivo.*

Importantly, when a '*Drug*' is duly administered *via* the *IV-route* (*i.e., intravenous injection*) exclusively, the **distribution and elimination** are in effect perceptively [*DE-Kinetics*]. Hence, the respective study of the **DE-Kinetics of a drug substance** is usually known as:

"Drug Disposition phenomenon".

Points to Ponder: These essentially comprise:

1. The *actual site of administration* and the *characteristics* of the **dosage from** (or *drug product*) may critically and effectively influence the so-called **Bioavailability of the Administered Drug.** Hence, once absorbed the respective '*Drug*' is being subjected only to the **DE-Kinetics** perceptively.

2. Besides, either any or all of the ensuing **ADE rate phenomena** could be largely influenced by the following *two* **cardinal aspects,** namely:
   - **Physiochemical characteristics of the Drug**; and
   - **Age, health and sex of the patient.**

Another school of thought refers **Biopharmaceutics** to the study of **the relationship between physical, chemical and biological properties of matter specifically in relation to drug substances, dosage forms (or drug products), drug availability *in vivo* (or Bioavailability) and the overall therapeutic actions'.**

It has been experimentally proven that the occurring '**therapeutic response of a drug**' is dependent on the following *two* **important aspects,** namely:
   - **sufficient concentration of the acting drug,** and
   - **sustained presence of the drug either at a particular site or at several sites of action simultaneously**.

In a border perspective, the '**Drug Substances**' which exert their action systematically are considered to be **most preferred for clinical purposes exclusively** because there exists a '**Dynamic Equilibrium**' between the *two* **under-mentioned entities,** such as:
   - **critical concentration of drug in circulating blood,** and
   - **specific concentration of drug at its site(s) of action.**

In other words, there exists a so-called '**Linear Relationship**' between the *drug-concentration in blood* and *drug-concentration at the site of action.* Obviously, one may easily predict-'**the exact and precise drug-concentration at the site of action based upon the presented concentration of drug in the blood'.**

However, it is pertinent to state here that the actual concentration of drug in **plasma water***: dose serve as a more reliable index of drug concentration prevailing at the site(s) of action compared to the actual concentration of drug occurring in whole plasma. Hence, it may be concluded that only such drug, which is unbound, *i.e.,* practically dissolved in plasma-water, may exhibit a tendency to release from plasma *via*
   - **capillary endothelium** and
   - **various adjoining tissues,**

and virtually approach other body fluids; and, therefore, gain a viable entry to the site(s) of action appropriately.

To carry out the precise measurements (*i.e.,* determination) of a specific 'unbound drug substance' in protein-free plasma (or plasma water) definitely requires a more sensitive and complex assay techniques rather than estimating the total concentration of both *bound* and *unbound drug* substance in the '**whole plasma**'**.

---

*   **Plasma Water**: It refers to the protein-free plasma

** **Whole Plasma**: It contains plasma protein which has a tendency to bind the drug in a reversible manner.

2.1.1. *Alternative Distinctness of Biopharmaceutics*

Biopharmaceutics may also be defined as 'the intensive and extensive study of various factors that critically influence the rate and amount of drug reaching the systematic circulation; and the subsequent usage of this extremely valuable information so as to optimize the therapeutic efficaciousness of the Drug Product (or Dosage Forms)'.

2.1.2. *Important Modalities Encountered by a Drug*

In other words, there are *four* **important modalities** which are eventually encountered by a **Drug inside a human body,** namely:

- **Absorption**: It usually refers to the process of movement of the '**drug substance**' from its site of administration to the systemic circulation.
- **Distribution**: It refers to the particular movement of drug substance between one compartment and the other (*viz.* blood and extracellular tissues). Nevertheless, as the site of action is strategically located in the extracellular tissues, the ultimate accomplished onset, intensity and duration of the action of drug depends exclusively on the behavioural distribution pattern of the drug substance.
- **Elimination**: it may be defined as '**the critical phenomenon during which the body tends to remove the drug and terminate its action completely'.**

In fact, **Elimination** comes into play *via* *two* **well-recognized processes**, such as:

- **Biotransformation (or Metabolism)-that normally renders the 'drug' inactive, and**
- **Excretion-that is responsible for the complete exit of the 'drug' or its 'respective' metabolites from the human body.**

Earlier it was believed that the **therapeutic response of a 'drug substance'** is attributed to its intrinsic pharmacologic activity. However, as-to-date, it is absolutely clear that the ensuing **dose-response relationship** is accomplished after **'drug administartion'** *via* **different routes,** such as:

- **Oral Administration,** and
- **Parental Administration** (*viz.* IV, IM, SC etc.),

are not found to be of the same level

Besides, wide variations in drug products may also be noticed predominantly when produced by different manufacturers, which could be caused due to critical factors, such as:

- **Physiochemical characteristics features of the drug substance,**
- **Excipients incorporated in the drug product,**
- **Formulation technique adopted,** and
- **Route of administration engaged.**

On the basis of these facts, one has to take cognizance of factual information(s) and data pertaining to the **Optimal Administration of Drugs** so as to accomplish:

- **Fully understand the inherent mechanisms of drug-absorption-distribution-metabolism-and excretion (ADME), and**
- **Evaluate the kinetics (rate) at which ADME takes place,** *i.e.*, **the 'Pharmacokinetics'.**

2.1.3. *Pharmacokinetics*

Pharmacokinetics may be referred to 'the study of the quantitative relationships of the rates of drug absorption, distribution and elimination processes, *i.e.*, data used to establish dosage amount and frequency for desired therapeutic response'.

In a rather simpler version, **Pharmacokinetics** represents the ensuing **kinetics of ADME or more precisely, KADME.**

2.1.4. *Clinical Pharmacokinetics*

It refers to 'the application of Pharmacokinetics to the safe and effective therapeutic management of an individual patient'.

Shargel and Yu (1999)* emphasized that **Biopharmaceutics'** makes use of both **Quantitative Methodologies and Theoretical Models** to evaluate the effects of the *four* **aspects,** namely:

- **Drug substance,**
- **Dosage form,**
- **Routes of drug administration upon the therapeutic needs of the 'drug'**, and
- **Critical role of drug products in a typical physiological environment.**

Table 2.1 records the various aspects of **Biopharmaceutic** considerations in the specific design of **Drug Product** (or **Dosage Form**) which is entirely based on the following characteristics features:

- **Physiochemical properties of the 'active drug'**,
- **Desired 'dosage form' (or drug product),** and
- **Anatomical and Physiological considerations of the human body.**

Importantly, the meticulous design of an appropriate **Dosage Form** requires in-depth knowledge of **Pharmacodynamics**** of the drug substance including the following *four* **important criteria,** namely:

- **Onset time of drug product,**
- **Duration of the drug product exhibiting its action.**
- **Observed intensity of clinical responses,** and
- **Pharmacokinetics of the drug. *e.g.*, absorption pattern, distribution profile, elimination mode and the ultimate target-drug concentration.**

Shargel and Yu (1999)* put forward a descriptive scheme, as shown in Figure 2.1, demonstrating the ensuing dynamic correlation prevailing among the **Drug Substance**, Drug Product, and **Pharmacologic Effect**. Interestingly, **Biopharmaceutics** embraces the factors which influence the following **four aspects,** such as:

---

*   **Shargel and Yu (1999)** ABC: **Applied Biopharmaceutics and Pharmacokinetics**, 4th ed., McGraw Hill Medical Publishing, New York, 1999

**   **Pharmacodynamics**:It refers to the study of absorption, distribution, metabolism and excretion of a drug substance, besides its mechanism of action and its biochemical and physiological effects

S. No.	Various Considerations Factors	Characteristics Features	Special Remarks
	Table 2.1. Various Aspects of Biopharmaceutic Considerations in the Specific Design of Drug Product (or Dosage Form)		
1	**Active Pharmaceutical Ingredient (API)**	Stability; solubility; pH and pK; polymorph (crystalline form; excipient interaction; compatibility).	Presence of impurities; particle size; salt form; and complexation.
2	**Dosage Form (or Drug Product)**	Types of secondary pharmaceutical product (dosage form), *viz.* tablet, capsule, parenterals; immediate or modified drug release profile; dosage strength variability; and bioavailability.	Stability profile; excipient variants; and manufacturing variable criteria.
3	**Physiological Factors**	Various routes of administration; permeation of drug across the cell membranes; and binding of 'drug' to macromolecules (*viz.* proteins).	Blood-flow pattern; surface area; and **Biotransformation.**
4	**Pharmacodynamic and Pharmacokinetic Factors**	Bioavailability; therapeutic aim and objective; and adverse drug reactions.	**Pharmacokinetics**; dose; and toxic effects.
5	**Manufacturing Aspects**	Production methods; latest technological adaptation; quality assurance; and raw material specifications.	Cost-effective measures and product stability testing.

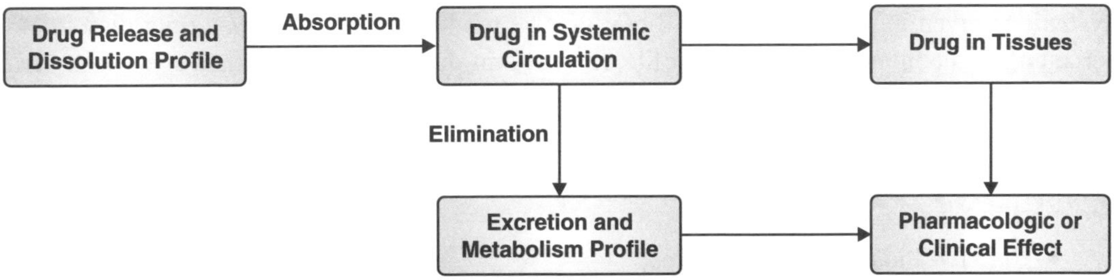

Fig. 2.1: A Descriptive Scheme Showing the Dynamic Correlation Prevailing Among Drug Substance, Drug Product and Pharmacologic Effect.

[*Adapted From*: Shargel L, Yu ABC. Applied Biopharmaceuties and Pharmacokinetics, 4th ed. Mc Graw Hill Medical Publising, New York: 1999.]

- Adequate protection and sufficient stability of the active drug present duly within the Dosage Form (or Drug Product),
- Rate of drug release profile emanated from the drug product,
- Rate of dissolution of the Drug Substance at the specific, absorption site, and
- Critical and precise availability of the drug at the very site of action.

2.2. BIOPHARMACEUTICS CLASSIFICATION SYSTEM (BCS)

Amidon *et al.* **(1995)*** made an excellent breakthrough by establishing the remarkable correlation between:

- *In Vivo* **drug dissolution studies,** and
- *In Vivo* **bioavailability studies,**

that are designed solely upon the theoretical basis. The broader perspective and systematic approach is relied exclusively on following *two* **important aspects,** namely:

- **Aquenous solubility profile of the 'active drug',** and
- **Critical permeation of the 'active drug'** *via* **GIT.**

The **Biopharmaceutics Classification System (BCS)** is particularly based upon the **Fick's first law** as applicable to a **Biological Membrane** by the following expression:

where,

J_w = Drug flux (mass/area/time) *via* the intestinal lumen (inner wall) at any position and material time,

P_w = Permeability of the membrane and

C_w = Drug concentration at the surface of the intestinal membrane.

Assumptions: It is necessary to state here that the aforesaid logical suggestion assumes that no other components in the formulation do affect the following *two* **aspects,** namely:

- **Membrane permeability,** and/or
- **Intestinal transport.**

Amidon *et al.* **(1995)*** carried out an extensive investigative study regarding the solubility and permeability characteristics features of a host of representative drug substances) belonging to different categories). Thus, they successfully established a **Biopharmaceutics-Drug-Classification System,** as given in Table 2.2, of solid-oral precise prediction of the *in-vitro* drug dissolution pertaining to the immediate-release profile of solid-oral drug products having a specific *in-vivo* absorption.

In short, it may be added that **US-FDA:** Guidelines for Industry-Bioanalytical Method Validation,** 1997 may help in the waiver towards the requirement for carrying out the following *two* **specific aspects,** such as:

- *In-Vivo* **Bioavailability studies,**
- **Bioequivalence studies pertaining to certain immediate release solid oral dosage forms.**
- **Solubility,**
- **Permeability,** and
- **Dissolution of drug substance.**

---

  *   **Amidon** *et al.* **(1995)** *Pharm. Res.,* **12:**413-420,1995

**   **US-FDA: Guidance for Industry-Bioanalytical Method Validation,** 1997.

Table 2.2. Biopharmaceutics Drug Classification System				
Biopharmaceutics Drug Class	Solubility Profile	Permeability Pattern	Special Remarks
Class 1	High	High	Drug gets dissotved quickly and is well absorbed; remote chances of any probable bioavailability problems for immediate release drug products.
Class 2	Low	High	Drug offers restricted dissolution profile and is well absorbed systematically; drug product (dosage form) controls both bioavailabilty and rate of release of drug.
Class 3	High	Low	Drug exhibits limited permeability; bioavailability may be rendered incomplete provided drug never gets duly released and dissolved very much within the absorption phase (window).
Class 4	Low	Low	Drug product formulation encounters serious problem(s) which may deliver consistent drug bioavailability; may indirectly suggest an alternative route of administration, *e.g.*, SC, IM, IV.

* **US-FDA Guidance for Industry:** Waiver of *in-vivo* Bioavailability and Bioequivalence studies for Immediate Release Solid Oral Dosage Forms containing Certain Active Moieties/Active Ingredients: Based on a Biopharmaceutics Classification System (2000).

which may fulfill some highly critical and specific criteria, such as:

Besides, these properties essentially comprise the *in vitro* dissolution of the respective Dosage Form in different media, information(s) regarding drug permeability, and above all the anticipated ideal behavior of dosage form-dissolution profile absorption in GIT.

2.3. *IN VITRO-IN VIVO* CORRELATION (IVIVC): AN INTROSPECTION

Jorgensen and Bhagwat (1998)* evaluated the urgency and priority for the much needed requirement of a pharmaceutical industry towards a rapid-drug development and its due approval from a competent authority (*viz.* respective **Government Agency**); whereas, the drug-regulatory agencies (*viz.* US-FDA) essentially and primarily ask for the following *two* **cardinal pre-requisite** namely:

- **Assurance of 'Product Quality'** and
- **Optimized Performance of 'Drug Product' (or Dosage Form).**

This has led the researchers across the globe to establish a **fool-proof, feasible and achievable 'link'** between the so-called **'Dissolution Testing'** and **'Bioavailability'**. Nevertheless, the aforesaid concept and ideology have remarkably paved the way for the much talked about *in vitro-in-vivo* correlation (IVIVC). In our day-to-day drug development activities in the Research and Development (R & D) wing of a pharmaceutical industry, *e.g.*, Dr. Reddy's Laboratory, Hyderabad; Ranbaxy Laboratories, New Delhi; Glaxo Smith Kline, London (UK); Pfizer Laboratories, New York.

* Jorgensen ED and Bhagwat D: **Development of Dissolution Tests for Oral Extended Release Product**, PSST, **1** (3): 128-135.1998

2.3.1. *Genesis of IVIVC*

Early 1980s witnessed vigorous initiative and well-organized collaborative research focused on **IVIVC (duly sponsored by US-FDA/American Drug Industries)** putting forward useful findings , such as:

- **Extended Release (ER) Product**, and
- **Encouraged more meaningful intensive research in this direction (Skelley *et al*.1987)*.**

Skelley *et.al*.(1993)** reported an unusual unique trend depicting enhanced level of confidence in **IVIVC for ER-Oral Drug Products [USP XXIII (1995)]** which specifically included this aspect as a **USP chapter (1088)**. Soon after, **US-FDA (1997)** established elaborated guidelines for industry under the head:

'ER-Oral Dosage Forms: Development–Evaluation-Application of IVIVC.'

In short, it may be appropriate to have comprehensive details with respect to **IVIVC *vs*. dissolution factors in:**

- **Development of IVIVC,** and
- **Critical progress in IVIVC**

2.3.2. *FDA Definition for IVIVC*

US-FDA defines- IVIVC as a **"predictive mathematical model describing relationship between in vitro properties of a drug product and its relevant response in *vivo*".**

Obviously, an **in vitro property** reveals explicitly the rate-degree of drug dissolution-drug release profile; whereas, the **in *vivo* response** represents adequately the plasma-drug concentration or exact quantum of drug absorbed systematically.

2.3.3. *Important Factors for Development of IVIVC*

It has been duly established that there exists *two* **important factors for the development of IVIVC,** namely:

- **Stereochemistry,** and
- **First-Pass Effect**.

(a) Stereochemistry: It refers to that branch of chemistry which deals with the atoms in their spatial relationship, and the effect of such a relationship on the action and effects of the molecule.

In other words, the observed difference is caused duly in the '**Pharmacokinetics; or 'Pharmacodynamics'** behavior profile of *two* **enantiomers** (*i.e*., **stereoisomers**). Evidently, the overall applicability of in vitro dissolution retrieved data of a **racemic mixture** (or *dl*-**mixture**) alone may not perhaps be quite useful for the **development of IVIVC; and, therefore, the correct prediction of *in-vivo* availability of the active enantiomer.**

---

   * Skelley JP *et al.*: *Pharm. Res.*, **4**(1): 75-77,1987.

 ** Skelley *et.al. Dosage Forms*, **10**(12): 1800-1805, 1993.

(b) **First-Pass Effect**: It refers to the dosage form having an exceptionally **high hepatic-extraction ratio**. This dosage form undergoes critical **Biotransformation** before entering the ensuing systemic circulation thereby lowering the usual availability of the '**parent drug**'.

In this manner, the precise quantum of drug actually available in the systematic circulation may not match up to the amount of **drug-released in GIT.**

Sirisuth and Eddington (2002)* Showed that the observed influence of the **First-Pass Effect upon the development and validation of IVIVC** was established justifiably between:

- **Fraction of 'metaprolol' dissolved,** and
- **Fraction of 'total drug absorbed' due to altogether differed drug release-rate formulations.**

2.3.4. *IVIVC Utilization in Novel Dosage Forms*

The excellent usage of **IVIVC** has been largely exploited in the following *six* **novel dosage forms,** namely:

1. **Controlled Release (CR) or Sustained Release (SR) drug delivery syst**em,
2. **Transmitted Drug Delivery System (TDDS),**
3. **Nasal Drug Delivery System (NDDS),**
4. **Enteric Coated Multiple Unit Dosage Form,**
5. **Buccal Tablets** and
6. **Suppositories**

2.3.5. *Applications of IVIVC*

These essentially comprise the following: *two* **aspects,** such as:

1. Recommended and suggested to **use in vitro dissolution studies as surrogate for the human Bioequivalence (BE) studies** in order to accomplish specifically the following *two* **aspects,** namely:

   - **Reduction in the number of human bioequivalence (BE) studies,** and
   - **Minimize the cumbersome task of initial approval process, and certain 'scale up post approval changes (SUPAC)'.**

2. Spectacular success in the early development of **'Drug Product'** (or **Dosage Form**) together with its critical optimization criteria.

Venkatesh and Lipper (2000)** studied thoroughly the development of drug products which are solely characterized by certain *in-vitro* **systems.** Besides, some *in-vivo* **studies** in animal models to address the following *two* **aspects** critically:

- **Toxicity features,** and
- **Efficacy studies.**

---

* Sirisuth N and Eddington ND: *Eur. J. Pharm. Biopharm.*,**53**:301-309,2002.

** Venkatesh S and Lipper RA:J. *Pharm. Sci*, **89**(2): 145-154, 2000

These researchers also emphasized that if the preliminary relationship existing between in *vitro* and in-vivo characteristic features may be established appropriately, it might substantially provide the following *two* **critical criteria,** for instance:

- **Better visionary in drug design,** and
- **Crucial development of drug product**

Consequently, the **valid IVIVC developed formulation may be optimized based upon the in vitro dissolution studies** meticulously.

3. **Bio Waiver for Minor Formulation and Process Changes**: The critical and specific relationsip established duly between the intended so-called:

- **Very important manufacturing variants**; and
- *In-vivo* **dissolution rate,**

has been spelled out explicitly for both **Controlled-Release (CR) Formulation** and **IVIVC** perceptively, that eventually enables the utilization of *in-vitro* **Dissolution Data** extended appropriately to both:

- **Minor Formulations,** and
- **Process changes,**

comprising significantly of an array of typical and vital aspects, such as:

- **Colour**
- **Size**
- **Shape**
- **Flavour**
- **Preservative**
- **Coating**
- **Technique**
- **Composition of Materials**
- **Ingredients (Active and Inactive)**
- **Equipments and**
- **Manufacturing Site**

2.4. PASSAGE OF DRUGS ACROSS BIOLOGICAL BARRIER

Biological Barrier refers to a-**'selective boundary, or separation pertaining biology'.**

It has been duly observed that a **membrane** (or *a barrier*) having highly specialized structural features may cause undesirable permeability restriction with respect to the **distribution of drugs to certain tissues in a human body.** Following are some typical examples of simple and specialized **Physiological or Biologic Barriers,** namely:

- **Capillary Endothelial Barrier (CEB),**
- **Cell Membrane Barrier (CMB),**
- **Blood-Brain Barrier (BBB),**
- **Blood-Cerebrospinal Fluid Barrier (BCSFB),**
- **Placental Barrier (PB),** and
- **Blood-Testis Barrier (BTB).**

These **Physiological Biological Barriers** *solely responsible for the passage of drugs across certain tissues shall now be treated individually in the following sections:*

2.4.1. *Simple Capillary Endothelial Barrier (CEB)*

The ability of **Drug Substances** to get diffused *via* capillary walls into tissue spaces is usually termed as **Capillary Permeability.** It is influenced by **Hypoxia*, Adrenocortcal**

---

* **Hypoxia:** A decreased concentration of oxygen in the inspired air.

Hormone* and **concentration of Ca^{2+} ions present in the blood.** However, it is pertinent to state here that the **membrane of capillaries, which supply blood to most tissues, does not serve as a barrier to drug molecules.** Therefore, most drug substances, *unionized form or ionized form,* **having a Molecular Size lower than 600 Da get eventually diffused** *via* the capillary endothelium right inside the intestinal fluid.

> **NOTE** **Interestingly, only such drug molecules that gets critically bound to the respective blood components (*viz.* blood proteins) are usually restricted by the capillary endothelial barrier due to its distinct 'larger molecular size' of the resulting drug-protein complex so formed by the interaction of drug and protein.**

2.4.2. *Cell Membrane Barrier (CMB)*

The 'Cell Membrane' (or **Plasma Membrane**) refers to-the **'Membrane that forms the outer boundary of a Cell and is made up of protein, carbohydrates and phospholipids on its outer surface (as shown in Figure 2.2)'.**

The **Cell Membrane** may be viewed as a 'Dynamic Biomolecular Layer of phospotipids with scattered protein molecules floating in them as ieberg in sea'.

In Figure 2.2 one may observe the following characteristics features, namely:

- **Lipid layers are represented as more or less arranged in a orderly fashion, packed compactly, lamellar array of phospholipid entities located strategically tail-to-tail.**
- **Each tail being an alkyl-chain or a steroidal moiety,** and
- **Each head is designated as a polar moiety,** *viz.* glycerate groups-having their polar functional segments as ether, carbonyl-oxygens and phosphates with intimately attached polar moieties.

Salient Features: These predominantly comprise (see Figure 2.2) the following **Salient features:**

1. The **Lamellar** ** **segment** is not arranged in an orderly manner because its inherent composition seems to be quite complex.
2. The **'Chains of Fatty Acids'** of different degrees of saturation and **'Cholesterol'** do not usually array themselves in rather simple parallel arrangements.
3. Interestingly, the aforesaid **Lamellar Segment** is duly penetrated by means of large globular proteins, the inner portion of which essentially processes a **high hydrophobicity** (*very much akin to lipid layers*), and **certain typical fibrous proteins:**

> **NOTE** **Differences have been observed between the membrane of the endoplasmic reticulum and the cell membrane (or plasma membrane), even though they are co-extensive.**

---

* **Adrenocortical Hormone:** A group of hormones secreted by the adrenal cortex that are duly classified by biological activity into **glucocorticoids, mineralocorticoids, adrenogens, estrogens and progestine**

** **Lamellar**: That is, arranged in this plates or scales.

4. The **Cell Membrane** could be seen as perforated duly by water-filled pores of various sizes, ranging between **4 and 10Å**, but mostly they are **~7Å.**

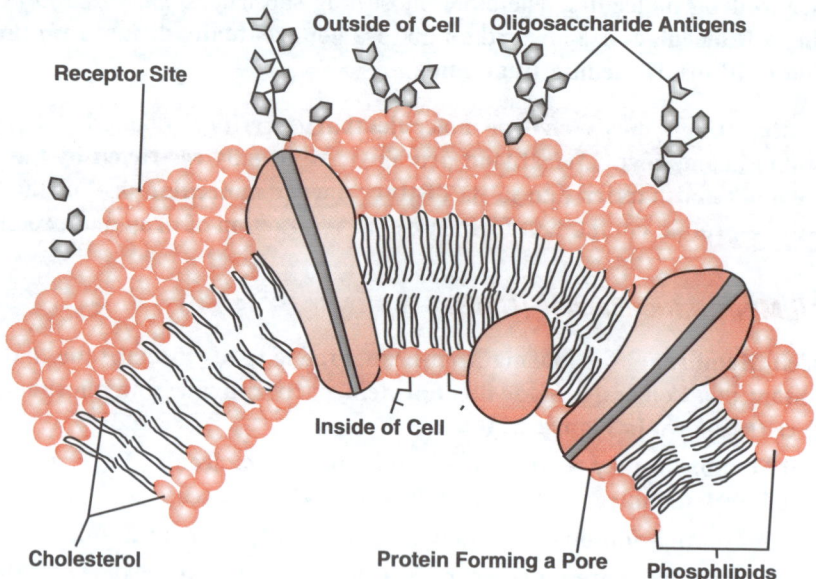

Outside of Cell   Oligosaccharide Antigens

Receptor Site

Inside of Cell

Cholesterol   Protein Forming a Pore   Phosphlipids

Fig. 2.2: Diagrammatic Illustration of a Cell Membrane.

5. Importantly, all major **Ion-Channels** do exist *via* the **Large Globular Proteins** which eventually traverse the **Cell Membrane,** and though these pores, several **Inorganic Ions** together with **Small Organic Molecules pass** ultimately.

Examples

Na^+ **ions** are relatively bigger than the corresponding K^+ **ions and Cl⁻ ions,** since the former gets more hydrated than the latter; and, therefore, cannot pass across the pores as freely as the K^+ and Cl⁻ ions.

6. **Vascular Endothelium have pores ~40A**; however, these invariably do serve as **Interstitial Passages*** rather than **Transmembrane Pores.**

The physiochemical characteristics features which normally exert their direct influence upon the **Permeation of Drug Substances** very much across the **Simple Cell Membrane Barrier (CMB)** may be illustrated explicitly in Figure 2.3.

Passive Diffusion: It may be defined as-'**movement of drug molecules from a region of higher concentration to a region of lower concentration *via* a membrane that does not participate in the process'.**

In this particular instance, the **Membrane** is referred to as-'**the cell membrane (or plasma membrane).** Importantly, one may express explicitly the passive diffusion quantitatively by **Fick's first law of diffusion.**

---

* **Interstitial Passages:** Refer to passages pertaining to spaces within an organ or tissue

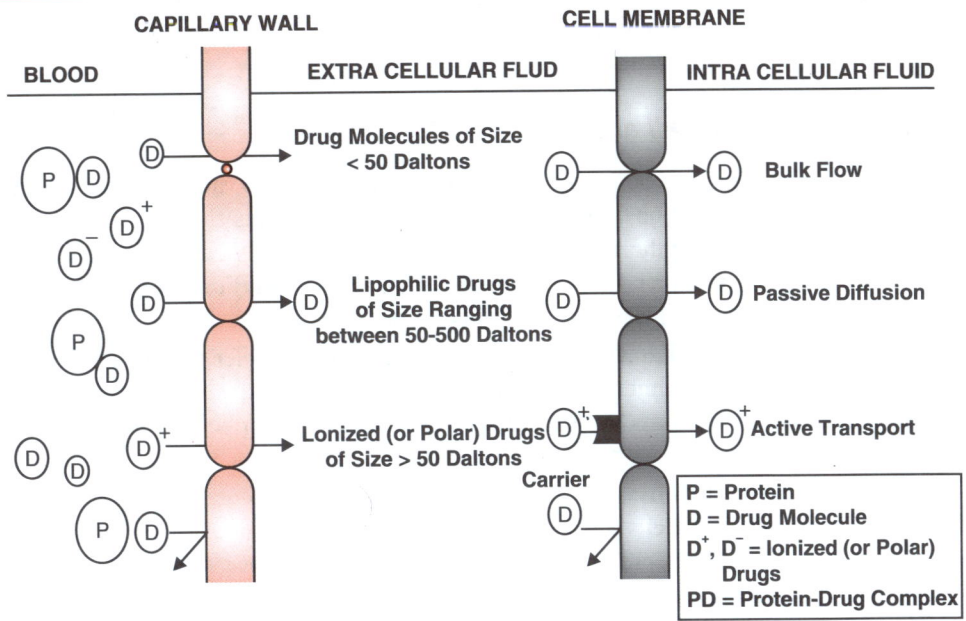

Fig. 2.3: Cell Membrane Barrier and Diffusion of Drug Molecule

Active Transport: It refers to 'the specific biological process by which drugs and other substances are critically transported across body membranes, *e.g.*, intestines, skin, cells.'

Explanation

The various aspects of Figure 2.3 may be explained easily as given below:

1. **Drug Molecules having particle size less than 50 Da** may pass through blood into the **Extracellular Fluid (ECF)**, which may sail across the **Intracellular Fluid (ICF) as the major bulk flow.**

2. Most **Lipophilic Drugs** (*viz.* **Steroids) having a particle ranging between 50 and 500 Da** easily pass through the blood right into **ECF**, and subsequently, *via* **passive diffusion into ICF through the Cell Membrane.**

3. The **Ionized (or Polar) Drugs having a particle size either equal or more than 50 Da** exhibit a tendency to sail across to **ICF** *via* **Cell Membrane** due to the active transport phenomenon.

4. Interestingly, the **Protein-Drug Complexes** formed duly, being bulkier in size *vis-a-vis* **Normal Drug Molecules, Lipophilic Drugs, and Ionized Drugs,** distinctly remain floating in the circulating blood only.

2.4.3. *Blood-Brain Barrier (BBB)*

Blood-Brain-Barrier (BBB) may be defined as-'the specialized capillary membrane existing between circulating blood and the brain so as to prevent harmful substances from entering the brain'

BBB invariably allows fat-soluble, but not water-soluble drug substances to pass across the brain.

2.4.3.1. *Permeability of Cell and Capillary Membranes*

It has been amply proven and demonstrated that **Cell Membrane** do vary in their permeability characteristic features depending on the tissue exclusively. However, it may be further substantiated and exemplified by the fact that the **Capillary Membranes** specifically confined to the **kidneys** and **liver** are observed to be rather, more permeable to the **Transmembrane-drug Movement'** *vis-a-vis* the ensuing capillaries located strategically in the brain.

1. **Role of Sinusoidal Capillaries:** The **Sinusoidal Capillaries** refer to a large, permeable capillary, often lined with microphages, usually found in organs, *e.g.*, **liver, spleen, bone marrow and adrenal glands**. Nevertheless, their permeability explicitly allows either large protein or cells to gain an easy access or prompt departure from the blood.

2. **Capillary Endothelial Cells:** The **Capillary Endothelial Cells** are critically surrounded by a **Thin-layer of Glial Cells** (*i.e., concerning the non-nervous or supporting tissue of the brain and spinal cord*), that predominantly comprise enough **tight intercellular functions**. Obviously, the aforesaid *additional layer of cells* intimately present around the so-called capillary membranes does exert its effective activity profile by slowing down the **Rate of Drug Diffusion inside the brain by acting as a distinct Thicker Lipid Barrier.** Eventually, the resulting **'Lipid Barrier'** that largely retards the penetration as well as diffusion of:

   • **water-soluble drug substances** and
   • **polar (or ionized) drug**

right inside the **brain** and **spinal cord** is invariably termed as the **Blood-Brain Barrier (BBB):**

3. **Typical Pathophysiological Parameter**: The specific and crucial permeability of cell membranes (including the capillary cell membranes) usually get changed under the influence of certain typical pathophysiological parameters.

Examples

There are *two* **marked and pronounced specific examples**, as given below:

1. **Meningitis**: It essentially involves the inflammation of the membranes located in the brain or spinal cord, thereby enhancing the ensuing drug-uptake right into the brain.

2. **Severe Burns:** In the particular instance of severe burns, one may evidently notice an apparent change with respect to:

   • **Permeability profile of skin layer,** and
   • **Passage of drug substances plus relatively larger molecules to permeate either inward or outward**.

   Figure 2.4. depicts the diagrammatic representation 1 of BBB.

Explanation

The various aspects of **BBB** may be explained as under:

1. **Blood-brain barrier (BBB)** designates a vital and important **Line-of-Control (LOC)** between the **peripheral and CNS** invariably by means of a critical **'permeability barrier'** to the ensuing **'passive diffusion'** of various drug substances right from the blood stream into different segments of the CNS.

2. Nevertheless, the crucial existence of the aforesaid ; **'permeability barrier'** may be observed explicitly due to the **appearance of relatively large reduced rate of access of chemical entities from the plasma to the brain.**

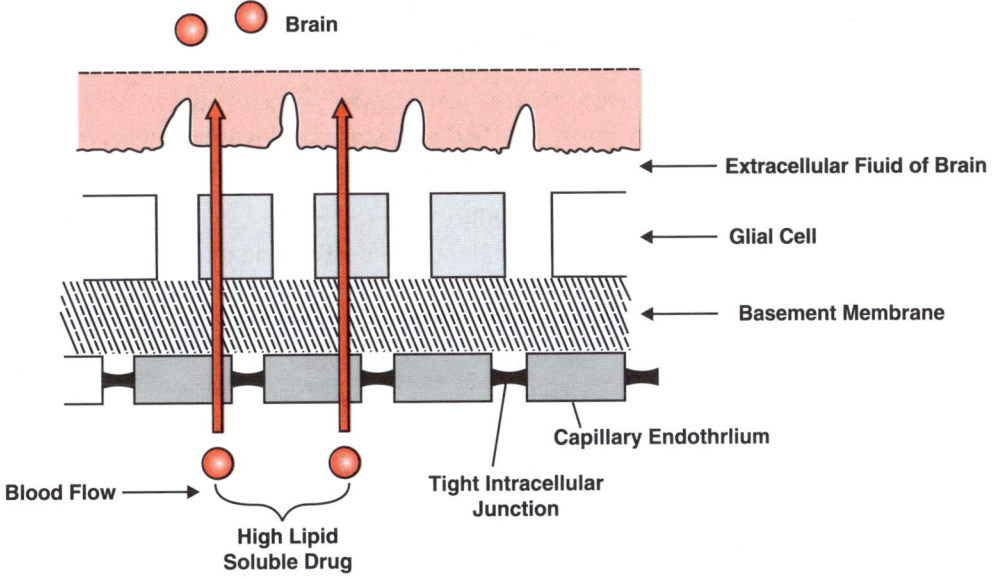

Fig. 2.4: Diagrammatic Representation of Blood-Brain Barrier (BBB).

3. Generally, the lipid-soluble drugs may obviously get specifically diffused very much inside the **'interstitial fluid'** of the brain and spinal cord exclusively.

4. The critical presence of highly specialized cells usually termed as **astrocytes*** do form a sort of **solid-envelope around the brain-capillaries**. This consequently causes blockade of the intracellular passage (see the lower part of Figure 2.4). Therefore, for enabling a 'drug' to have a proper access from the ensuing capillary circulation in the brain, it may have to get across through the cell instead of between them.

NOTE	There exist certain specific sites strategically located in the brain, wherein BBB has virtually no role to play, such as:
	• **trigger area and** • **median hypothalamic zone.**

2.4.3.2. *Highlights of BBB as a Lipoidal Barrier*

Following are some of the **highlights of BBB as a lipoidal barrier:**

---

* **Astrocytes**:It refers to the elements of the supporting issue located strategically at the base of the endothelial membrane

1. **BBB** permits solely the passage of such drug substances with a distinctly **high o/w partition coefficient** in order to cause an **effective 'Passive Diffusion';** whereas, both partially ionized drug molecules and moderately ionized drug molecules (see Figure 2.4) do penetrate at a **slow rate**.

Example

Thiopental, a *hypnotic drug*, which being an *extremely lipid-soluble drug*, shows an effective partition coefficient that is almost 50 folds in comparison to **Pentobarbital**; and, therefore, gets across the **BBB** rather **more readily and efficaciously.**

> **NOTE**   It has been observed duly that a host of other structurally similar foreign molecules may also get across the BBB almost *via* the identical mechanism, *e.g.,* carbohydrates, amino acids (derived from in vivo protein hydrolystates).

2. Importantly, the highly **'Selective Permeability'** of specific lipid-soluble functional moieties do exhibit an appreciable tendency to sail through the **BBB;** and thus, definitely ascertain the most credible and appropriate choice towards the **'selection of a drug'** so as to treat the disorders of CNS efficaciously as an **essential component of the therapeutic armamentarium.**

Example

Parkinsonism* may be treated effectively by **'Levodopa'** (a *prodrug*) that can penetrate CNS to get converted to dopamine via metabolism.

3. The genuine attempt for targeting a **Polar Drug** (or **Ionized Drug**) directly into the brain, in some serious and acute conditions, *viz.* **cancerous tumour in the brain**, had always been a matter of deep concern in the medical profession. The advent of **scientific advancement** in the past few decades have actually introduced *three* **different and important approaches** that virtually enabled the successful utilization to induct drug(s) across the **BBB** namely:

   (a) **Permeation enhancers, *i.e.*, dimethysulfoxide (DMSO), in conjunction with the drug substance,**

   (b) **Osmotic imbalance of BBB, *i.e.*, to disrupt/imbalance the ensuing osmotic pressure across the membranes (BBB) by carrying out the careful infusion of the carotid artery with mannitol solution, and**

   (c) **Drug carrier, *i.e.*, adaptation of dihydropyridine redox system, as a drug carrier to the brain.**

Mechanism of Dihydropyridine: In this particular instance, **Dihydropyridine** (a *lipid-soluble compound*) gets intimately hooked on as a perspective **'carrier'** to the **Polar Drug** (or *Ionized Drug*) to give rise to the formation of a **'Prodrug'** which crosses the **BBB** rapidly. Importantly, in the brain the presence of distinct **CNS-enzymes** helps in the critical **oxidation of the ensuing dihydropyridine molecule to the corresponding Polar Pyridinium Ion state that may not be able to escape out of the brain anymore.** Consequently, the **'drugmolecule'** gets eventually trapped into the brain.

---

* **Parkinsonism** It refers to a group of neurological disorders characterized by **tremor, hypokinesia and rigidity**

2.4.4. *Blood-Cerebrospinal Fluid Barrier (BCSFB)*

The **Cerebrospinal Fluid (CSF)** is generated in the **Choroid Plexus***, specifically at the lateral, third and fourth ventricles. However, it is similar in composition to the **Extracellular Fluid (ECF)** of the brain. It has been duly observed that the strategically located **capillary endothelium** that critically lies the **choroid plexus do have several open gaps** (or *junctions*) through which the drug substances may flow without any hinderance (*i.e., freely*) right into the **extracellular space** prevailing between the so-called:

- **Capillary Walls,** and
- **Choroidal Cells**

Nevertheless, the **Choroidal Cells** are joined meticulously to one another by means of the tight junctions that crucially give rise to the information of the said **Blood-CSF Barrier** that predominantly exhibits the permeability characteristics features very much akin to the **blood-brain barrier (BBB)** (see Figure 2.4).

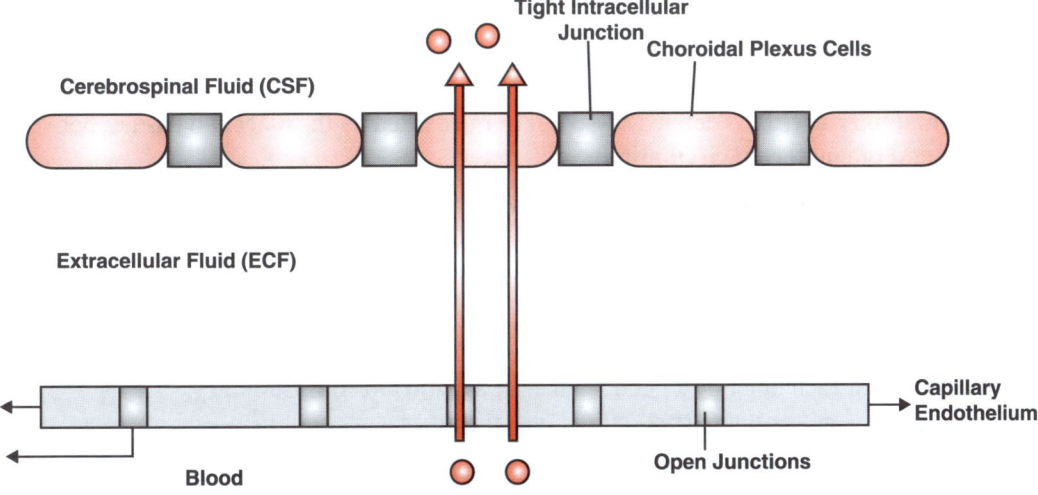

Fig. 2.5: Diagrammatic Representation of the Transport of Lipid Soluble Drug Across Blood-Cerebrospinal Fluid Barrier.

However, Figure 2.5 illustrates the **Blood-Cerebrospinal Fluid Barrier (BCSFB)** through which the transport of the lipid-soluble drug takes place.

Modus Operandi: As one may observe in the particular instance of **BBB**, the highly lipid soluble drugs would sail across the **BCSFB** without any obstruction; whereas, the corresponding moderately lipid soluble drugs and partially ionized drug entities permeate rather sluggishly and

---

* **Choroid Plexus:** It refers to the dark blue vascular layer of the type between the **sclera and retina**, extending duly to the optic nerve.

slowly. Obviously, a specific drug substance that enters the **CSF** gradually would never accomplish a distinctly high concentration due to the fact that the usual **'bulk flow of cerebrospinal fluid (CSF)'** will remove continuously the **'drug substance'** from the circulating blood. Importantly, at any point in time, any administered **'drug substance'** shall explicitly show its concentration in the brain invariably at a higher level *vis-a-vis* in the **CSF**.

Mechanism of Action: Evidently, the precise mechanism pertaining to the *critical diffusion of drugs right into the* **CNS** *and* **CSF** *are almost at par with each other*. However, the extent of drug uptake may vary appreciably.

Examples

Following are some typical examples:

1. **Sulphamethoxazole and Trimethoprim [Septran®]:** This specific drug combination (used as **anti-bacterial agent**) clearly shows higher drug concentration in the **Cerebrospinal Fluid (CSF)** *vis-a-vis* its **Cerebral Concentration.**

2. **Phenytoin,** an ***anti-epileptic agent***, exhibits a six-fold higher activity in epileptic patients particularly in the temporal lobe than in the **CSF.**

3. **A-Blockers** (*e.g.,* **Timolol®, Propranolol®, Oxyprenolol®, Nadolol®, Pidolol®**) *show lower drug concentration in the* **CSF**.

2.4.5. Placement Barrier (PB)

Placental Barrier (PB) is defined as – **'a barrier provided by the placental tissues, between the foetal and the maternal circulation'.**

It has been duly observed that the relatively **small substances,** *excluding the* ***Blood Cells,*** may eventually across Barrier easily and conveniently:

Besides, it has also been established that:

- **maternal blood vessels**, and
- **foetal blood vessels,**

are separated from each other by a good number of **Membrane and Capillary,** such as:

- **tissue layers made up of foetal trophoblast basement membrane***
- **endothelium capillary,**

that eventually in combination give rise to the formation of the so-called **'Placental Barrier'.** Importantly, the critical and usual flow of blood takes place through: **(a) the maternal vein, and (b) the foetal vein and arteries (blood vessels)**, as illustrated vividly in Figure 2.6.

Modus Operandi: Various steps essentially comprise the following:

1. The mean thickness of **the 'Human Placental Barrier'** in the early stages of pregnancy stands at **25μ,** which eventually gets reduced to only **2μ in full pregnancy. Importantly, the said variance in the thickness of Human Placental Barrier (HPB) hardly reduces its efficaciousness.**

---

* **Foetal Membrane**: It is one of the membranous structures that protects and supports the embryo and provides in nutrition, respiration and excretion.

2. Several drug substances having:
   - **molecular weight less than 1,000 Da,** and
   - **moderate to high lipodial solubility,**

actually do cross over the **Placental Barrier** almost readily by means of *simple diffusion phenomenon,* for instance:

   - **anaesthetics,**
   - **antibiotics,**
   - **anti-convulsants,**
   - **barbiturates,**
   - **narcotic analgesics,**
   - **sulphonamides**, and
   - **steroids.**

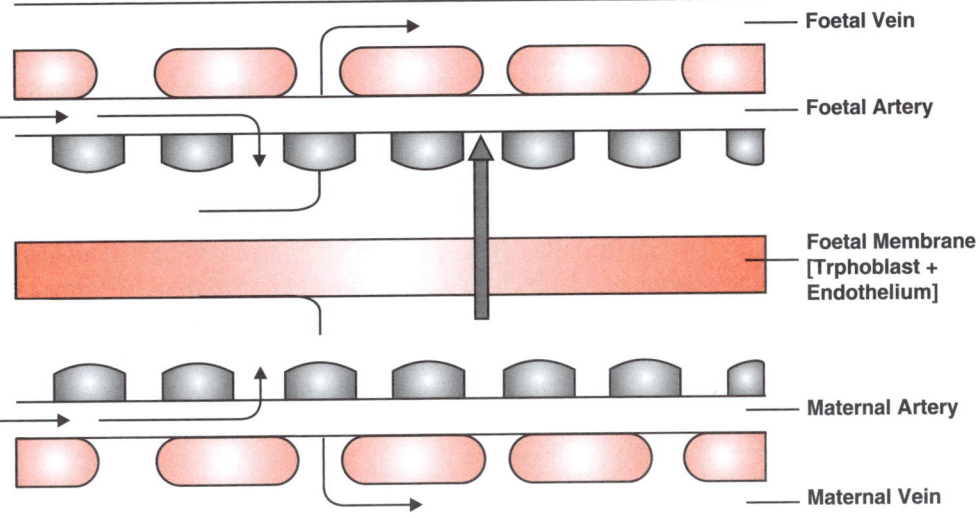

Foetal Vein

Foetal Artery

Foetal Membrane [Trphoblast + Endothelium]

Maternal Artery

Maternal Vein

Fig. 2.6: Diagrammatic Representation of the Placental Barrier (PB) and Flow of Blood Across Foetal Membrane

 NOTE The above observations ascertain the fact that the 'Placentral Barrier' does not prove to be as effective and useful when compared to the 'Blood-Brain Barrier (BBB)'.

3. The essential nutrients required urgently for the normal foetal growth are adequately membraul. transported by the specific and vital **Carrier-Medicated Phenomenon** in human body.

Example

Immunoglobulins (Ig) needed primarily for the **immuno-defensive mechanism** are duly transported by the **Endocytosis***

---

* **Endocytosis**: A method of ingestion of a foreign substance by a cell. The cell membrane invaginates to form a space for the material and then the opening closes to trap the material inside the cell.

Cautions: At *two* **critical stages**, certain drugs are found to be specifically **'dangerous'** in nature to the normal growth of the foetus in humans, namely:

Stage I: During the **'First Trimester'** when the foetal organs undergo development. Importantly, in this particular stage, most of the drugs do exhibit their inherent and typical characteristics teratogenic effects (*i.e.*, serious congenital abnormalities).

Examples

Thalidomide (a *banned drug*), **Phenytoin** (*an anti-epileptic agent*), **Isotretinoin** (*an anti-acne drug*), **Testosterone** (*a male sex hormone*), and **methotrexate** (*an anti-neoplastic agent*).

Stage II: During the **latter stages of pregnancy,** *i.e.*, when the drugs do show their typical known physiological functions, *e.g.*, **respiratory depression caused by Morphine'** (*a narcotic analgesic).*

NOTE	It is, therefore, always advised to restrict heavily the usage of 'all drugs' during pregnancy, based on the fact that the hazardous/adverse effects (of drug) are not known due to their uncertainty or unpredictable physiological action in humans.

2.4.6. *Blood-Testis Barrier (BTB)*

It has been duly established that the **Somniferous Tubules** (*i.e.*, *sleep-producing tubules*) are distinctly isolated from the general circulation by a definite *Blood-Testis Barrier (BTB)* which is regarded to be fairly comparable to **BBB**. Importantly, the **BTB** is strategically located not at the **Endothelium Capillary** level but at the specific Sertoli Cell* junction. In fact, it is the **Tight Intracellular Junctions** prevailing at the neighbouring **Sertoli Cells** which act predominantly as the **BTB**.

Interestingly, the **Barrier (BTB)** restricts prominently the free flow and passage of drug substances to the following *two* **vital and important sites,** namely:

- **Spermatids** and
- **Spermatocytes.**

2.5. FACTORS INFLUENCING DRUG ABSORPTION

Drug Absorption may be defined as–**'the critical phenomenon related to movement of unchanged drug substance from the specific site of administration to the systemic circulation'.**

In other words, the prevailing absorption process is duly developed in the ensuing biological system for obtaining the much required **organic as well as inorganic chemicals** (*being utilized as nutrients*) right inside the **'Systemic Circulation'** so as to maintain and sustain life.

In usual practice, the drug substances are **administered orally, or injected parenterally** (*i.e.*, ***IV, IM, SC or intra-arterially***), whereby the drug gains entry directly into the **Systemic**

---

* **Sertoli Cell**: It refers to one of the supporting elongated cells of the **Somniferous Tubules of the Testis** to which the spermatids get attached to be nourished duly till such time they become mature spermatozoan. The sertoli cells do produce the **hormone 'inhibin'**. It is also termed as **Sustentacular Cell**

Circulation and exerts the desired pharmacologic effect(s). The **Extravascular Administration of Drugs** invariably show up their therapeutic effect only in a situation when they come in contact with the circulating blood right from very site of application; and, therefore, absorption of drugs serves as a vital and important pre-requisite step.

Nevertheless, it is rather tedious and almost difficult to measure exactly the concentration of drug at such a 'site'. Alternatively, one may, therefore, measure the actual drug concentration accurately in plasma. Obviously, it is feasible and possible to establish a fairly acceptable correlation between the following *two* entities, namely:

- **plasma-concentration of a drug substance**, and
- **therapeutic response of the drug substance.**

Figure 2.7 illustrates explicitly the following *two* **most vital aspects,** such as:

- **quantum of drug that gains entry to the systemic circulation,** and
- **rate at which the drug gets absorbed ideally.**

2.5.1. *Rate-Limited Stages in Oral Drug Absorption*

It has been duly observed that a **'Drug Product'** (or **Dosage Form**) undergoes the **systemic drug absorption** *via* **an array of** *successive rate processes*, as depicted in Figure 2.8. Importantly, the **solid oral immediate release dosage forms** (*viz.* **Tablet, Capsule**) the various rate processes involved essentially comprises the following cardinal stages, such as:

- **disintegration of the dosage form and subsequent release profile of the drug,**
- **dissolution of the drug in an aqueous environment,** and
- **critical absorption *via* the cell membranes into the systemic circulation.**

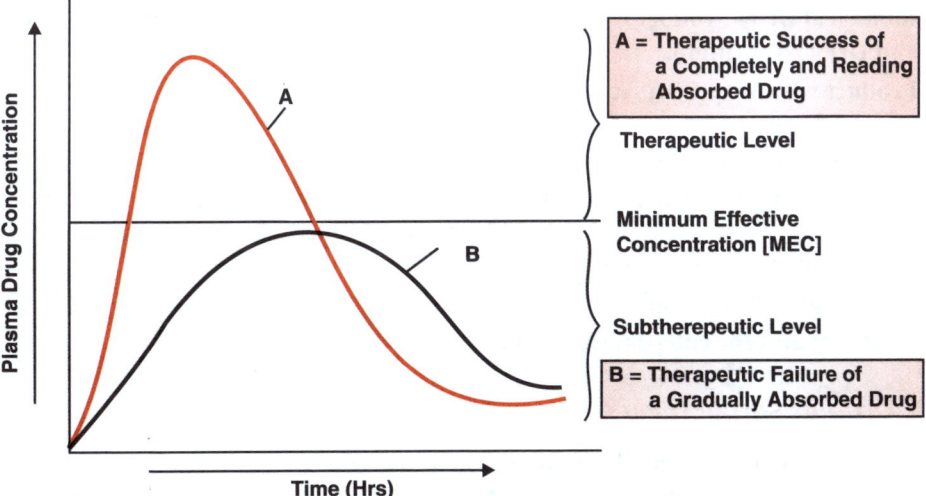

Fig. 2.7: A Plot between Time (hrs) and Plasma Drug Concentration Exhibiting Significance of Rate and Degree of Absorption in Drug Therapy.

Thus, one may take cognizance of the fact that in the critical phenomenon comprising **Drug: Disintegration, Dissolution,** and **Absorption,** the slowest step in the sequence signifies the **Rate-Determination Step** at which the drug reaches the ensuing **circulatory system.**

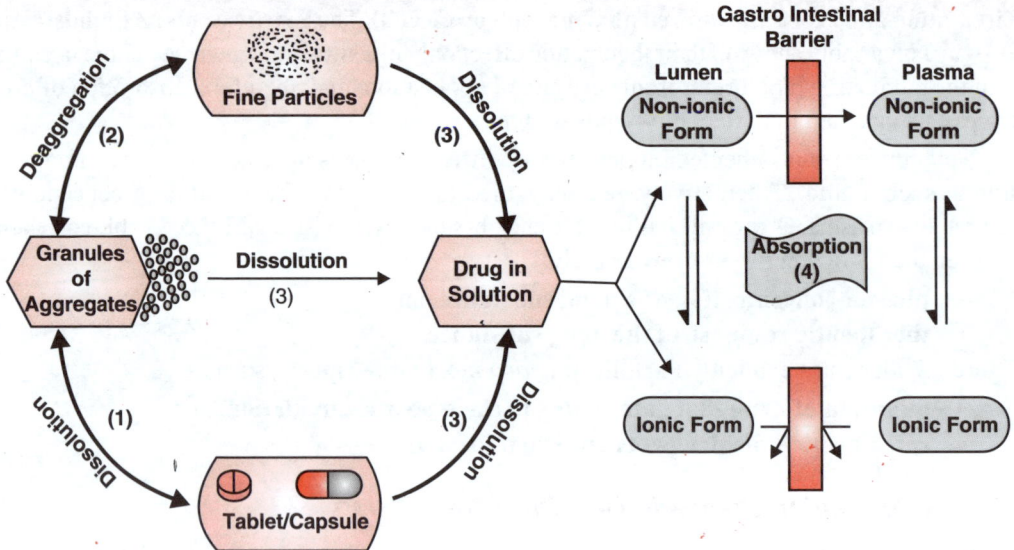

Fig. 2.8: Summary at a Glance of Various Processes Involved Following Oral Administration of a Drug in Tablet/Capsule Form.

[**Adapted From**: Blanchard **J. Am. J. Pharm.**, 150, 132-151, 1978]

Rate-Limiting Step: Amazingly, in an on-going '**Kinetic Process**', the slowest step is designated as the '**Rate-Limiting Step**'.

Usually, one may come across *three* **drug product variants,** namely:

1. **Controlled Release Product:** In this particular instance, the observed **disintegration of a solid Oral Drug Product is found to be more fast and rapid** *vis-a-vis* **Drug Dissolution and Drug Absorption.**

2. **Product with Very Poor Aqueous Solubility**: In this case, the rate at which the **drug gets dissolved** (*i.e., undergoes dissolution*) is often the slowest-observed step; and, therefore, exhibits a **Rate-Limiting Effect** *upon* **Bioavailability of a Drug Substance.**

3. **Drug Product with a High Water Solubility**: In this specific instance, the observed **Rate of Dissolution is fast and rapid**. Besides, the rate at which the drug sails across or permeates cell membranes is found to be:

   • **The slowest step,** and
   • **Designates the rate-limiting step.**

2.5.2. *Drug Absorption via Gastrointestinal Tract (GIT)*

It is widely known that the '**Oral Administration**' of a '**Drug**' is recognized to be the most common route usually adopted for systematically acting drug substances. Perhaps, one would expect to lay more emphasis on the **Gastrointestinal (GI) Absorption of Drugs**. Besides, it essentially embraces almost a broad spectrum of the so-called **Observed Drug Absorption Variability**.

In order to understand the in-depth intricacies of the various aspects of **GI Drug Absorptions**, it will be worthwhile to have a brief and comprehensive description of:

- **cell membrane structure,** and
- **GI physiology.**

2.5.2.1. *Cell Membrane Structure*

The **Cell Membranes** do form the barriers between various innumerable aqueous compartments present in the human body. Importantly, even a single layer of membrane is sufficient to cause an effective separation of the '**Intracellular Compartments**' from the '**Extracellular Compartments**'.

Salient Features: They essentially consist of the following:

1. The presence of an **Epithelial Barrier**, such as:

    (a) **gastrointestinal mucosa,** and

    (b) **renal tubule.**

Invariably comprises a '**Layer of Cells**' packed and connected tightly to each other in order that '**Drug Molecules**' should critically pass across at least *two* **Cell Membranes** (*viz. inner and outer*) to sail through from one side to the other easily and conveniently.

2. Importantly, the **Vascular Endothelium** appears to be rather more complex and complicated as well with regard to its so-called:
   - **critical anatomical disposition,** and
   - **variance in permeability from one tissue to another.**

3. Prevailing gaps between the particular **Endothelial Cells** are usually packed with a loose matrix of proteinous matter which more or less acts as '**filters**', thereby helping largely to
   - **retain large molecules,** and
   - **allow smaller ones to pass through.**

4. The actual '**cut-off Molecular Size**' appears to be not '**exact**':
   - **water molecules get transferred rapidly,** and
   - **drug molecules having molecule size ranging between 80-100 KD_a usually get transferred very sluggishly and gradually.**

5. Exceptionally, in **CNS** and **placenta**, one may normally come across **Tight Intracellular Junctions** existing between:
   - **membrane cells,** and
   - **endothelium**

which is encased adequately in an **Impermeable Layer of the 'Periendothelial Cells' (or 'Pericytes').**

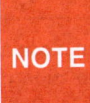

NOTE   In fact, these observed critical features do help in the prevention of potentially harmful and disastrous molecules from being leaked from the circulating blood right into these aforesaid organs (*viz.* placenta) and, hence, contribute to much desired major pharmacokinetics consequences for drug distribution.

6. Interestingly, in **liver** and **spleen**, the **Endothelium** is found to be discontinuous, which eventually permits **free passage between the cells.** Besides, in **liver** one may observe critically

the occurrence of **'Hepatocytes'** formed duly that serves as the **barrier between intra-and extravascular compartments.** The above phenomenon ultimately gives rise to an array of *several* **Endothelial Cell Functionalities**.

Routes Adopted by Small Drug Molecules in Crossing Cell Membranes There are in all four major variants by which the relatively **small drug molecules may be able to cross the ensuing cell-membranes** (as *shown in Figure 2.9*): *viz.*,

- effective diffusion directly *via* the lipid layer,
- critical diffusion *via* the inherent aqueous pores duly formed by specific proteins (*viz.* 'aquaporins'*) which pass through the lipid,

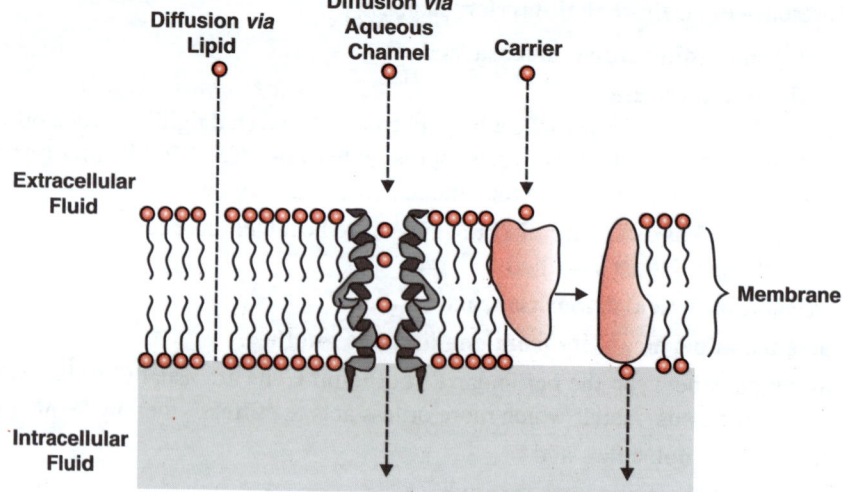

Fig. 2.9: Various Routes *via* Which Solutes ('Drugs') Can Pass Across Cell Membranes.

- crucial combination with a specific transmembrane-carrier protein which usually binds a drug molecule on one side of the membrane, and subsequently alters the prevailing conformation and finally release it on the other side of the membrane, and
- by means of 'Binocytosis' *i.e.*, the process by which cells absorb or ingest nutrients and fluid.

2.5.2.2. Pathways of Drug Absorption

The **Oral Administration of the Drug** releases it in the **Gastrointestinal (GI) Fluids** in the form of a solution, which essentially has the inherent potential of getting absorbed.**

---

* **Aquaporins:** They refer to a group of integral membrane proteins that usually function as molecular water channels to facilitate osmotic movement of water across the plasma membrane. Isolation of Aquaporin-1 from human erythrocytes/renal tubules [Denker BM *et al.*: J.Biol.Chem., **263**: 15634,1988].

** **Absorbable Form of Drug**: It solely depends upon the Physiochemical characteristic feature of the 'drug' besides such other environment physical properties, *viz.* pH, interfering substances and type of absorbing membrane.

Obviously, in the absence of any **'Interfering Materials'**, which may directly or indirectly affect its absorption, ultimately ascertains the diffusion from the respective **GI fluid to the corresponding Absorbable Membrane Surface.** In fact, **drug absorption overwhelmingly indicates the penetration of the drug substance very much across the intestinal membrane.** Thus, it subsequently appears in an unaltered form in the ensuing oozing blood flow from the **Gastrointestinal Tract (GIT).**

Important Points The above statement of facts suggests *two* **important points** *vis-a-vis* **drug absorption** phenomena, namely:

- As a common practice, it is assumed that the specific disappearance of a **'drug'** from the ensuing **Gastrointestinal (GI) Fluids** designates drug absorption predominantly; and its immediate appearance in the **circulating blood**. However, the aforesaid phenomenon does not hold good for such drug substances that:
  - ➤ **gets duly degraded in GI fluids**, or
  - ➤ **gets adequately metabolized in intestinal cells.**
- In true sense, the terminology **'Intestinal Membrane'** seems to be a **misnomer**, because the said **'membrane'** does not represent a *unicellular structure* but an array of unicellular membranes strategically positioned parallel to one another. Obviously, for a **'drug molecule'** to approach the blood stream,
  - ➤ **It should penetrate the critical mucous layer,** and
  - ➤ **It must reach the glycocalyx fully covering the gastrointestinal (GI) lumen, apical cell surface, fluids within cell, basal membrane, basement membrane, tissue segment of lamina propria, external capillary membrane, cytoplasm of capillary cell and inner capillary membrane.**

In short, it may be added that a particular **'Drug Molecule'** to enable its due absorption from the **GIT** and to sail across to the **Systemic Blood Circulation,** it should by all means penetrate efficaciously all the vital and important segments of the intestinal tract cited above.

There are, in fact, *three* **cardinal factors**-which predominantly govern the very **phenomenon of absorption,** namely:

1. **physiochemical properties of 'drug molecule',**
2. **characteristic features and components of 'GI fluid',** and
3. **nature of the 'absorbing membrane'.**

2.5.2.3. *Gastrointestinal (GI) Physiology*

In order to understand the **'Gastrointestinal Physiology'**, one needs to get familiarized with the major components of the **GI tract-stomach, small intestine** and **colon** (or *large intestine*). Besides, the small intestine essentially comprises such vital segments as: **duodenum, jejunum** and **ileum.** Interestingly, the *major segments of the GIT* mostly differentiate from one another in the following *four* aspects, such as:

- **anatomic variance,**
- **morphologic variance**,
- **emanated secretions,** and
- **preventing pH.**

Figure 2.10 clearly shows the following *three* **most prominent and vital aspects**, for instance:

1. **human gastrointestinal (GI) tract,**
2. **anatomy of stomach**, and
3. **anatomical regions of small intestine showing its relatively large surface area.**

Explanation

It essentially includes:

For Figure 2.10(a): The **GI Tract** compromises **stomach (pH 1-3)** having a **Pylorus** (*i.e.*, the lower portion of the stomach that opens into the duodenum) extending to **duodenum (pH 5-7), jejunum, ilenum, and finally to the ascending colon (pH 7-8).**

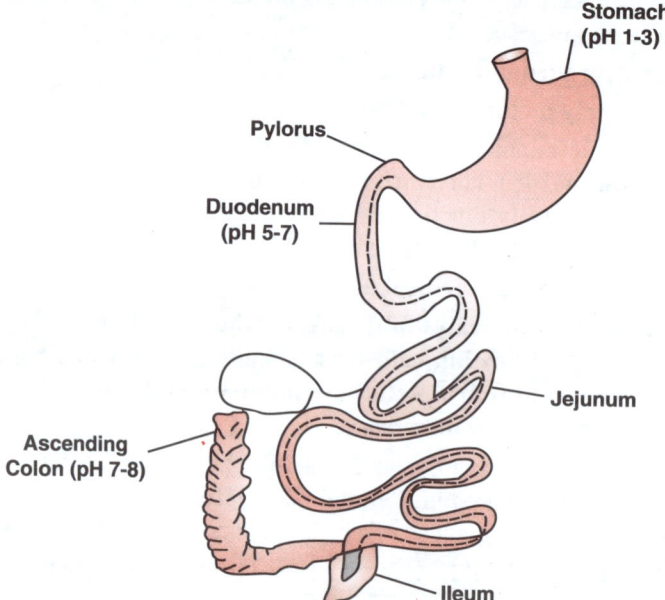

Fig. 2.10 (a): Diagram of a Human Gastrointestinal (GI) Tract.

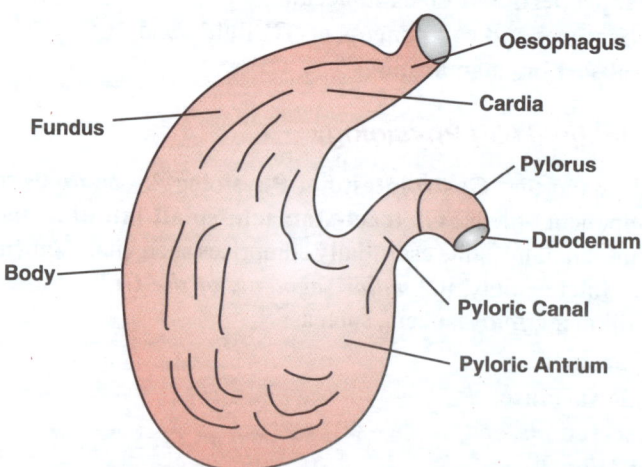

Fig. 2.10 (b): Anatomical Regions of the Human Stomach.

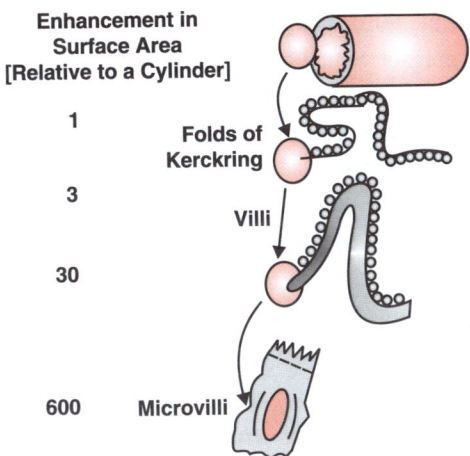

**Enhancement in
Surface Area
[Relative to a Cylinder]**

1

**Folds of
Kerckring**

3

Villi

30

600   **Microvilli**

Fig. 2.10 (c): Anatomical Details of Human Small Intestine Depicting its Large Surface Area
(extending from 1-600).

 NOTE   The main vital and important segments of GI tract critically differ from one another with respect to anatomical details, morphological specification, secretion pattern and pH.

For Figure 2.10(b): Stomach Looks like a pouch-resembling structure lined with a more or less smooth epithelial surface. Obviously, under certain experimental parameters, it may accomplish the following absorptions reasonably viable, such as:

- **weakly acidic drug substances,**
- **non-ionized drugs,** and
- **some weakly basic drug substances.**

Examples

Some typical examples have been duly reported by **Crouthamel *et al.* (1971)*** *e,g.,* **Sulphaethidole** and **Barbital, in surgically altered albino rats.**

Besides, under usual normal conditions, *viz.* a situation when **Gastric Emptying Phenomenon** is not impede, one may critically observe a rather modest drug absorption profile in the stomach. **Cooke and Hunt (1970)**** and **Cooke and Brichall (1969)***** demonstrated that the absorption of **Aspirin** and ethanol from the human stomach, after due oral administration of aqueous solutions in healthy subjects, has been determined to be **nearly 10% and 30%** of the normal dose, respectively. Nevertheless, in each of the above cite instance, the actual '**balance of the administered dose**' gets absorbed very much from the small intestine.

Figure 2.10(c): It may be observed that ensuing **Epithelial Surface Area**, *via* which the absorption may come into play in the small intestine, happens to be *extraordinary large*

---

* Crouthamel W G et al.: *J. Pharm. Sci.,* 60: 1160,1971.

** Cooke AR and Hunt JN: *Am. J. Dig. Dis., 15:*95,1970

*** Cooke AG and Birchall A: *Gastroenterology, 57:* 269,1969

(*i.e.,* **extending from 1 to 600**) by virtue of the critical presence of **Villi** and **Microvilli** that eventually give rise to typical characteristic **Finger-Like Projection(s)** emanating from and forming several folds in the **intestinal mucosa.**

Interestingly, the observed **irregularities in the mucosa surface** invariably produced by the **Villi, Microvilli,** and **Submucosal Folds** perceptively help in the enhancement of the specific area available for the absorption by almost 30-folds *vis-a-vis* the one would have gotten of a small intestine with a smooth surface in the tube (**Granger and Baker, 1950**)*

NOTE	It has been reported that the surface area in humans has been duly determined to vary between 80 cm cm serosal length just beyond the duodenojejunal flexure to nearly 20 cm^2 cm^{-1} serosal length just before the ileococal value.

2.5.3. *Fluid-Mosaic Model for Transcellular Diffusion of Polar Molecules*

The '**Fliud-Mosaic Model**' refers to '**the currently accepted model of cell membrane in which the membranes is a lipid bilayer with integral proteins buried in the lipid and peripheral proteins more loosely attached to the membrane surface**'.

Singer and Nicolson (1972)** proposed duly that the said '**Model**' explains explicitly the cell membrane which comprises the **globular proteins embedded intimately in a dynamic fluid** and a **lipid bilayer matrix** as illustrated in Figure 2.11.

Modus Operandi : The various steps consist of:

1. Importantly, the **Globular Proteins** critically give rise to the pathway responsible for causing the selective transfer of certain **Ionized (or Polar) Molecules and Charged Ions** *via* the **Lipid Barrier.**

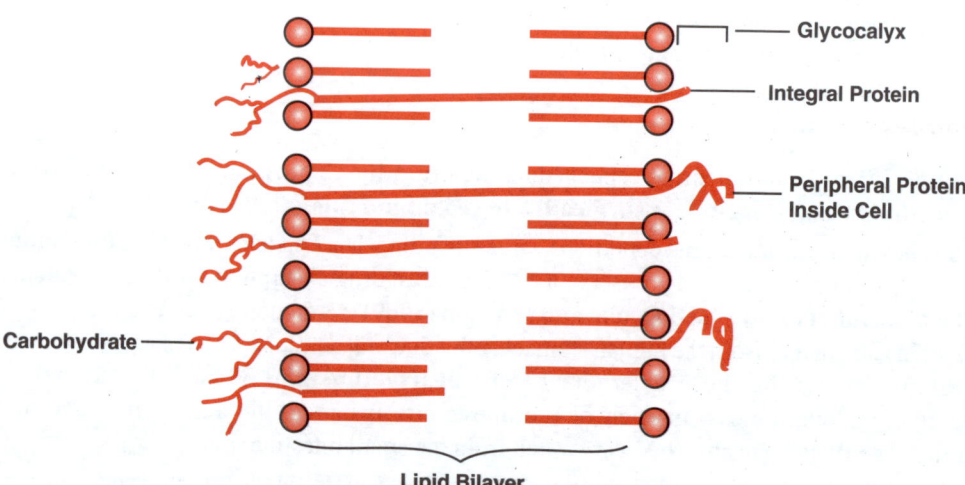

Fig. 2.11: Diagrammatic Representation of Various Cell Membrane Components.

*   Granger B and Baker RF: *Anat. Rec.,* **107**: 423,1950.
** Singer SJ and Nicolson GL: *Science,* **175**: 720-731, 1972.

2. From Figure 2.11 one may vividly observe that the **Transmembrane Proteins do get interdispersed particularly in the entire membrane.**

It has been observed that there exists two different types of pores: (a) ~10 nm, and (b) 50-70 nm, which were duly presented in the said membranes*.

3. These small inherent pores do provide a distinct channel *via* which **cations (Na, K), anioms (CI), urea, water may move across the Cell Membrane.**
4. Interestingly, the **movement of other Proteins,** *duly embedded in the membrane,* **fails to cross the entire membrane effectively.**
5. Besides, there are certain **Surface Glycoproteins** that do carry out vital and important function both as **'Drug Receptors'** and **'Biological Entities'.**

2.5.4. *Gastrointestinal Physiology*

Gastrointestinal Physiology may be expatiated adequately with the help of the following *two* **cardinal aspects,** namely:

- **gastrointestinal blood flow**, and
- **gastrointestinal pH.**

2.5.4.1. *Gastrointestinal Blood Flow*

It has been established beyond any doubt that the **blood perfusing the entire GI tract does play a vital and important role in the crucial absorption of drug by maintaining and modulating the ensuing. 'Concentration Gradient of the Drug' very much across the epithelial membrane.** Winne (1980)** pointed out that the predominant dependence of intestinal absorption upon the blood flow rate from the respective **'Blood-Flow Dependent'** to **'Blood-Flow Limited',** *which Is due to the enhanced absorbability* of **'drug substance'.**

Important Features: Following are some of the important features, namely:

1. **Polar Drug Molecules**, which usually get absorbed rather gradually, exhibit categorically little dependence upon the observed **Blood-Flow-Profile;** whereas, the following *two* aspects, namely:
   - **absorption pattern of lipid-soluble drug molecules (***viz.* **steroids), and**
   - **drug molecules which are tiny enough to pass through the 'aqueous pores' conveniently,**

are dependent exclusively upon the **Rate of Blood Flow** perceptively.

2. Importantly, the observed rate of most drug substances invariably demonstrates an **'Intermediate Dependence'** with regard to the **Rate of Blood Flow.** Nevertheless, it further suggests that a substantial lowering from the normal **'Mesenteric-Blood-Flow-Rate'** *is needed absolutely to cause a predominant change in the observed absorption rate of drug.*

---

* These studies were critically based upon the **Capillary Membrane Transport Mechanism.**

** Winne D: **Influence of Blood Flow upon Intestinal Absorption of Xenobiotics,** *Pharmacology,* **21**:1,1980

3. Generally, one may observe that the **Rate of Drug Absorption** is not affected at all by normal variability in critical **Mesenteric Blood Flow**.

4. Commonly, the apparent changes in **Mesenteric Blood-Flow** which usually come into play due to:

   - **disease conditions,** and/or
   - **drug effects**

should be sufficient and sustained to influence significantly the **absorption of drug.**

Mechanism of GI-Blood Flow: The following are some of the various important steps, namely:

1. The whole of blood supply invariably drawing most of the **GI tract** gets returned to the **Systemic Blood-Circulation** via the **'Liver'**. Perhaps, therefore, the **'Total Dose of a Drug'** being administered orally gets absorbed almost completely due to exposure to the **'Liver'** before reaching the **circulating blood-stream.**

2. As **'Liver'** serves as the most vital and important organ in the human body responsible for performing the **'Drug Metabolism'**, hence it helps in the **fast and rapid metabolization of certain drugs**. The latter prominent step duly suggests that a relatively **large segment of the dose shall never be able to reach the so-called 'Systemic Circulation' by virtue of its 'Hepatic Metabolism' during absorption process** *in-vivo.*

NOTE	The aforesaid phenomenon is usually termed as the 'Hepatic First-Pass-effect' which is eventually responsible for the less-than complete bioavailability of several drug substances being administered orally.

3. Besides, the critically observed metabolism of a **'Drug'** in the course of absorption by *certain enzymes duly present in the gut-wall may also cause an appreciable reduction in the bioavailability profile of the drug.*

2.5.4.2. *Gastrointestinal pH*

Amazingly, there exists predominantly almost a **10 million times** *the actual difference in the level of H ion concentration between the:*

   - **stomach,** and
   - **colon (large intestine),**

Importantly, an exceedingly large **10,000 times difference in the** *level of H ion concentration occurs between:*

   - **stomach,** and
   - **duodenum**.

Importance of GI pH: The prevailing **pH** at the very site of absorption seems to be a vital and important factor in the actual observed absorption profile due to the cardinal fact that several drug substances fall into the category of either **weak organic acids or weak organic bases**.

1. Mostly, in solution state, the typical **'Organic Electrolytes'** do exist in *two* **distinct forms,** namely:

   - **non-ionized form (***i.e.***, usually lipid-soluble),** and
   - **ionized form (***i.e.***, usually sparingly lipid-soluble),**

whereby the fraction of each species specifically depends upon the **ensuing pH of the solution**

2. **Observed variance from one segment to another:** Interestingly, as the particular **GI barriers*** are found to be definitely more permeable to the following *two* **solute variants**, namely:

- **unchanged solutes**, and
- **lipid-soluble solutes,**

a **'Drug Molecule'** may eventually get well absorbed from one segment of the GI tract wherein prevails a congenial (favourable) pH; whereas, it gets sparingly absorbed from another segment when it encounters a comparatively less favourable pH.

Examples

The following are a few *typical examples:*

(a) **Weakly Basic Drugs:** Such as **Anti-histaminies (Meclozine, Antazoline, Methapyrilence,) and 'Anti-depressants' (Amitriptyline, Buspirone) are usually favoured in the small-intestine where these drugs are largely present in a non-ionized form. Besides, the acidic gastric juice** has a tendency to reduce the particular absorption of the aforesaid **weakly basic drugs.**

(b) **Weakly Acidic Drugs**: Such as **'Sulphonamides' (Sulphadiazine, Sulphathiazole) and NSAIDs (Paracetamol, Aspirin, Ibuprofen),** where they would alter the pH of the fluids in a *given portion of GI tract which may improve or impede the ultimate absorption of a 'Drug' (as mentioned above).*

3. **Wide Variance in pH of 'Gastric Juice':** It has been duly recorded that the **gastric secretions invariably exhibit a pH less than 1;** whereas, the **pH of the gastric contents normally ranges between 1 and 3 due to the incurred dilution and food intake.** In addition, the pH of stomach contents is significantly and transiently elevated after a normal meal; however, attained **pH values at 5** are not at all regarded to be an **unusual/abnormal range.**

Some Typical Condition *vis-a-vis* **pH Variance GIT:** These essentially comprise the following.

(a) **Fasting condition in humans do help in the drastic lowering of pH of gastric juices.**

(b) **Certain disease conditions may also cause a noticeable reduction in the pH of the stomach.**

(c) **Patients having a history of 'duodenal ulcer' exhibit a marked and pronounced lower average gastric pH** *vis-a-vis* **the healthy humans.**

(d) **Excessive supplement of 'fats and fatty acids' in the regular diets do give rise to a distinct inhibition in gastric secretions.**

(e) **Clinical effect of certain specific class of drugs cause prominent reduction in the ensuing gastric secretions.**

---

* Besides other barriers and membranes present in the human body.

Examples

Some typical examples are given below:

- **Anti-spasmodic drugs,** *e.g.,* **Atropine, Propantheline,**
- **H-Blockers,** *e.g.,* **Ranitidine, Cimetidine,**
- **Several other drugs also show such pharmacologic actions,** *e.g.,* **suppression of gastric secretions and anti-cholinergic activity,** and
- **Antacids,** *e.g.,* **Aluminium Hydroxide, Magnesium Hydroxide are used abundantly in accomplish**
  - ➤ **neutralization of gastric hydroxide,** and
  - ➤ **enhancing the pH of gastric contents.**

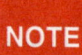 **NOTE**   **It is, however, pertinent to state here that the two critical situations that may arise due to (a) drug-influenced changes and (b) disease conditions may predominantly influence the stability or dissolution profile and/or some specific drug absorptions.**

2.5.5. *Gastric Emptying*

Theoretically, one would expect the weakly acidic drugs to exhibit essentially much improved absorbability from the stomach *vis-a-vis* from the intestine, since a major segment of the **'Dose'** is usually present in the state of:

- **non-ionized,** and
- **lipid-soluble.**

Besides, there are *two* **more logical and conceptualized beliefs** that govern and regulate the balance in influencing the ensuing **pH for determining the exact and precise site of 'Optimized Absorption',** such as:

- **restricted residence span of the 'drug' in the stomach,** and
- **comparatively smaller available surface area of the stomach.**

Thus, it may be duly concluded that several factors, in fact, do help in the **promotion of gastric emptying process; and thereby, enhance critically the rate of absorption of all drugs.** One may come across *two* divergent situations, for instance:

- **prompt gastric emptying-leading to faster onset of effect of 'drugs' that are eventually 'unstable in stomach juices' perhaps on account of:**
  - ➤ **low pH level,** and/or
  - ➤ **unavoidable enzyme activity.**

Examples

Penicillin G undergoes degradation after oral administration that solely depends upon *two* **cardinal factors: (a) residence time in stomach,** and **(b) pH of stomach fluid.**

- **Delayed gastric emptying causes delay in the onset of effect of orally administered drugs,** for instance:
  - ➤ **NSAIDs (Analgesics),** and
  - ➤ **Hypnotics and Sedatives (Barbiturates),**

which essentially need a rather fast and rapid clinical response to the patient

2.5.5.1. *Mechanism of Gastric Emptying*

There are several recognized and well-known mechanism that have been put forward for the gastric emptying phenomenon. A few vital and important examples are briefly discussed in the following sections.

Gastric Emptying- An Exponential Phenomenon

First-Order Reaction, *i.e.*, the ingested low-bulk meals and liquids are duly transferred right from the stomach to the duodenum [*see Figure 2.10(a)*] pre-dominantly exhibits a **biological half-life ($t_{1/2}$) extending from 20 to 60 minutes** in a healthy adult. Importantly, there are an array of factors that may directly affect the aforesaid **First-Order Reaction**, namely:

- **reduction of gastric emptying by means of fats and fatty acids in the regular food-intake, and**
- **relatively higher concentration of H ions, electrolytes, high viscosity or bulk, lying on the left-side, mental depression, disease conditions, *e.g.*, Crohn's disease, gastric ulcer, gastroesophageal reflux, gastroenteritis, pyloricstenosis, celiac disease, hypothyroidism, and in the course of the luteal phase in the menstrual cycle.**

Example

A host of drug may also reduce the phenomenon of gastric emptying, such as **Atropine, Amitrypline, Aluminium hydroxide, Chlorpromazine, Despiramine, Imipramine, Propantheline,** and Narcotic Analgesics.

NOTE	1. **Gastric emptying process is potentiated by an array of specific conditions, for instance hunger, fasting, alkaline, buffer solutions, anxiety, and lying on the right-hand side.** 2. **It may also be caused by several disease conditions, such as hyperthyroidism.** 3. **Due to certain typical drug actions, namely metaclopramide (*i.e.*, a dopaminergic blocker) frequently used for combating nausea and vomiting linked with cancer chemotherapy medicaments.**

Gastric Emptying of Liquids *vs.* Solid Drug Products or Foods

It has been established beyond any reasonable doubt that the observed gastric emptying of liquids is definitely much faster than that of the corresponding solid drug products (*e.g.*, Tablets, **Capsules**) and **Food Products**.

Examples

Horton *et al.* (1965)* reported that soon after the administration of 1.5 g of paracetamol (= three tablets) to 14 convalescent hospital patients, the observed plasma-drug concentration varied between 7.4 and 37 mcg mL, whereas the necessary time (minute) actually needed to attain the maximum plasma concentration ranged between 30 and 180 minutes.

Figure 2.12 depicts both these aforesaid indices of absorption explicitly indicating thereby that there prevailed a linear relationship between the rate of absorption and the gastric emptying half-life observed in each individual subject.

---

* Horton R E et al: *Br Med.J.*,**1**:1537, 1965.

Influence: Irrespective of the observed variability in rate of absorption, almost no noticeable difference could be recorded in the *degree of absorption of Paracetamol* among the subjects.

Gastric Emptying Designates a Simple Mono-Exponential Process

In certain specific instances, the **gastric emptying phenomenon** may be regarded as a **'simple mono-exponential process'**. Nevertheless, there existed a more or less complete agreement between

- **apparent absorption rate constant***, and
- **gastric emptying rate constant**.

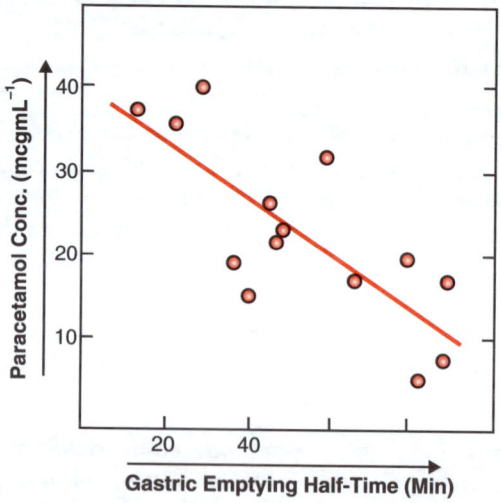

Fig. 2.12: Diagrammatic Representation Showing Relationship between Peak Concentration of Paracetamol in Plasma and Gastric Emptying Half-time (min) after a Single Oral Administration. (Rapid gastric emptying results in high-peak levels)**

Figure 2.13 illustrates the critical relationship existing between the apparent absorption rate constant (min) soon after a single oral dosage of **Paracetamol** in healthy human subjects who eventually emptied the '**Drug**' (**Paracetamol**) from their stomachs individually in a **mono-exponential manner**. Thus, one may also distinctly observe the so-called '**Line of Identity**'. However, under certain specific experimental parameters, the observed **Absorption Rate of a Drug** is designated by the respective **Rate-limited Gastric Emptying Process.**

Inference: Thus, one may conclude that instead of the **'Gastric Emptying'**, it is in reality the actual **'Transmucosal Transfer'** originating from the lumen of the small intestine that happens to be the **Rate-limiting Step** in the **Paracetamol absorption when administered in solution orally.**

In Figure 2.13 the distinct line of identity is duly depicted. However, under some typical experimental parameters, the *exact and precise Absorption Rate of a Drug is found to be Rate limited critically by Gastric Emptying Process.*

Besides, it has been observed that in most cases, the so-called **Calculated Rate Constant for Transfer of Paracetamol from the small intestine to the Circulating Blood Stream was**

---

*   Clements JA *et al.: Clin. Pharmacol. Ther.*, **24**: 420,1978.

** Based on Actual Data obtained from: Heading R C *et al*: *Br. J. Pharmacol*, **47**:415, 1973.

apparently more *vis-a-vis* the specific Rate Constant for Gastric Emptying.* Further more, once the drug approached the small intestine legitimately, the **Absorption was Fast and Rapid,** *i.e.,* **having the mean absorption plasma half-life of approximately 7 minute.**

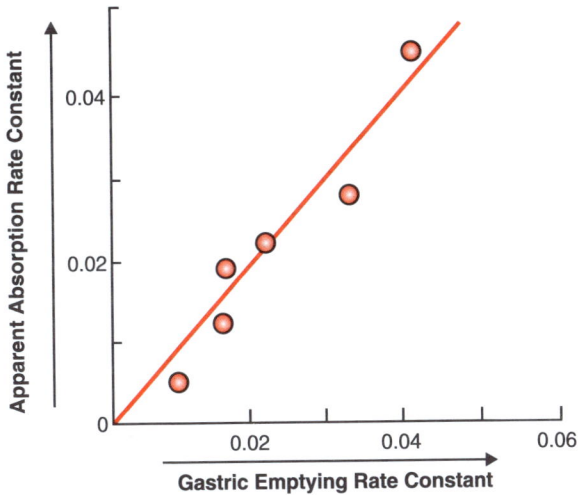

Fig. 2.13: Diagrammatic Representation of Critical Relationship between the Apparent Absorption Rate Constant (min) *vs* Gastric Emptying Rate Constant (min) After a Single Dose of Paracetamol in Healthy Patients in whom the 'Drug' Paracetamol was Emptied duly in a Mono-exponential Way**.

2.5.6. *Gastrointestinal (GI) Motility*

The observed critical **GI-Motility** of the small intestine, as evidently indicated by the **Small-Bowel Transit Time**, does exert a pivotal role in **Absorption of Drug. Eve (1966)** advocated that the mean transit time of the following *two* **components**, namely:

- **unabsorbed food residues**, and
- **insoluble granules**,

via the small intestine is **determined to be almost 4 hours. Davis *et al.* (1988)*** reported that intestinal-transit of pharmaceutical **Dosage Forms** (or **Drug Products**), *e.g.,* **small pellets, solutions, tablets, non-disintegrating capsules** *etc.,* remarkably varied between 3 and 4 hours and were found to be independent of:

- **type of drug product**, and
- **fasting or feeding of the subjects.**

Following are some of the observed values *per se* of a **Constant Release-Rate Tablet:** for its **gastrointestinal transits, 7.6 hours,** and **stomach emptying time averaged 3.1 hours**. Therefore, the **Intestinal Transit Time** is determined to be **(7.6-3.1) = 4.5 hours.**

Important Highlights: There are several important highlights with regard to the effects of **Gastrointestinal Motility**, namely:

---

* **Gastric Emptying Rate:**It refers to the average time required for the stomach to empty its contents into the intestine; invariably, once every 2-4 hrs.

** Eve IS: *Health Phys*, **12**: 131, 1966

*** Davis SS *et. al.*: *J Clin Pharmacol.*, **26**: 435,1988.

1. The degree of absorption of drugs which are absorbed quite incompletely could be solely due to its dependence on the **Intestinal Motility.**

Example

Both intensive and extensive '**clinical investigative studies**' have revealed duly that the drug **Propantheline** (an **antispasmodic**) critically enhances the absorption of:

- **Riboflavin (Vitamin B)* beyond two times in healthy human volunteers,**
- **Hydrochlorothiazid** (a diuretic)-by nearly one-third,.**
- **Nitrofurantoin ***(an antimicrobial)-by almost 50%,** and
- **Digoxin****** Manninen **It augments the steady-state serum concentration of digoxin (a cardioactive agent particularly in patients already put on a maintenance digoxin therapy.**

2.6. MECHANISM OF DRUG ABSORPTION

In a broader perspective, it would be understood fairly that for initiating and accomplishing specific and critical '**Systemic Absorption**', a drug substance should pass from the *absorption site via or around one or more than one layers of cells to enter the overall general circulation in a human body*. Importantly, perhaps one of the most vital and crucial aspects could be ideally the **permeability of a 'drug' at the very absorption site based upon the following** *two* **cardinal aspects, namely:**

- **Systemic circulation being closely associated with the molecular structure of the ensuing drug molecule,** and
- **Biochemical and physical characteristic features of the requisite cell membranes.**

However, it is pertinent to mention at this point in time that to afford the critical absorption right inside the cell, **the drug entity should have the ability and potential to transverse the cell membranes squarely.** Quite often, we may come across the following *two* **types of absorption phenomenon perceptively** *viz.,:*

1. **Transcellular Absorption**: It refers to the phenomenon of a **Drug Movement Very Much Across a Cell.**
2. **Paracellular Drug Absorption**: In certain polar molecules, we may observe their inability to transverse the cell membrane; however, instead they pass via the '**right junctions**' or '**gaps**' existing between the cells commonly known as **Paracellular Drug Absorption.**

NOTE	**A few drug substances do have a tendency to get absorbed by means of a 'mixed mechanism' that essentially involves either one or more processes.**

A survey of literature would reveal meticulously that the so-called '**Principal Mechanisms**' for the particular and crucial transport of drug molecules duly **Across the Cell Membrane** based strictly upon their *inherent fundamental importance* are as stated under sequentially:

---

   * Levy G *et al.*: *J. Pharm.Sci.*, **61**: 789, 1972

  ** Beermann B and Groschinsky-Grind M: *Eur. J. Clin. Phamacol.*, **13**:385, 1978

 *** Jaffe JM:*J. Pharm. Sci.*, **64**:1729, 1975.

**** Manninen V *et al.*: *Lancet*, **1**:398, 1973

1. **Passive Diffusion,**
2. **Pore Transport (or Convective Transport),**
3. **Carrier-mediated Transport,**
4. **Active Transport,**
5. **Facilitated Diffusion,**
6. **Carrier-mediated Intestinal Transport,**
7. **Ionic or Electrochemical Diffusion,**
8. **Ion-pair Transport,** and
9. **Endocytosis.**

All the aforesaid variants pertaining to the '**Principal Mechanisms**' shall now be treated individually in the sections that follow:

2.6.1. *Passive Diffusion*

Passive Diffusion relates to-'**the movement of drug molecules from a region of higher concentration to a region of lower concentration** *via* **a membrane that does not participate in the actual process'.**

However, it may be **expressed quantitatively by Fick's First Law of diffusion.**

In other words, this typical phenomenon is exclusively '**Passive**' *in nature since no external energy is expended virtually*. It may be observed explicitly that the drug molecules do exhibit a tendency to move randomly forward and backward specifically across a membrane as illustrated vividly in Figure 2.14.

In actual practice, *two* **typical situations may arise distinctively** as stated under:

1. **Two Regions Having Same Drug Concentration**: Here, the forward-moving drug entities shall be balanced by molecules moving backward, thereby giving rise to absolutely little overall net transfer of drug.
2. **A Region Having Higher Drug Concentration** *vis-a-vis* **Other Region:** In this instance, the actual number of the forward-moving drug molecules shall be higher than the number of backward-moving drug molecules, thereby resulting in an obvious glaring transfer of molecules to the particular region having the critical lower-drug concentration, as shown by the '**Big-Arrow**' in Figure 2.14.

Explanation

The various essential aspects essentially comprise the following:

1. Drug molecules in solution have a **tendency to diffuse randomly in all directions equally and squarely.**
2. Since the drug molecules undergo diffusion from **LHS to RHS** and *vice versa* (as indicated by small arrows in Figure 2.14), one may evidently visualize and observe an overall net diffusion taking place from the **high-concentration region to the low-concentration region perceptively.**

3. The aforesaid sequence of fateful event results in a net '**Flux**'* designated as J, to the RHS. In fact, the resulting '**Flux**' **is duly measured in mass per unit area (***viz*.**mg cm^{-2})****

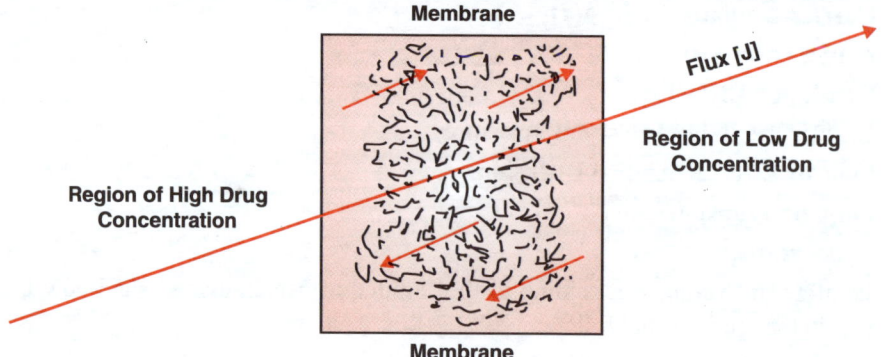

Fig. 2.14: Diagrammatic Representation of Passive Diffusion of Drug Molecules.

2.6.1.1. *Fick's Law of Diffusion*

It has been duly established that a majority of drug molecules obviously undergo '**Passive Diffusion**' *via* the most ***common and major*** **Transmembrane Phenomenon**. Nevertheless, the critical and main driving force for causing the **Passive Diffusion** being the virtual difference prevailing in the drug concentrations on either sides of the **Cell Membrane** (*see Figure 2.14*).

Thus, according to **Fick's Law of Diffusion**, the drug molecules do undergo critical diffusion right **from a region of high drug concentration to the region of low drug concentration, which is given by the following expression:**

$$\frac{dQ}{dt} = \left[\frac{DAK}{h} \right] (CGI-Cp)$$

where,

dQ/dt = Rate of drug diffusion (amount/time),

D   = Diffusion coefficient of drug via the membrane (area/time),

A   = Surface area of membrane for drug diffusion (area),

K   = Partition coefficient (of the drug between the lipoidal membrane and the aqueous GI fluids has no units),

h   = Thickness of membrane and

CGI-Cp relates to-'**the difference between the concentrations of drug in the gastrointestinal (GI) tract and in the plasma [also known as the concentration gradient (amount/volume or mg mL^{-1}]**'.

---

*   '**Flux**': It refers to the rate of drug transfer and is usually represented by a vector to indicates its actual direction.

**   Shargel L and Yu ABC: **Applied Biopharmaceutics and Pharmacokinetics**, 4th ed., McGraw-Hill Medical Publishing, New York, 1999.

2.6.1.2. *Characteristic Features of Passive Diffusion*

Following are some of the **Characteristic Features of Passive Diffusion:**

1. Drug molecule distributes rapidly into a relatively large volume soon after gaining an access to the circulating blood thereby resulting in an extremely **Low Plasma-Drug Concentration** *vis-a-vis* **the observed concentration at the very site of drug administration.**

2. Drug substance is invariably administered in 'mg' doses; whereas, the recorded **Plasma-Drug Concentrations** are **often expressed as mcg mL or ng mL ranges.**

3. The **Orally Administered Drugs** (*viz.* **Tablets, Capsules**) the **CGI > Cp**, which obviously indicates that a definitely large concentration gradient is duly maintained and sustained thereby driving the drug molecules very much into the **plasma** from the ensuing **GI Tract**.

4. **Fick's Law of Diffusion** obviously expatiates such cardinal aspects as:
   - **lipoidal solubility of the drug molecule,**
   - **surface area of the membrane,** and
   - **thickness of the membrane,**

   do influence enormously the observed **Passive Diffusion of Drug Molecules.**

5. **Partition Coefficient 'K'** evidently designates the *lipid-water partitioning of a drug molecule*. It may be observed that *lipid-soluble drugs* (*viz.* **Steroids**) *do exhibit a definite greater* **'K' values, which enhance theoretically the specific rate of systemic drug absorption.**

> **NOTE**   In usual practice, the absorption of drug is generously influenced by an array of physical factors possessed by the drug; and, thus, restricts its practical application of 'K'.

6. The critical **Surface Area of the Cell Membrane** *vis-a-vis* the drug gets normally absorbed influences more or less directly the **Actual Rate of Drug Absorption.**

7. Most **drug substances get duly absorbed** from several region located strategically along the **GI Tract**.

8. Incidentally, the particular **duodenal region of the small intestine** clearly displays the most **rapid drug absorption** perhaps under the influence of such obvious anatomic features as: *Villi* and **Microvilli,** that distinctly afford a large surface area [see Figure 2.10(c)].

> **NOTE**   Importantly, one may not come across these villi such a huge quantum in other regions of the GI tract.

9. Interestingly, the **Cell Membrane Thickness 'h'** remains constant at the very site of **absorption;** however, it *may get changed due to certain disease conditions perceptively.*

10. The *Capillaries are more thickly lined with the* **Glial Cells in the brain thereby creating a Denser Lipid Barrier** [also know as **blood-brain barrier (BBB)**] *which may cause a drug substance to undergo diffusion in a more sluggish manner into the brain.*

> **NOTE**   In 'meningitis' (*i.e.,* inflammation of the membranes of the brain), the cell membranes may become either more permeable to drug diffusion or get disrupted profusely.

2.6.1.3. *Fate of Lipophilic and Hydrophilic Substituted Drugs*

There are a good number of **Lipophilic and Hydrophillic Substituted Drugs** available abundantly in the therapeutic armamentarium.

Lipophillic-Substituted Drugs: Sodium salt of novobiocin, tolbutamide, testosterone palmitate;

Hydrophillic-Substituted Drugs: Crystalline Penicillin G, Chloramphenicol succinate; Lipid-Soluble Drugs: They usually traverse across the cell membranes more easily and conveniently than the relatively less lipid-soluble ones (more water-soluble drugs).

There are *two* **types of drugs,** namely:

1. **Weak-Electrolyte Drugs [or Weak acids Bases]:** In this particular instance, the degree of ionization influences, *viz.,*
   * **solubility of drug,** and
   * **rate of drug transport.**

2. **Ionized Drugs:** Mostly the **Ionized Drugs** (or polar drugs) are found to be **More Water-Soluble** *vis-a-vis* the **Non-Ionized Drugs that are More Lipid Soluble in nature.**

It is, however, pertinent to mention here that the **Degree of Ionization of a 'Weak Electrolyte'** [see (1) above] solely depends upon:

* **pK value of the drug substance,** and
* **pH (*i.e.,* partition hypothesis) of the medium where the 'Drug' remains in a dissolved state.**

2.6.1.4. Implication of Henderson and Hasselbalch Equation

According to the **Henderson and Hasselbalch Equation,** the prevailing *ratio of charged state of drug to uncharged form of the drug depends exclusively upon the following factors,* such as:

* **pH conditions,** and
* **pK value of 'Drug Substance'.**

Thus, we may have *two* **different ratios** for **'Weak Bases'** as given under:

For 'Weak Acids':

$$\text{Ratio} = \frac{\text{(Salt)}}{\text{(Acid)}} \quad \frac{[A^-]}{HA} = 10^{(pH-pK_a)}$$

For ;'Weak Bases':

$$\text{Ratio} = -\text{(Base) (Salt)} = [RNH]_2\,[RNH^{3+}] = 10^{(pH-pK_a)}$$

Examples

Following are *two* **typical examples** to exemplify the **Weak Acids and Weak Bases:**

1. **Salicylic Acid** (*i.e.,* a **'Weak Acid'):** As per the **inherent pH of salicylic acid,** it is expected to get absorbed readily right from the **stomach (pH 1.2)** by virtue of a congenial and favourable

existence of a concentration gradient of the unionized (*i.e.*, more lipid-soluble) state of the drug from the stomach into the **circulating blood***.

2. **Quinidine (*i.e.*, a 'Weak Base'):** The drug gets highly ionized in an environment of acidic pH and gets absorbed rather sluggishly right from the stomach. Importantly, majority of drugs are duly governed by the prevailing pH; however, in actual practice most of the drugs get absorbed abundantly in the **duodenum**** *perhaps due to the availability of a relatively large and extended surface area plus a high blood-flow.*

2.6.2. *Pore Transport (Convective Transport)*

Pore Transport (or **Convective Transport**) refers to-'**the smooth passage of large molecules or small particulate colloids *via* a minute opening in a cell membrane tissue (serving as a filtration membrane)'**.

It is also known as a **Bulk Flow or Simple Filtration.**

Importantly, **Pore Transport** predominantly aids in the following *three* **critical and specific drug variants**, namely:

- **low molecular weight drugs (with values <100),**
- **low molecular size drug (having lesser diameter than the pore itself), and**
- **usually water-soluble drugs via narrow aqueous-filled channels or membranes duly present in the membranes structure.**

NOTE   The *three* most common components are Urea, Carbohydrates and Water.

2..6.2.1. *Highlights of Pore Transport*

These essentially consist of

1. **Linear or Chain-like drug molecules having Molecular Weight up to 400 Da** which may eventually also get absorbed by filtration.
2. In true sense, the driving force is meticulously caused by *two* **physical characteristics features,** namely:
   - **hydrostatic pressure,** or
   - **osmotic differences,**

prevailing across the membrane due to which the *bulk flow of water along with small solid molecules comes into being via such aqueous channels.*

Water Flux: Water Flux normally refers to –'**the excessive flow or discharge of water across a membrane'**. It promotes prominently via the aqueous channels and is frequently termed **'Solvent Drag'**.

The specific importance and advantageous benefits due to the **'Drug Permeation'** *via* the water-filled channels are as stated under:

---

*   This is on account of the fact that almost '**all the drug**' present duly in the blood compartment get entirely **ionized (or dissociated) at pH 7.4.1**

**   That is, small intestine

- **renal excretion,**
- **critical removal of 'Drug' from the cerebrospinal fluid (CSF),** and
- **access of Drug Substances into the liver**.

2.6.3. *Carrier-Mediated Transport*

On the basis of theoretical aspects, one may take cognizance of the underlying fact that a-**'lipophilic drug substance would be able to pass *via* the cell or even go around it'**. Importantly, in case, a drug possess a *low molecular weight* and also is *lipophilic in nature*, it may be safely noted that the **ensuing lipid-cell membrane fails to pose as a stiff barrier to afford the desired:**

- **drug diffusion,** and
- **drug absorption.**

Interestingly, in the entire length of the small intestine, such drug molecules that are *smaller than 500 MW may eventually get absorbed particularly by the so-called* '**Paracellular Drug Absorption**'.

In other words, there exists a host of '**Polar Drugs**' or '**Ionized Drugs**' that do have a tendency to cross the cell membrane more rapidly *vis-a-vis* based on the prediction from their respective inherent:

- **concentration gradient values**, and
- **partition coefficient values**.

In a broader perspective, the aforesaid concepts and ideas suggest overwhelmingly the prominent and critical presence of *certain highly specialized* '**Transport Mechanism**' without which an array of ***water-soluble essential nutrients**, e.g.,* **Vitamins**, **Amino Acids**, and **Monosaccharide (Glucose)**, shall undergo absorption rather slowly and sluggishly. The most preferred and logical mechanism that explains the above may be the specific component of the membrane invariably termed as the '**Carrier**' which gets duly bound to:

- **reversibly,** and/or
- **noncovalently,**

In association with the **solute molecules** (*e.g.*, **drug molecules**) intended to be transported ultimately. It has been observed with enough evidential support that the emerging **Carrier-Solute Complex** does transverse very much across the membrane to the other side, **where it eventually dissociates and discharges the intended drug molecule**. After playing its pivotal role, '**Carrier**' gets back to its so-called '**Original Site**' so as to go ahead with the completion of the cycle by promptly accepting another fresh/new drug molecule of the solute. Interestingly, the said '**Carrier**' could be critically either:

- **an enzyme**, or
- **certain other integral constituent belonging to the membrane**.

2.6.3.1. *Important Characteristic Features of Carrier-Mediated Transport System*

Following are the *five* vital and important characteristic features of the Carrier-Mediated Transport System, namely:

1. importantly, the critical **'Transport Process'** turns out to be highly structure specific, which means that the ensuring carriers do possess not only a specific affinity for, but also has the ability to transfer a **'Drug'** with a particular chemical structure only. In general, the carriers exhibit a special affinity for certain essential nutrients.

2. As the **Carrier-Mediated Transport System** happens to be a *structure-specific one*, **such drug substances do have a close structural resemblance to the essential nutrients** (*viz.* **Amino acids, Glucose, Vitamins** etc.) invariably termed as the **'False Nutrients'** are adequately absorbed by the *Same Carrier System*.

Examples

Several **Anti-Neoplastic Drugs**, *e.g.*, **5-Fluoracial [or 5-FU], 5-Bromouracil [or 5-BU]**, do serve as **false nutrients**, thereby indicating the importance of their *mechanism of action*.

3. Since the exact and precise number of 'Carriers' is usually restricted, the **Transport System** is invariably subjected to **encounter a sort of competition between such drug molecules possessing intimately identical structures.**

4. Furthermore, as the actual number of 'Carriers' is found to be limited in quantum, the **Transport System** is regarded to be a **Capacity-Limited System.** In other words, **at higher level of drug concentration, the aforesaid system is rendered almost saturated; and, therefore, ultimately approaches an asymptomatic state**. Nevertheless, it is important to note that for a drug substance being suitably absorbed by

   - **Passive Diffusion Processes**- where by the rate of absorption gets enhanced linearly with the ensuring concentration of **'Drug'** and

   - **Carrier-Mediated Processes**- whereby the absorption of the **'Drug'** increases almost linearly with its concentration till such time the resulting carries get duly saturated after which it is rendered:

     ➤ **Curvilinear**, and

     ➤ **Accomplishes a 'Constant Value' at specific higher dose levels**.

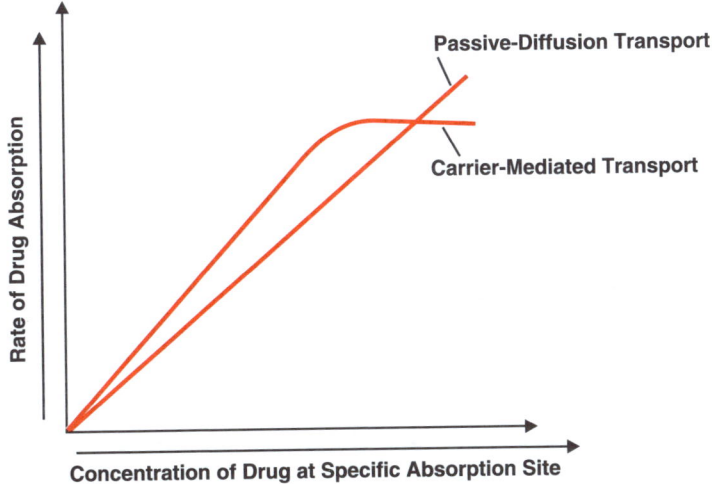

Fig. 2.15: A Typical Comparison between the Actual Rate of Absorption of Drug *vs.* Drug Concentration Plots due to Passive Diffusion and Carrier-mediated Transport Processes.

Figure 2.15 illustrates the typical comparison in the **Actual Rate of Absorption** *vis-a-vis* the **Drug Concentration Plots** duly obtained for:

- **Passive Diffusion Transport Process**, and
- **Carrier-mediated Transport Process**.

Explanation

Various steps essentially include:

1. A **Capacity-Limited Process** may be expatiated duly by means of the **Mixed-Order Kinetics**, which is also known as: **Non-Linear Kinetics** or **Michaelis-Menten Saturation**.

2. The phenomenon is termed as '**Mixed-Order Kinetics**' by virtue of the following *two* **glaring facts**, namely:

   - **It remains First-order at the sub-saturation drug concentration levels exclusively,** and

   - **It attains Zero-order at as well as above saturation levels ultimately.**

3. Besides, the ensuring **Capacity-Limited Specialized Features** of such a system do suggest that the **Observed Biovailabilty of a Drug Substance being absorbed meticulously *via* such a system retard with an increasing dosage regimen.**

Example

A typical example includes administration of **Water-Soluble Vitamins**, *e.g.*, **Vitamins B_1, B_2 and B_{12}**.

NOTE	Therefore, the administration of a 'single large oral dose' of the vitamins B_1, B_2 and B_{12} appear to be absolutely irrational and uncalled for.

4. The **Carrier-Mediated Absorption Processes** (or-**Specialized Absorption Phenomenon**) invariably comes into play from the specific sites located strategically in the intestinal tract that are found to be abundantly richer in the availability of requisite carriers.

Concept of Absorption Window: It refers to –'**an area wherein the particular carrier-system is observed to be highly dense**'.

Incidentally, all drugs that are duly absorbed *via* these types of absorption windows do represent as *poor candidates* (drugs) usually required for the **Controlled-Release Formulations** perceptively.

2.6.4. Active Transport

The **Active Transport** may be defined as –'**the process by which a cell membrane moves molecules against a concentration or electrochemical gradient**'.

It is indeed a *metabolic work*. A glaring example being the *very low observed concentration of K^+ ions present in the* **Extracellular Fluid (ECF)**. Besides, there are **other ions that are transported actively**, *e.g.*, Na^{2+}, Ca^+, H, Fe^{2+}, CI, I^- and H^+NCONH_2 **(Urate)**. Interestingly, there are quite a few *amino acids* and *carbohydrates* that also transport actively.

Another school of thought believes that **'Active Transport'** is more or less a **Carrier-Mediated Transport membrane Process** which is found to be absolutely essential for:

- **GI absorptions of certain drug substances**, and
- **Active participation in both renal and biliary secretion of several drug molecules and their respective metabolites.**

Mechanism of Action: The precise **Mechanism of Active Transport** may be explained judiciously when a **'Carrier'** gets bound to the **drug molecule** to give to the formation of a **Carrier-Drug Complex** which carefully carries out the following *two* activities, namely:

- **Pushing the drug across the membrane**, and
- **Subsequent dissociation of the drug on the other side of the membrane as depicted in Figure 2.16(a) and (b).**

Figure 2.16 (a) and (b) clearly explains the following related aspects pertaining to the **'Active transport'** such as:

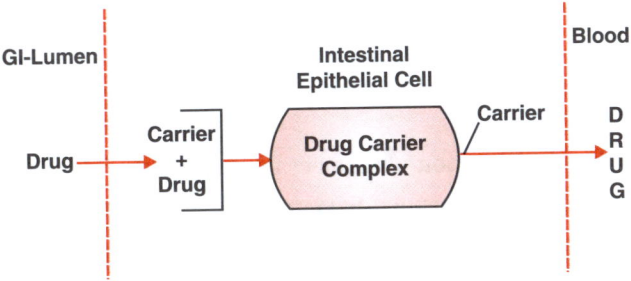

Fig. 2.16: (a) Representation of a Hypothetical Carrier-Mediated Transport Phenomenon. [Adapted from: Shargel L, Yu ABC. Applied Biopharmaceutics and Pharmacokinetics, 4th ed. McGraw Hill Medical Publishing, New York, 1999]

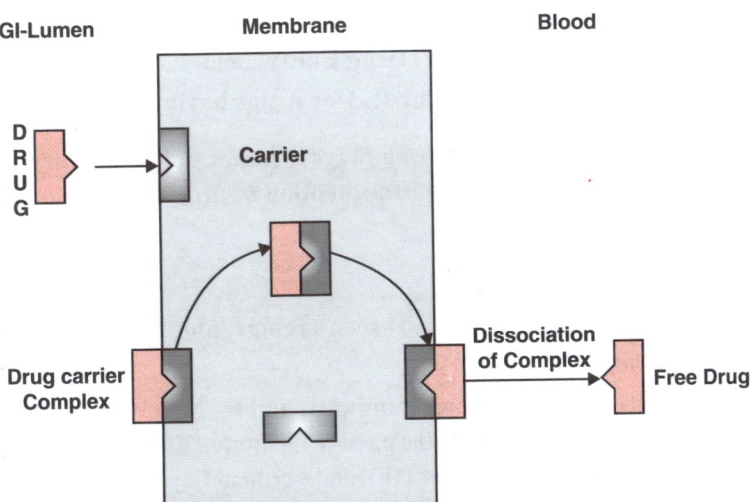

Fig. 2.16: (b) Diagrammatic Representation of an Active Absorption of a Drug (ATP = Adenosine triphosphate).
[*Adapted From*: **Shargel L, Yu ABC.** Applied Biopharmaceutics and Pharmacokinetics, **4th ed:** McGraw Hill Medical Publishing, New York, 1999].

- Candidate **'Drug'** is duly transported from a region of lower concentration to a region of higher concentration, *i.e.*, a sort of **'Uphill Transport'** or sometimes also referred to as **'Against a Concentration Gradient'**, without attaining a state of equilibrium.

- As the ensuring phenomenon engages a **'Uphill Transport'**, it essentially needs **energy for the necessary-job-done by 'Carrier'**.

- Since the entire phenomenon requires prominently the critical utilization of energy, it may be inhibited duly by the incorporation of certain **'Metabolic Poisons'**, *viz. lack of O,F, CN⁻ and dinitrophenol*, which directly interfere with the **vital function of energy production**.

2.6.5. *Facilitated Diffusion*

The **Facilitated Diffusion** may be defined as-**'the movement of molecules (drugs) across a membrane barrier in which a carrier protein is required'**.

It essentially involves the movement of drug molecules from a region of higher concentration to a region of lower concentration, and the most entrusted driving force being the **concentration gradient.** Besides, no other energy input is ever required beyond that necessary for carrying out the normal cellular function.

In short, the **'Facilitated Diffusion'** designates predominantly:

- **a Non-Energy Needed Transport System,** and
- **a Carrier-Mediated Transport system,**

wherein the **'Drug Substance'** moves critically and essentially very much along a **concentration gradient. Facilitated Diffusion** does possess the following *three* **major characteristic features,** namely:

- **process entails a 'Saturable One',**
- **remains selective structurally for 'Drug Entity',** and
- **exhibits distinct 'Competition Kinetics' for drugs having a similar structure.**

 NOTE   **Generally, the facilitated diffusion plays a rather not-so important role in the entire phenomenon related to the absorption of drug molecule.**

Examples

Some typical examples engaging essentially such a **remarkable transport system** comprise:

1. Entry of **'Glucose'** into the **RBCs**.

2. Intestinal absorption of **Water-soluble vitamins B_1 and B_2.** Nevertheless, one may expatiate the probable mechanism with respect to the **passive facilitated diffusion in the GI absorption of vitamin B.** Thus, an **Intrinsic Factor (IF),** and a critical **Glycoprotein** generated duly by the **Gastric Parietal Cells,** ultimately gives rise to the formation of a **Complex with Vitamin B_{12} (Cyanocobalamine),** that eventually is transported across the so-called **'Intestinal Membrane'** with the help of a **Carrier System** *in-vivo*.

Figure 2.17 depicts the diagrammatic representation of the **Facilitated Diffusion of Vitamin B$_{12}$ (Cyanocobalamine)**.

2.6.6. *Carrier-Mediated Intestinal Transport*

It has been duly observed that there exists a plethora of **Carrier-Mediated Systems (Transporters)** located strategically at:

- **intestinal brush border,** and
- **basolateral membrane,**

serving specifically for the critical absorption of certain **Specialized Ions and Nutrients required urgently for the human body.** An array of drug substances get absorbed meticulously by the aid of these **Carriers due to their close structural similarly to the naturally occurring substrates.**

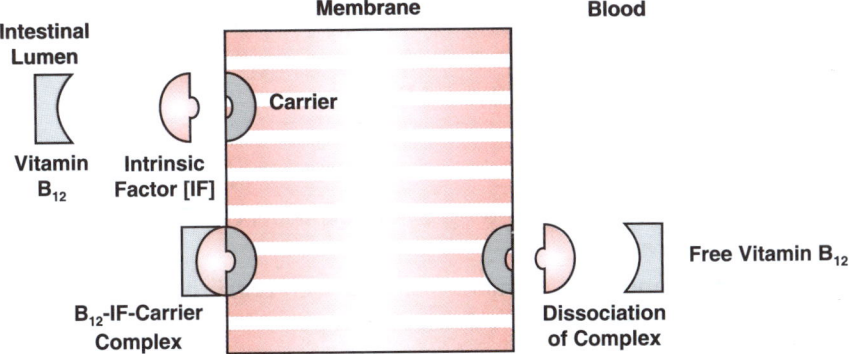

Fig. 2.17: Diagrammatic Representation of Facilitated Diffusion of Vitamin B$_{12}$.

Examples

Following are some of the typical examples of **Carrier-Mediated Intestinal Transport Process,** *viz.,*

1. **P-Glycoprotein [or P-Gp]: P-Glycoprotein** is an intestinal transmembrane protein that causes the specific reduction of the ensuing **intestinal epithelial cell permeability from lumen to the circulating blood for a good number of Cytotoxic** and **Lipophillic Drugs**.

2. **Amino Acid Transporters:** These are duly present in the intestines. A number of **Oral Cephalosporins** are adequately *absorbed via the amino acid transporters perceptively.*

2.6.7. *Ionic Diffusion (or Electrochemical Diffusion)*

One may take cognizance of the fact that the inherent charge residing on the membrane influences the actual permeation of drug substances. Nevertheless, the usual **molecular forms of solutes** (or **Drug Molecules) are found to be quite unaffected by the corresponding membrane charge;** and, therefore, permeate even faster *vis-a-vis* the **Ionic Forms**. Interestingly, it has been duly observed that the **anionic solute permeates more rapidly than the cationic solute.**

Hence, at a given pH, the observed rate of permeation will be of the following order:

Unionized Molecules > Anions > Cations

2.6.7.1. *Permeation Profile of Cationic Drug Molecules*

The **Permeation Profile of Cationic Drug Molecule** solely depends upon either the ensuing **'Electrical Gradient'** or the prevailing **'Potential Difference'** as the critical *driving force occurring across the membrane.* Obviously, a **Cationic Drug** gets dully repelled because of the *specific positive charge residing firmly on the outer region of the membrane.* Consequently, only such particular **Cationic Drug Molecules having a distinct 'High-Kinetic Energy Status' would be able to penetrate the ionic barrier with great ease and fervour.** Importantly, once the cations have an access inside the membrane, they usually get attracted to the **Negatively Charged Intracellular Membrane** thereby raising a distinct **'Electrical Gradient'.**

Thus, in the above situation it may be said that the **'Drug'** is moving towards the **'downhill direction' along with the Electrical gradient.**

Electrochemical Diffusion: It refers to a situation when the –**'drug moves from a higher to a lower concentration, *i.e.,* the drug moving down the electrical gradient'.**

The **Ionic or Electrochemical Diffusion** continues till such time an *equilibrium is accomplished* (*viz.* **very much akin to Passive Diffusion**).

2.6.8. *Ion-Pair Transport*

The **Ion-Pair Transport Mechanism** rightly and explicitly clarifies and explains the *critical absorption of drugs,* such as:

- **quaternary ammonium compounds,** *e.g.,* **Demecarium Bromide-a quaternary ammonium anti-cholinesterase drug; Pilocarpine Nitrate-a quaternary ammonium cholinomimetic drug,** and
- **sulphonic acids.**

The above-mentioned **Drugs** do have a tendency to undergo **Ionization Under All pH Conditions** perceptively.

Mechanism of Action: Though the **Quaternary Ammonium Compounds** as well as the **Sulphonic Acids** essentially possess **Low *o/w* Partition Coefficient Values,** yet such typical drug entities do exhibit a tendency to penetrate the membrane by the formation of **Typical Reversible Neutral Complexes specifically with the Endogenous Ions of the GIT,** *e.g.,* **Mucins***

In fact, such **Neutral Complexes** do possess:

- **requisite lipophilicity,** and
- **aqueous solubility,**

in order to undergo **Passive Diffusion Efficaciously;** and, hence, such a phenomenon is invariably termed as the **'Ion-Pair Transport'** as illustrated in Figure 2.18.

2.6.9. *Endocytosis*

Endocytosis refers to a method of *ingestion of a foreign substance by a cell.* **The Cell Membrane enables to form a space for the material, and then the opening closes to trap the material inside the cell.**

---

*   **Mucins:** These are high molecular weight glycoproteins and form major constituents of gastric juice, saliva, intestine juice and other secretions.

In another words, **Endocytosis** is a *minor transport mechanism that essentially involves the critical engulfing of the extracellular materials very much within a specific region of the cell membrane to give rise to the formation of a* **'Saccule' or a 'Vesicle' that gets detached intracellularly at the end of the phenomenon as depicted in Figure 2.19.** It is, therefore, also known as **'Vesicular Transport'** or **'Corpuscular Transport'** alternatively.

Pinocytosis refers to-**'the engulfment of the small solutes or fluids'**, 'whereas, **Phagocytosis** refers to-**'the Engulfment of larger macromolecules or particles invariably by means of the respective macrophages'**. Besides, **Endocytocis** and **Exocytocis** are the specific processes related to moving the **'macromolecules' either into or out of a Cell**, respectively.

Mechanism of Action: These essentially include the following *two* **sequential steps,** *viz.,*

1. First of all, in the course of **Pinocytosis** or **Phagocytosis**, the respective cell membrane duly invaginates to crucially surround the material; and subsequently, **engulfs the material right inside the cell.**

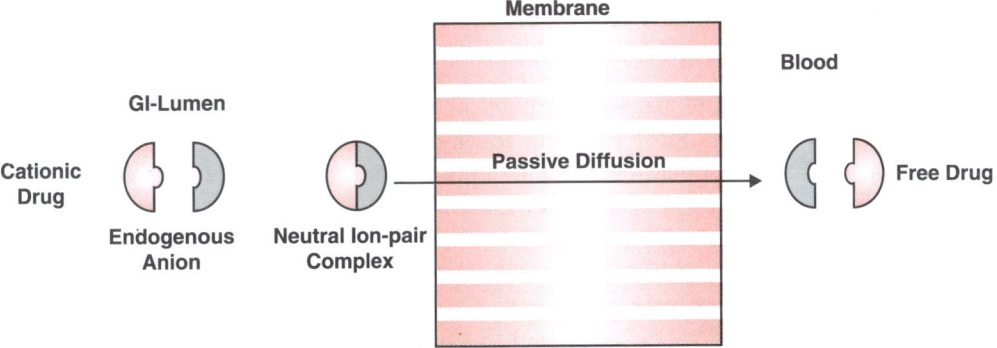

Fig. 2.18: Diagrammatic Representation of Ion-pair Transport of a Cationic Drug.

2. Consequently, the cell membrane comprising the material duly **generates a Vesicle (or Vacuole) within the Cell.**

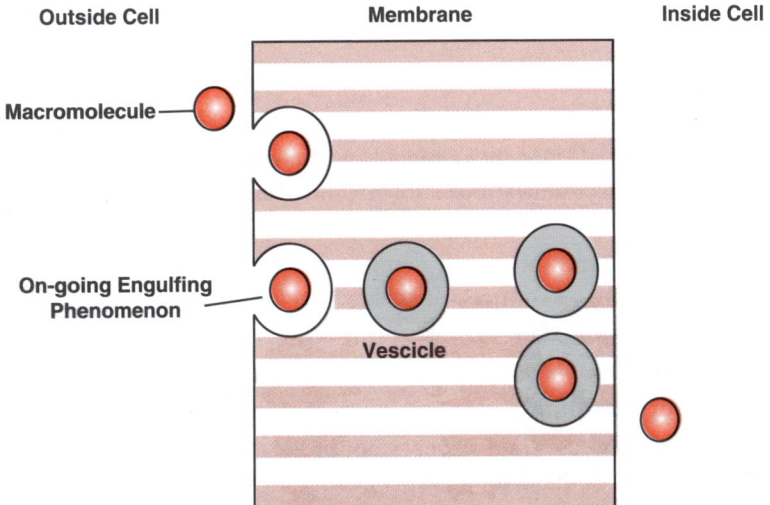

Fig. 2.19: Diagrammatic Representation of an Endocytic Uptake of Macromolecules.

Examples

Following are *two* **typical examples:**

1. **Sabin Polio Vaccine and other Large Proteins:** The proposed process for the specialized products, *viz.* **Orally administered Sabin Polio Vaccine, Sub-cutaneously Administered Erythropoietin 4000 U, are accomplished duly *via* the Vesicular Transport (or Endocytosis).**

2. **Insulin:** The transport of **'Insulin'** (a *protein*) from the respective **Insulin-Producing Cells of the Pancreas occurs due to Exocytosis,** into the *specific Extracellular Space.* The probable mechanism of action may be expatiated by the following *two* **cardinal steps in a sequential manner:**

   • **insulin molecules being packaged** into the **intracellular vesicles,** and
   • **subsequent** *'Fusion'* **with plasma** membrane to **release insulin outside the cell.**

2.6.10. *Summary of Important Transport Processes vis-a-vis Critical Absorption of Drugs by Different Mechanism*

It is, however, pertinent to state at this point in time that a **Drug Molecule** may get duly absorbed *in vivo* by definitely **more than one mechanism**. This fact may be further expatiated and substantiated by the most glaring example of the well-known **Cardiac Glycosides**, such as **Lanoxin, Crystodigin** that are absorbed so meticulously by *two* **entirely different transport mechanism,** namely, **'Passive Diffusion'** [*see Section 2 (6.1)*] and **'Active Transport'** [(*see Section 2 (6.4)*)]. It has also been established that the ensuing **Transport Mechanism** solely depends on the actual site of drug administration.

Figure 2.20 records the summary of certain **Important Transport Processes** *vis-a-vis* **Critical Absorption Profile of a few specific categories of Drug Substances by different mechanism in an orderly manner.**

2.7. DRUG ABSORPTION *VS.* BIOAVAILABILITY

2.7.1. *Preamble*

After having studied the intricacies and critical aspects of **'Drug Absorption Mechanism'** [*under Section* 2 (6)], one would be rather tempted and inclined to have an exhaustive inquiry into the absorption profile of drugs from various known **Solid-Dosage Forms** (*viz.* **Tablets, Capsules, Dragees).**

Importantly, to understand thoroughly and accomplish the conceptualized therapeutic objective(s), the eventful **'Drug Product'** (or **Dosage Form**) should be able to deliver the **Active Drug** with a reasonable success both:

   • **at an 'Optimized Rate'** and
   • **at a 'Sufficient Quantum'.**

Nevertheless, these *two* cardinal aspects could be duly addressed by the meticulous **'Biopharmaceutic Design'** of the **drug product** bearing in mind the crucial rate and the degree of absorption, invariably termed as **'Bioavailability'**. Indeed, the so-called **'Systemic Delivery of a Drug Substance'** right inside a human body may be achieved in *two* ways, namely:

- **a fast, rapid and complete absorption of drug,** and/or
- **a slow, sluggish and sustained absorption of drug,**

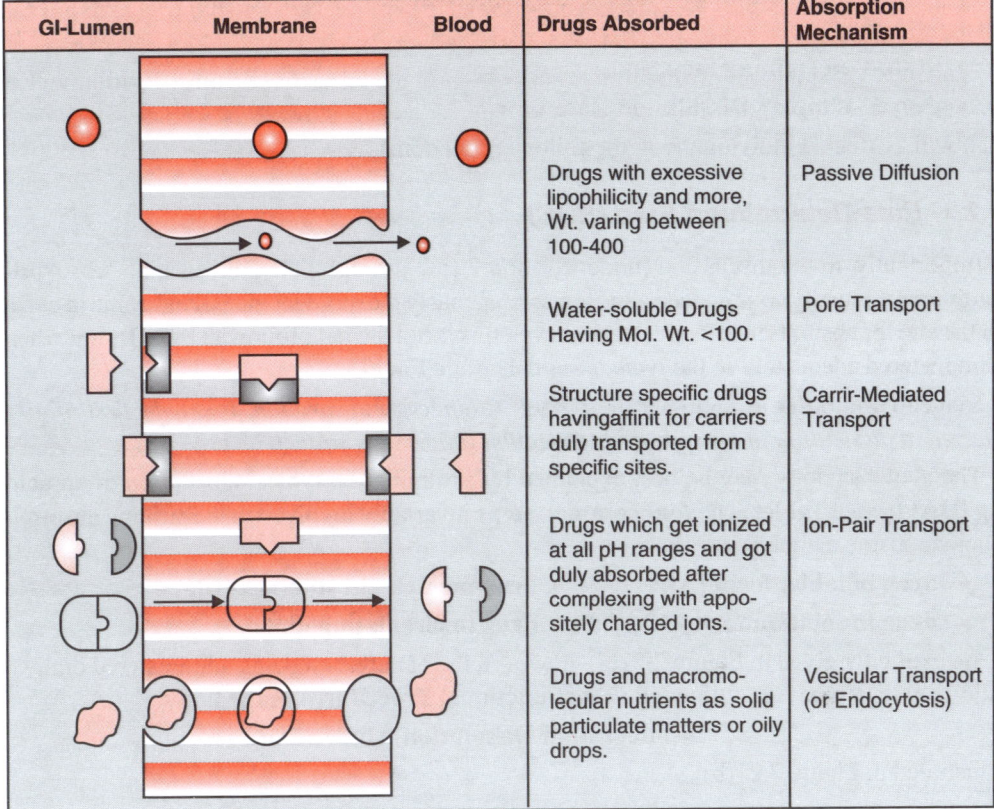

GI-Lumen	Membrane	Blood	Drugs Absorbed	Absorption Mechanism
			Drugs with excessive lipophilicity and more, Wt. varing between 100-400	Passive Diffusion
			Water-soluble Drugs Having Mol. Wt. <100.	Pore Transport
			Structure specific drugs havingaffinit for carriers duly transported from specific sites.	Carrir-Mediated Transport
			Drugs which get ionized at all pH ranges and got duly absorbed after complexing with appositely charged ions.	Ion-Pair Transport
			Drugs and macromolecular nutrients as solid particulate matters or oily drops.	Vesicular Transport (or Endocytosis)

Fig. 2.20: Diagrammatic Representation of the Summarized Status of Important Transport Phenomena and Drugs Absorbed *via* These Mechanisms.

that depends exclusively upon the **desired/predicted therapeutic aims and objectives** perceptively.

2.7.2. Pharmaceutical Factors (or Biopharmaceutic Considerations) Affecting Drug Bioavailability

The various **Pharmaceutical Factors** (or **Biopharmaceutic Considerations**) intimately associated with the ultimate design and judicious manufacture of **Drug Product** so as to enable the critical delivery of the **'Active Drug'** having the **desired** and **pre-empted Bioavailability characteristic features.** These are comprised essentially under the following *four* cardinal aspects, namely:

- **type of drug product** (*viz.* **solution, suspension, suppository**),

- nature of excipients used in the drug product,
- physicochemical characteristic features of drug molecules, and
- route of drug administration.

Importantly, the critical and important criteria for the adequate *absorption of 'Active Drugs'* from the **Solid-Dosage Forms** could be duly ascertained by the following *two* **vital aspects,** such as:

- **Rate-Determining Step,** and
- **Noyes-Whitney Dissolution Rate Law,**

which will be treated individually in the following sections:

2.7.2.1. *Rate-Determining Step (RDS)*

Importantly, in the discussion [under Section 2 (5.2 through 5.4)], the ensuing **Absorption Phenomenon** actually commenced almost instantaneously the moment the **'Drug'** came in contact with the site for absorption effectively. However, this is not the path followed by a **'Drug'** when it is administered adequately in the *typical* **Solid-Dosage Form.**

Evidently, in order to facilitate the **'Drug'** to *undergo absorption, it should first of all be subjected to dissolution in an appropriate medium (preferably water).*

The above analogy may be best explained by assuming the typical absorption of an **acidic drug [HA] from a Tablet.** The *four* **common steps** invariably involved in the ensuing absorption phenomenon are, namely:

- **drug in tablet form [A],**
- **drug particles in stomach [B],**
- **drug in solution form [C],** and
- **drug in circulating blood**

that are explicitly given in Figure 2.21(a). however, the **'Tablet'** on being administered orally (or swallowed) undergoes the following *three* **Functional Procedures in the body:**

Disintegration-Dissolution-Absorption

as illustrated in Figure 2.21(b):

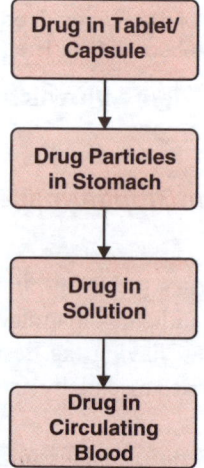

Fig. 2.21: (a) Four Common Steps Involved in Absorption Phenomenon of a Drug.

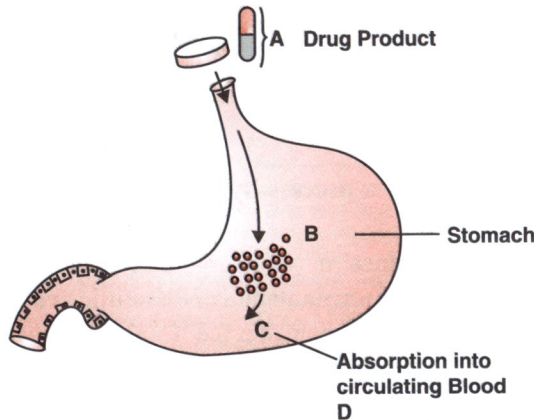

Fig. 2.21: (b) Diagrammatic Representation of Normal Steps Involved in Absorption of a Drug Following Oral Ingestion of a Tablet: Disintegration-Dissolution-Absorption.

At this point in time, it is absolutely necessary to have a clear distinction between the following *two* **important phenomena**, such as:

- **disintegration** and
- **dissolution.**

Disintegration : **Disintegration** may be defined as-'**the critical breaking apart of the compressed tablet into the respective primary particulate matters**'.

The incorporation of certain known **Disintegrants*** (or *disintegrating agents*) in the original formula, one may form a tablet which would eventually undergo a massive explosion on being submersed in an aqueous environment.

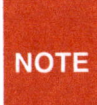

NOTE	It is worthwhile to mention here that though disintegration is an absolute prerequisite to the process of 'absorption' as well as fast and rapid disintegration, yet it certainly increase a speedy onset of action, however, it fails to ensure absorption.

Obviously, in case the '**Drug Particulate Matters**' never get dissolved adequately even after the disintegration comes into play, the '**Drug**' will never gain an access into the circulating blood stream.

Incidentally, *two* **different situations** may arise with respect to the **phenomenon of disintegration**, namely:

1. **Negative Disintegration**: The **Negative Disintegration Test** distinctly and certainly provides the evidence of a reasonably poor tablet, which is significantly based on the fact that:
   - **if the very 'first step' fails to materialize, and**
   - **the subsequent 'Dissolution' will be rather difficult, and under these circumstances, the follow up absorption process may not ever commence.**

---

* **Disintegrants**: It refers to a substance usually added to a tablet granulation during its preparation and after granulation to facilitate the breaking apart of the tablet into the granules, and splitting of the granules respectively when it is duly subjected to the fluids of the GI tract.

2. **Fast Disintegration**: It invariably helps in the appropriate prediction of a uniform behavioural profile from the **Tablets;** however, it may not ensure and ascertain, in itself, the overall effcaciousness ultimately.

Dissolution

Dissolution may be defined as-'a **process by which a solute is rendered homogeneous with a solvent'**.

In other words, a **'Drug Substance'** must undergo **dissolution** *before absorption* may take place. However, in actual practice, the **phenomenon of dissolution rate** is found to be usually the slowest and most sluggish step observed soon after the **'Oral Administration'** of a **solid-dosage form** (*viz.* **Tablets, Capsules, Dragees**).

NOTE	**A universal 'rule of thumb' suggests prominently that drug substance with an aqueous solubility < 1% of pH value 1-7 at 37± 1°C are critically predisposed to certain typical bioavailability problems.**

Predictor of Dissolution-Rate-Limited Absorption: Nevertheless, under the influence of *identical experimental parameters*, a typical and critical rate of dissolution which being <0.1 mg mL^{-1} cm^{-2} employing a rotating disk with a constant surface area represents the so-called **'Predictor of Dissolution-Rate-Limited Absorption'**.

Various Absorption Steps Immediately after Oral Ingestion of Coated Tablets or Capsules The following Scheme A illustrates explicitly the various absorption steps that are followed immediately after the oral ingestion of the coated tablets or capsules (see Figure 2.22).

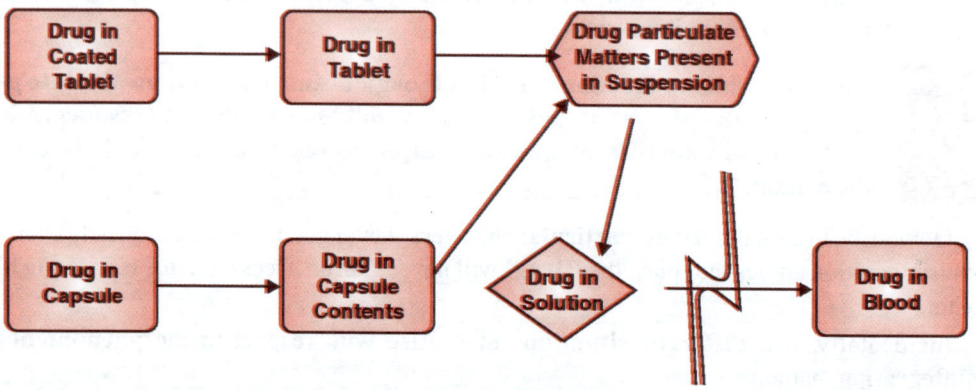

Fig. 2.22: Scheme A: Absorption Steps Involved Immediately After Oral Ingestion of Coated Tablets or Capsules.

It is, however, pertinent to state here that such **'drug entities whose solubility properties are observed to be distinctly less than the ideally required optimized formulations in order to skip over the exacerbation of an inherent Bioavailability Problem'**. Therefore, **Scheme A** may duly come into play in the steps immediately preceding the disintegration process so as to result in the requisite formation of –**'drug particulate matters in the ensuing suspension'**.

Rate-Limiting Steps *vis-à-vis* Risk for Incomplete Bioavailability: In a broader perspective, the **Drug Bioavailability** may be caused duly by the critical failure of the following *two* **vital and important features,** namely:

- **coating of tablet to expose the intended drug contents,** and
- **administered tablet to undergo rapid disintegration,**

Amazingly, if the aforesaid *two* **steps** are fairly and reasonably rapid, the observed **dissolution of particulate matters** duly present in the **'Suspension'** shall be expected to render into a **Rate-Limiting Feature**.

Interestingly, one may genuinely encounter greater hits in the **'Potential-Limiting Steps'** corresponding to the **'More Complex Nature'** of the **Drug Product** (or **Dosage Form**); and, therefore, entails greater risk for **'Incomplete Bioavailability'**. The most informative perception, knowledge and understanding with regard to the extent to which a desired formulation may exert overwhelmingly these criteria, such as:

- **typical influence upon the rate of absorption,** and
- **pivotal role in accomplishing bioavailability,**

are predictable effectively upon these fundamental basis.

Figure 2.23: **Scheme B** explicitly records the useful anticipated results pertaining to **'Absorption'** *vis-a-vis* **'Bioavailability Risk'** pertaining to an array of specifically **designed/formulated Drug Products.**

Explanation

The **various aspects of Scheme B essentially include the following** *eight* **cardinal points:**

1. **Solutions:** Drug substances that are administered usually in solution form, *viz.* **Elixirs, Syrups and Solutions,** do ascertain *fast and rapid absorption of the drug,* **since the rate-limiting dissolution gets eliminated almost completely by the drug product itself.**

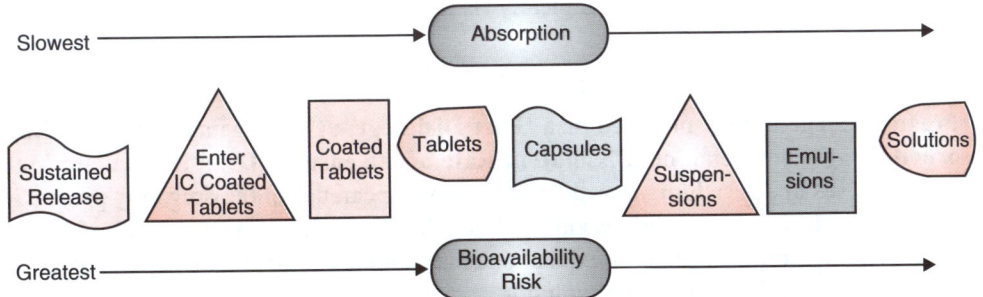

Fig. 2.23: Scheme B Shows Useful Anticipated Results Pertaining to Absorption *vis-a-vis* Bioavailability Risk.

2. **Sustained Release (or Prolonged Release or Delayed Release) Dosage Forms:** These drug products would be duly expected to exhibit the lowest level of absorption by virtue of the underlying fact that the **'Release Pattern of the Active Drug'** has been retarded intentionally.

3. **Enteric-Coated Tablets:** These specially designed dosage form are intended to check and prevent particularly the drug-release profile just prior to its arrival in the intestinal passage.

4. **Coated Tablet:** In this instance, first and foremost, the '**Coating**' should get dissolved, which is subsequently followed by the core tablet itself. Thus, the **rapid dissolution of the Active Drug** contained in the **Core Tablet** will not commence till such time the *tablet itself undergoes disintegration*.

5. **Capsules:** They invariably do have the '**Capsule Shell**' (made up of **Hard Gelatin**) which must get dissolved before the active drug contents are duly available for dissolution. Nevertheless, the contents of a capsule more or less behave as:

   • **a 'Tablet' (very much akin to a compressed one),** and
   • **a 'Suspension' (resemblance more closer),**

   and get distributed rather quickly right inside the **GI Fluids**.

6. **Suspensions:** They essentially posses no coatings at all to be removed; besides, no tablet to undergo disintegration, and no capsule-shell to get dissolved. Importantly, the suspensions are observed to be distinctly slower and more sluggish in nature *vis-a-vis* the emulsion, due to the fact that suspended drug substance should still undergo dissolution process in the **GI fluids**.

7. **Emulsions:** They normally contain the dissolved drug substance that should critically undergo partition between the *two* **existing immiscible phases.**

8. **Solutions:** They ultimately present the drug almost directly upon the **Gastrointestinal (GI) Wall** for causing the necessary absorption.

Important Features: They essentially include the following:

1. Any one of the other drug products (or dosage forms), as discussed above **from (1) through (7),** may be bio available as speedily as the solutions provided the various steps preceding the absorption phenomenon are fast and rapid enough.

2. Importantly, an '**active drug**' presented in one of the **non-solution dosage forms** may not be absorbed more rapidly and completely *vis-a-vis* its respective solution form.

2.7.2.2. Noyes-Whitney Dissolution Rate Law*

Preamble: The critical presence of a '**Fast Disintegrant**' amalgamated with a '**Rapidly Absorbed Drug**', the overall net **Dissolution Rate of the ensuing Drug Particulate Matters** would themselves impose a limit upon the very rate of appearance of the drug duly present in the **circulating blood**. However, the aforesaid conditionalities may fall within the scope of a '**Normal Instance**'. Besides, it has been observed that one may suitably augment the rate of absorption of a drug simply enhancing the rate of dissolution.

As the rate of dissolution determines the '**Limiting Factor**', it follows obviously that one could *Control and Modulate the Absorption Profile of a Drug by Controlling the Dissolution Rate accordingly*. Interestingly, it accomplishes the ultimate goal and targeted objective of various aspects related to **Drug Development in a Methodical Way** so as to *control/monitor the ensuing behavioural profile of the* '**Product**' **under investigative studies in a clinic.**

---

* Noyes AA and Whitney WR: *J. Am. Chem. Soc.,* **19**:930,1997

Importantly, in the case of a **solid-dosage form,** it is required necessarily to look into the following criteria intimately, such as:

- **influence of dissolution rate,** and
- **design and applicability of the drug product,**

that must be able to control the desired **'Dissolution Rate of the Drug'** perceptively.

According to **Noyes-Whitney Dissolution Rate Law, dm/dt** is given by the following expression:

$$\frac{dm}{dt} = \frac{DA(C_s - C_g)}{h}$$

where,

dm/dt = Rate of dissolution of drug particles,

D = Diffusion coefficient of drug in solution in GI fluids,

A = Effective surface area of drug particles,

h = Thickness of the diffusion layer (*i.e.,* the stationary layer of the solvent) around the drug particles,

C_s = Saturation solubility of the drug in the diffusion layer, and

C_g = Concentration of the drug in solution duly present in the bulk of GI fluids.

Figure 2.24 shows the schematic representation of the ensuing relationship of the various terminologies, as per the **Noyes-Whitney Equation** stated above, to the ensuing **Dissolution Process.** It may, however, be reasonably emphasized that the present **'crude model'** fails to describe the entire dissolution phenomenon to the complete extent.

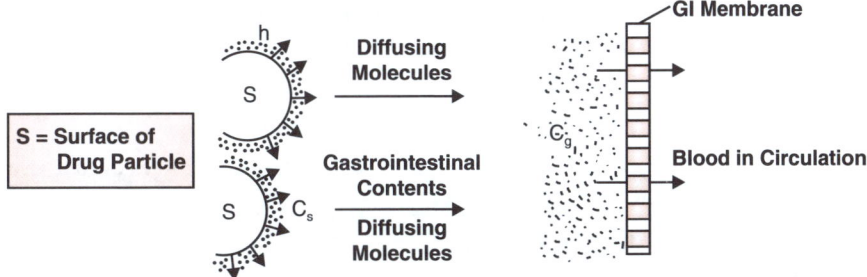

Fig. 2.24: A Schematic Diagram of Dissolution Phenomenon.

Explanation

These essentially comprise the following *three* aspects:

1. Each and every term in the aforesaid **Noyes-Whitney Expression** invariably influences the **Rate of Dissolution of a Drug in the GI Fluids.**

2. Since the **Dissolution of the Particles actually come into play,** one may also observe a *definite change in the following two physical characteristics:*

- **particle size,** and
- **surface area**.

3. **Hixson and Crowell (1931)** subsequently improvised and developed a **Modified Equation** to account for these changes adequately in the course of the **On-going Dissolution Process**. It is usually termed as **Hixson and Crowell's Cube Root Law of Dissolution*** and may be expressed as

$$W_0^{1/3} - W_t^{1/3} = kt$$

where,

W_0 = Original mass of the drug substance,

W_t = Mass of the drug remained at time 't', and

k = Constant pertaining to dissolution rate.

2.7.3. Factor Influencing GI Absorption of a Drug from Its Respective Dosage Forms

There are *two* **well-known and recognized factors** that perceptually influence the ensuing **Gastrointestinal (GI) Absorption of a Drug Substance** duly present in its respective **Dosage Form** (*viz*. **Tablets, Capsules, Dragees**), such as:

- **Pharmaceutical Factors,** and
- **Patient-related Factors.**

2.7.3.1. Pharmaceutical Factors

These predominantly consist of certain **Typical Factors** that are intimately related to the inherent corresponding **Physiochemical Characteristic Features of the respective Drug Substance; and also, the Dosage Form characteristics** together with the incorporated pharmaceutic ingredients.

Physiochemical Characteristic Features of Drug Substances

The various vital and important **Physiochemical Characteristic Features of drug Substance** essentially comprise the following; *eight* aspects:

- **drug solubility and dissolution rate,**
- **particle size and effective surface area,**
- **polymorphism and amorphism,**
- **pseudopolymorphism (hydrates/solvates),**
- **salt of the respective parent drug,**
- **lipophilicity of a drug (based on pH/partition hypothesis),**
- **pK_2 of a drug and its pH (based on pH/partition hypothesis),** and
- **stability of drug.**

---

*   Hixson A and Crowell J: *Ind.Eng. Chem.*, **23**:923, 1931.

Dosage Form Characteristics Features and Pharmaceutic Ingredient

The critical **dosage form characteristic features together with the respective pharmaceutic ingredients** are usually of *six* **variants** as stated under:

- disintegration time (*viz.* tablets/capsules),
- dissolution time,
- variability in manufacturing processes,
- pharmaceutic ingredients, *e.g.*, excipients, adjuvants,
- nature and type of dosage form, and
- product age and storage conditions.

2.7.3.2. *Patient-Related Factors*

Importantly, the **Patient-Related Factor** invariably comprises such aspects that are intimately related to the **anatomic, physiologic,** and **pathologic characteristic features of the patient,** namely:

- age factor;
- gastric emptying time;
- intestinal transit time;
- gastrointestinal (GI) pH;
- various disease conditions;
- passage of blood *via* GIT;
- gastrointestinal (GI) components, such as:
  - ➤ drugs,
  - ➤ foods,
  - ➤ fluids, and
  - ➤ other normal GI contents.
- pre-systemic metabolism accomplished by certain specific enzymes, for instance:
  - ➤ lumenal enzymes,
  - ➤ gut wall enzymes,
  - ➤ bacterial enzymes, and
  - ➤ hepatic enzymes.

2.7.4. *Physiochemical Nature of the Drug vis-a-vis Absorption*

The outcome of an array of **extensive and intensive investigative studies** have amply revealed and established that the inherent **Physiochemical Nature /Characteristic Feature of a particular Drug Substance significantly affords a change in its absorption profile** *in vivo*.

Following are the *six* **most important aspects** with regard to the *aforesaid relationship between the Physiochemical nature of the drug and its subsequent Absorption Profiles,* such as:

1. **Drug solubility and dissolution rate,**
2. **Theories of drug dissolution,**
3. **Particle size and drug absorption,**

4. **Polymorphic crystals, solvates and drug absorption,**
5. **Drug pK_2, lipophilicity and GI pH (or pH-Partition Hypothesis),** and
6. **Limitation of pH-Partition Hypothesis.**

The aforesaid *six* variants in the Physiochemical Nature of a Drug *vs.* its Absorption Profile shall now be discussed briefly in the following sections separately:

2.7.4.1. *Drug Solubility and Dissolution Rate*

Let us look into the sequence of events that eventually take place immediately followed by the 'Oral Administration' of a Solid Dosage Form (*viz.* **Tablet, Capsule, Dragee**) as illustrated in Figure 2.25.

From Figure 2.25 one may observe critically that the **Drug Substance** may *undergo* **Dissolution Effectively even before the actual Disintegration or Deaggregation of the solid dosage form commences (see LHS of Fig. 2.25), before or after approaching the absorption site in an efficacious manner.** Nevertheless, the **Drug Substance** shall never get absorbed appropriately into the *systematic circulation unless and until the former is dissolved completely:*

In true sense, Figure 2.25 prominently suggests *four* **cardinal steps sequentially,** such as:

- **disintegration of drug product (or dosage form),**
- **deaggregation followed by actual release of drug,**
- **dissolution of active drug in aqueous fluids strategically at the absorption site,** and
- **generous migration of dissolved active drug via GI membrane**
  - ➤ **right inside the systematic circulation,** and
  - ➤ **far away from the respective absorption site.**

Rate-Limiting Step (RLS): RLS refers to- **'the critical rate at which the drug approaches the systemic circulation as estimated meticulously by means of the slowest of the various observed steps involved actually in the entire sequence of events. It is also known as the Rate-Determining Step (RDS).**

Transmembrane Rate-Limited (TRL) or Permeation Rate-Limited (PRL)

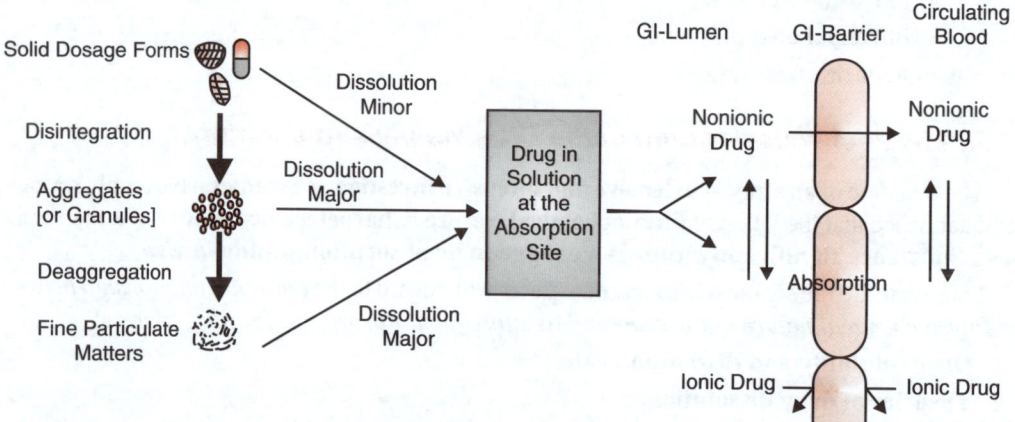

Fig. 2.25: Schematic Sequence of Events in the Absorption of Drugs from Orally Administered Dosage Forms.

In a broader perspective, **Dissolution** designates the **RDS** for highly specific drugs that are

- **hydrophobic in nature,** and
- **poorly water-soluble.**

Examples

The following are *two* **most typical drugs,** namely:

Spironolactone-a purely *synthetic steroid* having a '**natriuretic action**' thereby exerting its action as a '**Competitive Antagonist**' of the potent **Endogeneous Mineral-Corticoid; Adosterone.**

Griseofulvin-an *antibiotic substance* produced by **Penicillium grisefulvum** used as an **anti-fungal agent.**

Importantly, the *systematic absorption of* **Spironolactone** and **Griseofulvin** are regarded to be **dissolution rate-limited.**

In the same vein, if the drug is **hydrophilic in nature**, *i.e.*, having adequate aqueous solubility, one may predominantly observe:

- **rapid dissolution,** and
- **RDS pertaining to the absorption of such drugs is duly determined by the rate of permeation via the ensuing biomembranes.**

Examples

The *two* **typical examples are,** namely:

Neomycin-an *antibiotic* that usually gets absorbed very poorly from the digestive system; and, therefore, its oral administration primarily fails to cause a substantial systemic effect.

Sodium Cromoglycate- a *chromono derivative* that specifically inhibits the critical release of '**Histamine**' and **SRS-A in allergic reactions.**

It is, however, pertinent to state at this point in time that the remarkable absorption pattern of such drugs is usually termed as **Transmembrane Rate-Limited (TRL)** or **Permeation Rate-Limited (PRL)**. Figure 2.26 shows the *two* **Rate-Determining Steps (RDSs)** for (a) **lipophilic drugs** and (b) **hydrophilic drugs,** released duly from the **Orally Administered Formulations.**

The **Dissolution Rate** may be defined as–'**the quantum of solid drug substance that critically goes into solution per unit time under standard conditions of pH, temperature, solvent and constant solid surface area'.**

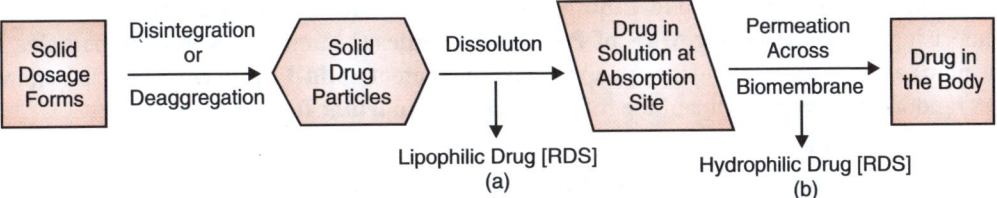

Fig. 2.26: Schematic Representation of Two Distinct Rate-Determining Steps (RDSs) for the Absorption of Drugs from Orally Administered Drug Products: (a) Lipophilic Drug, and (b) Hydrophilic Drug.

Besides, the **Dissolution Rate** serves as a dynamic phenomenon. There are a plethora of drugs that do exhibit noticeably poor aqueous solubility which essentially is responsible for showing abnormal **Dissolution Rate.** However, the situation becomes quite alarming and serious when the aqueous solubility becomes **lower than 1-2 mg mL^{-1} within the pH range 2-8.**

Exceptional Example of Cisapride: Cisapride, a **Gastrointestinal Prokinetic Agent** used as a *peristallic stimulant*, which in spite being poorly water soluble, remarkably exhibits **Sufficient Oral Bioavailability**. Importantly, such an exceptional behavioural pattern of **Cisapride** could be expatiated by means of the following *two* **cardinal reasons,** namely:

- **rapid rate of dissolution profile despite low inherent intrinsic solubility,** and
- **therapeutic effective dosage regimen being so small such that the actual prevailing GI transit duration in just enough for carrying out the desired dissolution and absorption effectively.**

NOTE	Obviously, it may be observed critically that contrary to the so-called 'absolute solubility', the excellent dynamic phenomenon of drug dissolution appears to be definitely better related to both drug absorption and bioavailability.

2.7.4.2. *Theories of Drug Dissolution*

In actual practice, **Dissolution** refers to – 'a process wherein a solid substance duly gets solubilized in a given solvent, *i.e.*, mass transfer occurs from the solid surface to the corresponding liquid phase'.

There are *three* **recognized and accepted Theories of Drug Dissolution,** namely:

- **Diffusion Layer Model (or Film Theory).**
- **Danckwert's Model (or Penetration/Surface Renewal Theory), and**
- **Interfacial Barrier Model (or Double Barrier or Limited Solvation Theory),**

which shall be discussed separately in the following sections.

Diffusion Layer Model (or Film Theory) In 1897, **Noyes and Whitney** examined the **Dissolution Rate** *of two almost insoluble compounds*, **Lead Chloride** and **Benzoic Acid*** based on an equation after the **Fick's Second Law to describe the dissolution phenomenon** [*see section 2(7.2.2)*]

Danckwert's Model (or Penetration/Surface Renewal Theory)

Danckwert obviously never approved the actual existence of a **Possible Stagnant Layer,** but instead suggested strongly that the turbulence prevailing in the ensuing **Dissolution Medium occurs prominently at the Solid-Liquid Interface.** Consequently, the agitated fluid essentially comprising the **Macroscopic Mass of Packets or Eddies** (*i.e.*, circularly moving particles in a medium) actually have a tendency to approach the inherent **Solid-Liquid Interface** in a more or less random manner by virtue of the following *three* **important functions;** namely:

- **Eddy Currents,**
- **Absorption of solute due to diffusion,** and
- **Migration of solute to the bulk of the solution.**

---

*   By carefully rotating a cylinder of each compound in water at a constant rate and subsequently sampling the solution for analysis at particular time intervals

Therefore, in this manner such **Solute Particles (Drugs)** consisting of **Eddies (or Packets)** are being replaced almost continuously with **newer supplies of 'Fresh Lots of Solvent'** on account of which the actual concentration of drug at the solid-liquid interface fails to retain 'C_s **level**' (*i.e.*, **concentration of drug at the stagnant layer**). Thus, it possess a distinct '**Lower Value** C_b' (*i.e.*, **concentration of drug present in the bulk of solution at time 't'**).

Importantly, one may evidently conclude that since the **solvent pockets** are adequately exposed to the new solid surface at each instance, the present theory is termed as penetration/surface renewal theory.

We may express the **Danckwert's Model** by the following equation:

$$\frac{dm}{dt} = S^{1/2}\, D^{1/2}\, (C_s - C_g)$$

where,

Dm/dt = Rate of dissolution of drug particles,

S = Mean rate at which a fresh surface gets generated,

D = Diffusion coefficient of drug in solution in GI fluids,

C_s = Saturation solubility of the drug in the diffusion layer and

C_g = Concentration of drug in solution present in the bulk of GI fluids.

Mechanisms of Dissolution: The Danckwert's Model: Figure 2.27 vividly shows the mechanisms involved in the **Dissolution Phenomenon**, otherwise known as the '**Danckwert's Model**':

Interfacial Barrier Model (or Double Barrier or Limited Solvation Theory)

We have examined that the **Diffusion Layer Model** [see **Diffusion Layer Model (or Film Theory)** in this section] and the **Danckwert's Model** [see **Danckwert's Model (or Penetration/ Surface Renewal Theory)** in this section] were exclusively based on the following *two* **assumptions**, namely:

- *First*, **the rate-determining step which controls/modulates the dissolution process concerned with the mass transport,** and
- *Secondly*, **the critical accomplishment of the solid-solution equilibrium prevailing at the solid-liquid interface.**

Importantly, the **Interfacial Barrier Model** provides prominently an **intermediate concentration** that may exist critically at the interface by virtue of **the Solvation Mechanism;** and, therefore, suggest largely that it is indeed a function of '**Solubility**' rather than '**Diffusion**'. Based on the above concept and analogy, the dissolution of a crystal shall essentially have on its each face an altogether different '**Interfacial Barrier**'. Hence, such a concept may be duly expressed by the following equation:

$$G = K_i\, (C_s - C_b)$$

where,

G = Dissolution rate per unit area,

K = Effective interfacial transport constant,

C_s = Concentration of drug in the stagnant layer (also referred to as the saturation or maximum drug solubility) and

C_b = Concentration of drug in the bulk of solution at time 't'.

Important Points: The limited salvation theory suggests *two* **important points,** namely :

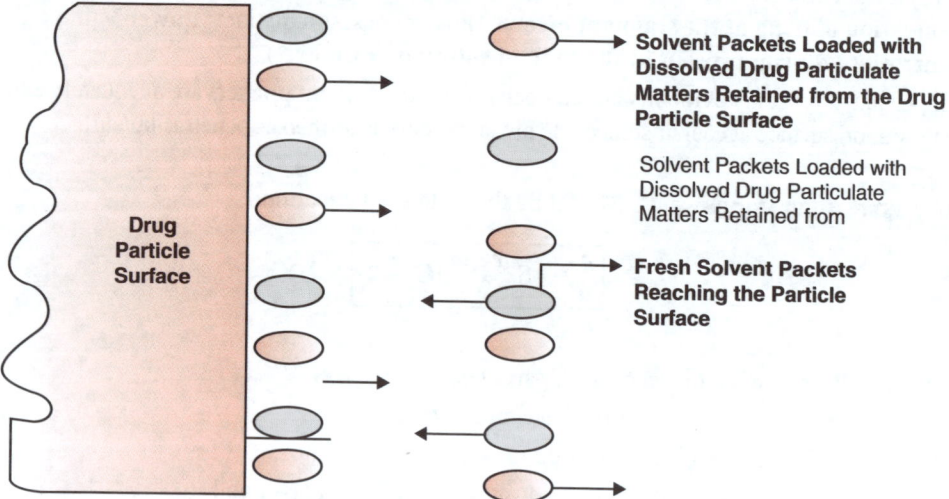

Fig. 2.27: Diagrammatic Sketch Showing Mechanisms of Dissolution Phenomenon of the Danckwert's Model.

- **D, *i.e.*, the diffusivity, may not found to be absolutely independent of the ensuring saturation concentration C_s, and**
- **the interfacial barrier model may be judiciously extended to either diffusion layer model** [see **Diffusion Layer Model (or Film Theory)** *in this section*] or **Danckwert's Model** [see **Danckwert's Model (or Penetration/Surface Renewal Theory)** *in this section*], *i.e.*, **specifically for *in vitro* Drug Dissolution Models.**

The **Interfacial Barrier Model** is depicted explicitly in Figure 2.28 for a specific situation wherein the acquired comparatively fast and rapid phenomenon takes place by critical diffusion through a so-called **Static Liquid Film.**

From Figure 2.28 one may observe that the prevailing **Saturation Solubility (C_s) of the Drug Substance duly present in the Diffusion layer and the respective Concentration (C_b) of the Drug Substance in solution is available in the bulk of GI Fluids after traversing the thickness of the Diffusion layer 'h'.**

2.7.4.3. Particle Size and Drug Absorption

It is quite obvious that the effective surface area of a drug gets enhanced enormously due to the reduction in the particle size. Since the dissolution of a drug invariably commences at the surface of the solute; and, therefore, **the availability of greater surface area would certainly ensure a faster and more rapid Rate of Drug Dissolution Process.** The **geometrical shape** of the drug particulate matter plays an important role with regard to these following *three* **important aspects,** such as:

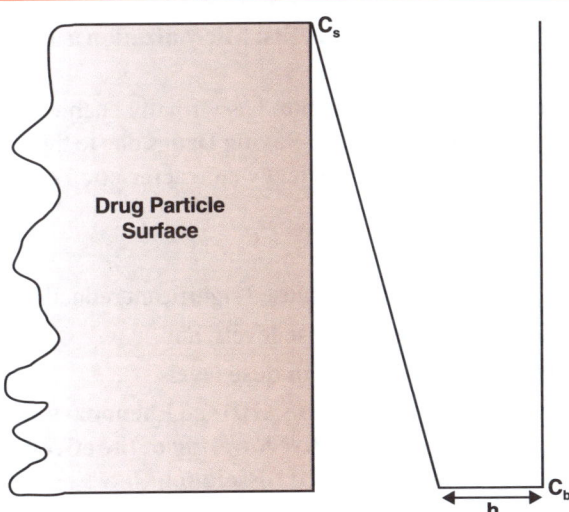

Fig. 2.28: Interfacial barrier Model Showing Mechanisms of Dissolution.

- **affect surface area,**
- **constant alteration of surface during dissolution,** and
- **solute particle(s) assumed to have retained its inherent Geometrical Shape for precise Dissolution Calculations.**

In addition, the *two* **vital and important aspects,** *i.e.*, **Particle Size** and **Particle Size Distribution** investigative studies, do play a critical role for such drugs with a low water-solubility. The **Diminution in Particle Size by milling up to a micronized form enhanced the crucial absorption criteria of an array of low-aqueous solubility drugs,** such as; **Testosterone, Progesterone, Griseofulvin, Nitrofurantoin** *etc.* Evidently, the accomplished smaller particle size invariably gives rise to the following *three* **advantageous plus points,** for instance:

- **substantial enhancement in the total surface area of the drug particles,**
- **increases significantly the water-penetration right into the drug particulate matters,** and
- **significant enhancement in the dissolution rates.**

NOTE   **In usual common practice, the solubility of the sparingly soluble drugs may be increased suitably by the incorporation of a 'disintegrant' into the formulation in order to ascertain fast and rapid disintegration of the duly 'compressed tablet', and subsequent release of the particulate matters.**

Types of Surface Area: In the domain of **Pharmaceutic Design,** one would normally come across *two* **different types of Surface Area,** namely:

1. **Absolute Surface Area:** It refers to the total area of a solid surface of any particulate matter.
2. **Effective Surface Area**: It implies to the area of solid surface being exposed effectively to the respective dissolution medium.

Micronization and Its Remarkable Benefits: Micronization actually means the reduction of particles to a micrometer diameter size.

In a broader perspective, the **Micronization** has virtually enabled the formulation expert to minimize the **dosage regimen of certain Life-Saving Drugs** due to the fact that it would give rise to an **Improved/Increased Absorption Efficiency characteristic Features.**

Examples

Micromization of Drug Particles have caused significant reduction in dosage regimen, *e.g.*,

- **Griseofulvin: 50% reduction in dose levels,** and
- **Spironolactone: 20-folds decrease in dose levels.**

In **Hydrophobic Drugs**, *viz*. **Aspirin** (an **NSAID**) and **Phenobarbitone** (a **hypnotic/sedative drug**), **Micronization gives rise to a perceptive lowering of the effective surface area thereby causing a remarkable** reduction in the observed **Dissolution Rate Following are the** *three* **logical explanations have been put forward to account for such a charge;** namely:

1. **The typical hydrophobic surface of the drug substances do have a tendency to absorb air onto the outer surface that predominantly cause an inhibition of their wettability; and, therefore, such powders usually float on ensuing dissolution medium.**

2. **Generally, the particulate matters undergo Reaggregation to generate relatively larger particles by virtue of their high surface-free available energy that:**
   - **are found to float on the surface, or**
   - **do settle at the bottom of the ensuing dissolution medium.**

3. **Nevertheless, an Excessive Reduction in the Particle Size may cause development of surface charges that:**
   - **would check and prevent wettability profile**, and
   - **electrically induced agglomeration would certainly prevent intimate and close contact of the drug specifically with the dissolution medium.**

Overall Net Result: The overall net result would be noticed largely in the shape of an appreciably decrease in the effective surface area genuinely available to the respective **Dissolution Medium;** and, therefore, result in the ultimate **Fall in the Dissolution Rate overwhelmingly.**

Conversion of Absolute Surface Area of Hydrophobic Drugs to Effective Surface Area: It may be gainfully accomplished by means of the following *two* **procedures adopted generally;** *viz.,*

- Judicious and intelligent application of a suitable surfactant serving as a 'wetting agent' which essentially lowers the prevailing surface tension and displaces the adsorbed air by means of the solvent.

Example

Tween-80 (a *synthetic surfactant*) critically enhances the bioavailability of acetaminophen by promoting its wettability directly.

- **Critical incorporation of 'Hydrophilic Diluents'** enables the coating of the surface of the hydrophobic drug particulate matters, and render them hydrophilic in nature ultimately.

Example

Dextrose, Polyvinylpyrrolidone (PVP) and **Polyethyleneglycol (PEG).**

CAUTION Such drugs that are either unstable or degradable in solution (*e.g.,* Erythromycin, Penicillin G), the reduction in particle size and suitable increase in surface area/dissolution rate may not be largely advisable.

The utility of an alternative mechanism which entails a reduction in particle size thereby categorically improving/modifying the **'Drug-Dissolution' profile** through a distinct enhancement in its solubility criteria is being practiced. Obviously, such an effect may be accomplished by diminution the particle size to the **'Sub-Micron Level'**, and this could be possible by the aid of the following *two* **available techniques:**

1. **Solid Solution (or Molecular Dispersion)**: The sparingly soluble drug is being trapped molecularly with great care right into the crystal lattice of a typical **Hydrophilic Agent,** *e.g.,* **Cyclodextrin.**
2. **Solid Dispersion**: In this instance, the **Drug** is duly dispersed in a **Specialized Soluble Carrier** *e.g.,* **PVP, PEG** and **Urea**.

2.7.4.4. *Polymorphic Crystals, Solvates and Drug Absorption*

Polymorphic invariably refers to-'**the arrangement of a drug in a variety of crystalline forms (Polymorphs)'**. It is worthwhile to mention here that the **Polymorphs** *do possess the same chemical structure, but altogether different physical characteristic features*, **for instance:**

- **solubility,**
- **density,**
- **hardness,** and
- **compression characteristics**.

Polymorphs are normally of *two* **types**, such as:

- **Enantiotropic Polymorph**: It may be defined as-'**the specific crystalline form that may be changed reversibly into another form by simply altering the pressure or temperature,** *viz.* **sulphur,** and
- **Monotropic Polymorph:** It is usually defined as-'**the particular crystalline form that remains to be unstable at all temperatures and pressures,** *viz.* **glyceryl stearates'**.

Aguiar *et al.* **(1967)*** observed that certain **Polymorphic Crystals** may exhibit distinctly *lower aqueous solubility vis-a-vis the amorphous forms*, **thereby rendering the product to get absorbed incompletely.**

Examples

Chloramphenicol shows several crystalline forms, and on being administered orally in the form of a suspension, the ultimate concentration of the drug in the human body solely depended upon the **exact and precise percentage of the available β-polymorph in the suspension.** Incidentally, the said β-form of Chloramphenicol is found to be *more soluble, better tolerated, and better absorbed in the body*, **as could be seen in Figure 2.29.**

---

* Aguiar AJ *et al: J. Pharm. Sci.*, **56**: 847-853, 1967

Highlights of Polymorphs: These essentially include:

1. The specific crystal form that exhibits the **'Lowest Free Energy'** gives rise to the **Most Stable Polymorph.**

2. Interestingly, the **Metastable Polymorphs** may over a certain period get converted to a **More Stable Form.**

3. **Polymorphism in crystalline form of Drug may pose a serious problem in the manufacturing of a Drug Product (or Dosage Form)** perceptively.

Examples

A distinct and perceptive change in the **Crystalline Structure of the Drug** may eventually:

- **develop a 'Crack' in a tablet,** and
- **cause a hurdle in the Granulation Process*.**

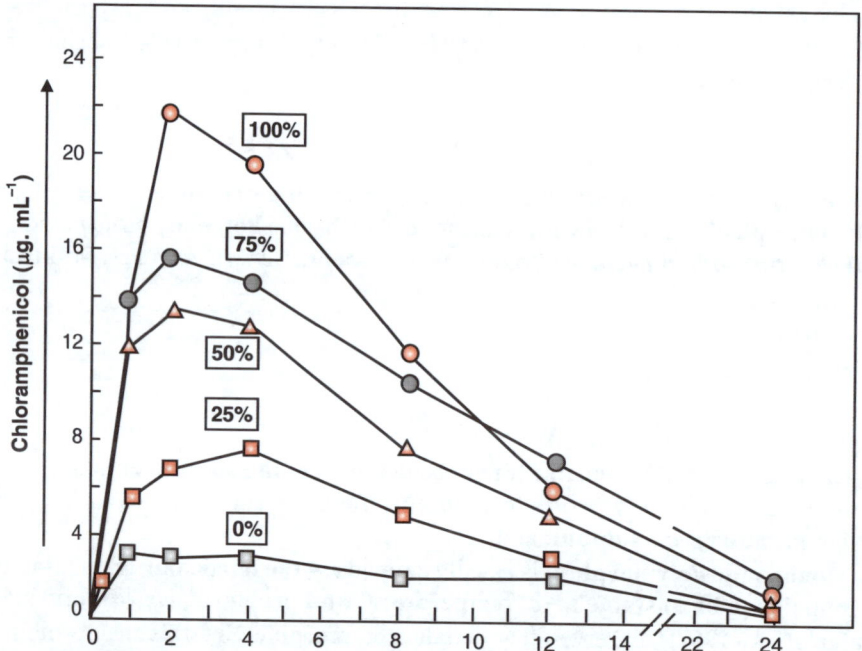

Fig. 2.29: Graphic Representation of Comparison of Mean Blood Serum Levels Duly Obtained with Chloramphenicol Palmitae Suspensions Comprising Varying Ratios of α-and-β-Polymorphs Following a Single Equivalent Oral Dose.
[Adapted from: **Aguiar Aj** *et al.* **J. Pharm.Sci., 56, 847-853, 1967].**

Solvates and Hydrates: There are some typical **Drug Substances** that do interact with 'Solvent' in the course of preparation to yield a crystal invariably termed the **'Solvates'.**

Likewise, **Water** also shows a tendency to form a *typical* and *specific* crystal with certain Drugs **Substances** usually known as **'Hydrates'.**

---

* That is, it may even prevent the compression into a 'tablet' which would otherwise require the entire reformulation of the product from ***ab initio.***

Allen *et al.* (1978)* remarkably demonstrated the – 'dissolution pattern of erythromycin dehydrate, monohydrate, and anhydrate in a freshly prepared 'Phosphate Buffer' having pH 7.5 at 37± 1°C, as illustrated in Figure 2.30.

It may be observed vividly from Figure 2.30 that the *two* aforesaid Hydrates do exhibit quite different solubility profile *vis-a-vis* the anhydrous state of the drug.

NOTE	Interstingly, ampicillin trihydrate has shown much less absorption vis-à-vis the corresponding anhydrous form of ampicillin perhaps on account of definite faster dissolution characteristics of the latter.

2.7.4.5. *Drug pK$_o$ Lipophilicity and GI pH (or pH-Partition Hypothesis)*

The pH Partition Theory (or pH-Partition Hypothesis): **Shore *et al.* (1957)**** carried out an elaborate and comprehensive investigation on the **pH Partition Theory** (or **pH-Partition Hypothesis)** that meticulously explains in rather simple terms the following *two* **critical on-going processes** *in vivo*, namely:

- **drug absorption from the gastrointestinal tract (GIT),** and
- **drug distribution very much across all the ensuing biological membranes.**

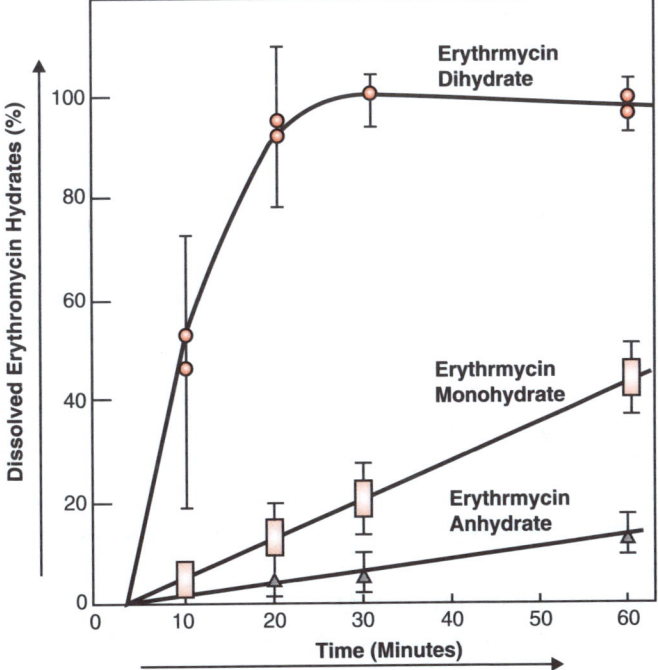

Fig. 2.30: Graphic Representation of the Dissolution Behaviour of Erythromycin Dihydrate Monohydrate and Anhydrate in Phosphate Buffer (pH 7.5) at 37± 1°C
[*Adapted from:* **Allen PV et al.:J.Pharm.Sci., 67, 1087-1093, 1978**]

---

* Allen PV *et al.: J. Pharm.* Sci., **67**:1087-1093, 1978.

** Shore PA *et al.: J. Pharmacol. Exp. Ther*, **119**:361, 1957

The **pH-Partition Theory** may be expatiated briefly as–'**for drug substances having molecular weight greater than 100, that are primarily transported critically across the biomembrane *via* Passive Diffusion specifically and generously**'.

In a broader perspective, the **Phenomenon of Drug Absorption** is critically governed by the following *three* **vital and important fundamental facts and observations,** such as:

1. **pK values (*i.e.*, the dissolution constant) of the drug,**
2. **lipid solubility profile of the 'Unionized Drug' (which designates the function of drug $K_{o/w}$), and**
3. **prevailing pH at the Absorption Site.**

In other words, the **pH Partition Theory** pertaining to **Drug Absorption** is actually based upon the **simple assumption that the GI tract more or less serves as a not-so-complicated Lipid Barrier to the critical and effective transport of drug molecules and chemicals.** Consequently, one may observe the following glaring facts, such as:

- An unionized form of an *acidic* or *basic* **Drug Substance, having enough Lipoidal Solubility Features,** gets absorbed adequately; whereas, the corresponding ionized form fails to do so.
- Interestingly, greater the fraction of drug in the **Unionized State at a Definite Particular Absorption Site, the more rapid would be the Absorption Profile** perceptively,
- Importantly, both *acidic* as well as *neutral* **Drug Substance would get absorbed from the stomach with great ease and fervor; whereas, the *Basic* Drugs may not undergo Absorption at all,** and
- Obviously, the exact and precise **Rate of Absorption is related intimately to the respective o/w partition Coefficient of a Drug**, *i.e.*, *the more lipophilic status of a drug, the faster shall be its absorption profile.*

It is, however, pertinent to state here that as **Most Drug Substances** do behave as **Weak Electrolytes (*i.e.*, Weak Acids or Weak Bases),** therefore, their *actual extent of Ionization* profile will solely depend upon the **inherent pH of the ensuing Biological Fluid** (*viz.* **blood, cerebrospinal fluid, urine** etc.). in case *the pH on either side of the Biological Membrane is found to be different, the compartment with a critical pH favouring more degree of ionization of the Drug Molecule shall comprise greater quantum of drug.* Alternatively, the respective Unionized or Undissociated Fraction of a Drug Molecule, with a reasonably sufficient lipoidal solubility, may have an access across the biological membrane passively, until such time an **'Equilibrium is Attained'** due to the ensuing **Concentration of the Unionized Drug on either side of the Biologic Membrane squarely.**

Drug pK and Gastrointestinal pH (or GI-pH)

In the beginning it may be understood that even the slightest fraction of a drug component in its solution state which does occur in the critical **Unionized Form (or Unionized state) truly** designates a function of both, *viz.,*

- **dissociation constant of the 'Drug', and**
- **pH of the prevailing solution (fluid) at the site of absorption.**

In usual practice, the **Dissociation Constant of both acidic and basic Drug Molecules is** expressed by pK values.

Salient Features: These essentially comprise the following:

1. **Lower pK$_a$ value of an acidic drug indicates that stronger will be acid, *i.e.*, availability of a definitely larger proportion of the ionized form (or polar form) at a specific pH.**

2. **Higher pK$_a$ value of a basic drug shows explicitly that stronger will be the base.**

Therefore, based on the aforesaid facts and observations, it is quite possible and feasible to determine the exact percentage of a **'Drug'** being ionized at the critical pH of the **Absorption site (or Biological Fluid)** by means of **Henderson-Hasselbalch Equations** elegantly:

For Weak Acids:

$$pK_2 - pH = \log\left(\frac{f_u}{f_i}\right)$$

where, f_u and f_i represent the fractions of a 'drug' duly present both in unionized and ionized states, respectively.

or

$$pH = pK_a + \log\left(\frac{\text{Ionized drug concentration}}{\text{Unionized drug concentration}}\right) \qquad \text{(a)}$$

or

$$\text{Drug ionized (\%)} = \frac{10^{pH-pK_2}}{1 + 10^{pH-pK_2}} \times 100$$

For Weak Bases:

$$pK_2 - pH = \log\left(\frac{f_i}{f_u}\right)$$

$$pH = pK_a + \log\left(\frac{\text{Unionized drug concentration}}{\text{Ionized drug concentration}}\right) \qquad \text{(b)}$$

$$\text{Drug ionized (\%)} = \frac{10^{pK_2-pH}}{1 + 10^{pK_2-pH}} \times 100$$

Thus, at a critical situation when the ensuing concentration of both **Ionized and Unionized Drug** equals each other, one may observe that the *second* term of Equations **(a)** and **(b)** gets eventually reduced to 'zero', because the value of 'Log 1' is 'zero'. Hence, we may have the following *revised version of the expression* as:

$$pH = pK_a$$

Nevertheless, the **pK$_a$ value** of a Drug always remains to be *typical characteristic feature of the Drug*.

Figure 2.31 records the **pK$_a$ value** of an array of important drugs together with their respective acid or base strengths of these selected drug molecules **(Rowland and Tozer, 1989)***

---

* Rowald M and Tozer TN: **Clinical Pharmacokinetics: Concepts and Applications**, 2nd ed., Lea & Febiger, Philadelphia (USA), 1989

Important Points

The various important points with regard to certain **selected acidic/basic Drug substances** are enumerated below:

1. Most acidic drugs are essentially unionized particularly at extremely low pH of the gastric juices; and, therefore, may be absorbed appropriately right from the stomach and the intestines.

2. The observed pH range in the GI tract specifically from the stomach to the colon ranges between 1 and 8.

3. Importantly, the very weak acidic drugs, having $pK_a > 8$, are found predominantly in an unionized state throughout the *entire GI tract*, e.g., **Glutethimide** (a *non-barbiturate sedative and hypnotic*), **Phenytoin** (a *hydration-based 'anti-convulsant'*), and **Theophylline** (a *CNS stimulant*).

4. Critical ionization of typical **'weak acids'** having **pK values** varying between **2.5 and 7.5 remains frequently sensitive to alternations in pH.**

Examples

Status of 'Aspirin' *vis-a-vis* **GI-Absorption Profile**: There **are** *two* **cardinal aspects** to be recognized, such as:

- **At pH 6.5, only 0.1% of 'Aspirin' remains in an uunionized form in the small intestine juices,** and

- **'Aspirin' plus other most weak acids do get absorbed quite adequately in the small intestinal canal despite the prevailing wide and unfavourable ratio existing between the unionized to Ionized Status of the Drug.**

NOTE

1. **The aforesaid goals and objectives are achievable due to the following** *two* **aspects:**
   - **large prevailing surface area and**
   - **long residence-time available in small intestine.**
2. **These crucial factors exclusively and mostly reduce the need for a relatively bigger fraction of the drug substance to be present essentially in an unionized state particularly in the small intestine.**

Predictions from the pH-Partition Hypothesis: Let us assume that there exists a **Membrane Barriers Located Strategically in a Biological System** which separates critically the aqueous solutions having altogether different pH values, such as:

- **GI-Tract Fluids** and
- **Plasma Fluids,**

so that the ensuing **Theoretical Ratio, 'R', of the prevailing Drug Concentration available usually on either side of the membrane may be expressed with the help of the following two typical equations derived intelligently by Shope** *et al.* **(1957):**

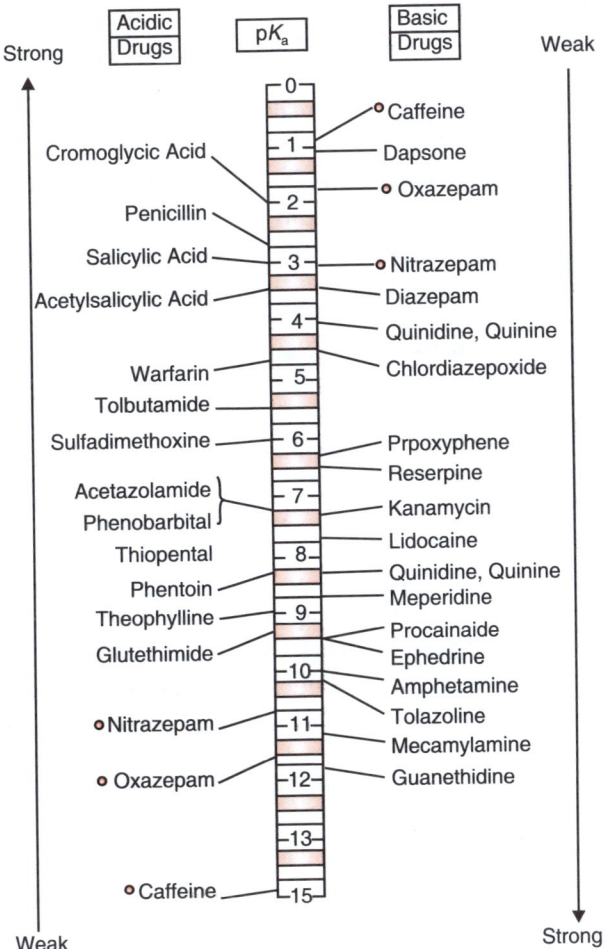

Fig. 2.31: The pK Values of Some Selected Acidic/Basic Drugs.

NOTE   **Drugs denoted with 'a' are amphoteric in nature.**

For Weak Acids

$$R_a = \frac{C_{GIT}}{C_{Plasma}} = \frac{1 + 10^{pHGIT-pK_a}}{1 + 10^{pPlasma-pK_a}}$$

(c)

For Weak Bases

$$R_b = \frac{C_{GIT}}{C_{Plasma}} = \frac{1 + 10^{pHpK_a-pHGIT}}{1 + 10^{pK_a-pH\,Plasma}}$$

(d)

From the above statement of actual experimental evidences and facts derived therefrom, one may arrive at a certain generalization with regard to **Absorption of Drugs and Ionization Based** entirely on the predictions from the pH-Partition Hypothesis, provided it is duly considered that the pH ranges from 1 to 8 in GIT; 1 to 3 in stomach and 5 to 8 in intestine (*i.e.*, Duodenum to Colon).

Two situations may arise with reference to the possible and logical predictions based upon the **pH-Partition Hypothesis**, namely:

1. **For Acidic Drugs**: There are *three* **different important aspects**; namely:

   - **Rapid absorption and independent of GI pH**: Mostly, the very weak acidic drugs having **pK$_a$ values > 8**, *e.g.*, **Ethosuximide, Phenytoin, Barbiturates**, invariably get unionized at all pH values thereby rendering *rapid absorption and remain independent of GI pH.*

   - **Unionized drugs show better absorption from stomach**: It has been duly observed that quite a **few acids, between the pK$_a$ range 2.5-7.5** are largely affected by definite alternations in pH; and, therefore, are subjected to a critical absorption in pH; and, therefore, subjected to a critical absorption absolutely independent of pH, *e.g.*, **NSAIDs** (*viz.*Aspirin, Ibuprofen, **Phenylbutazone**, an array of **Penicillin Derivatives**). In fact, such typical drug substances are obviously *better absorbed from the ensuing acidic conditions of stomach (where pH < pK$_a$)* besides their presence usually in Unionized State.

   - **Ionized form of drugs show poor absorption in GIT**: The *strongly acidic drug entities,* *e.g.*, **Cromolyn Sodium**, usually having **pK$_a$ values < 2.5** do remain in the ionized form throughout complete range of **GI-tract**; and, hence, show **poor absorption**.

2. **For Basic Drugs**: The *three* **most vital and important aspects** are as follows:

   - **Rapid absorption and pH independence in very weak basic drugs**: Interestingly, the very weak bases, having **pK values < 5**, *e.g.*, **Benzodiazepine structural analogues (Diazepam, Oxazepam, Nitrazepam), Xanthine Derivatives (Caffeine, Theophylline)**, *do get Unionized predominantly in the entire pH range; and, therefore, exhibit rapid absorption and pH independence completely.*

   - **Better absorption of unionized drugs from intestine**: Purely **Basic Drug Substances**, having **pK values varying between 5 and 11**, are mostly influenced by critical alterations in pH values; and, therefore, they do exhibit an **absolute pH-dependent absorption profile**.

Examples

The following drugs are definitely better absorbed from the intestinal passage (perhaps due to their alkaline conditions) *vis-a-vis* their existence as unionized state, *e.g.*, **Amitrypyline, Chloroquine, Imipramine, and Morphine Derivatives.**

   - **Poor absorption of strongly basic ionized form of drugs**: Mostly the strongly basic drugs, **having pK$_a$ values > 11** get duly ionized throughout the pH range in GIT, *e.g.*, **Guanethidine, and Mechamylamine;** and hence, remain poorly absorbed.

Table 2.3 provides the summarized form of a host of useful drug substances showing a distinct and explicit influence upon the ensuing **pK, values and GI-pH upon the Drug Absorption Pattern perceptively.**

Prediction the Degree of Absorption of Absorbable (Unionized)/Unobservable (Ionized) Forms of Drug at pH in GI Tract: Based on the **Equations (a) and (b),** it may be possible to calculate exactly and precisely the respective quantum of **Unionized** (absorbable) and **Ionized** (unabsorbable) **forms of the 'Drug Molecule'**. Nevertheless, it is also an easy and convenient task to predict, as closely as possible, the *degree of absorption pertaining to the aforesaid species (i.e., **Drug Variants**) at a given pH prevailing adequately in the gastrointestinal (GI) Tract.*

Figure 2.32 explicitly illustrates the manner whereby **pH directly influences upon the critical ionization of a Weak Acidic Drug, Ibuprofen** *designates as [HA]; and a Weak Basic Drug,* **Nitrazepam,** *represented as [BDH] vis-a-vis such species* as:

- **concentrations of unionized acid and base,** and
- **concentrations of ionized species [A⁻] and [B⁺].**

S. No	Drugs (pK$_a$ Profile)	pK$_a$	pH *vis-a-vis* Site of Absorption
	Table 2.3. Drug Absorption Influenced Significantly by Two Distinct Physical Charcateristics: pK$_a$ and GI-pH Values		
1	**Very weak acids (pK$_a$>8)**		
	Erthosuximide	9.1	* Unionized at all pH values
	Phenytoin	8.3	*Absorbed adequately along the total
	Hexobarbitone	8.2	stretch of GI tract
	Phenobarbitone	8.1	
2	**Moderately weak acids (pK$_a$ 2.5-7.5)**		
	Phenobarbitone	4.5	*Unionized in gastric pH
	Ibuprofen	4.4	* Ionized in intestinal pH
	Aspirin	3.5	*Better/improved absorption
	Cloxacillin	2.7	from stomach
3	**Stronger acids (pK$_a$ <2.5)**		
	Cromoglycate Disodium	2	*Ionized at all pH values
			*Poorly absorbed from GI
4	**Very weak bases (pK$_a$ <5)**		
	Diazepam	3.7	*Ionized at all pH values
	Oxazepam	1.7	*Poorly absorbed from GI
	Caffeine	0.8	tract
	Theophyllie	0.7	
5	**Moderately weak bases (pK$_a$ 5-11)**		
	Amitriptyline	9.4	*Ionized at ensuing gastric pH
	Codeine	8.2	*Relatively unionized at the
	Heroin	7.8	intestinal pH
	Reserpine	6.6	*Better/improved absorption
			from intestine
6	**Stronger bases (pK$_a$ >11)**		
	Guanethidine	11.7	*Ionized virtually at all pH values
	Mecamylamine	11.2	*Poorly absorbed from GI tract

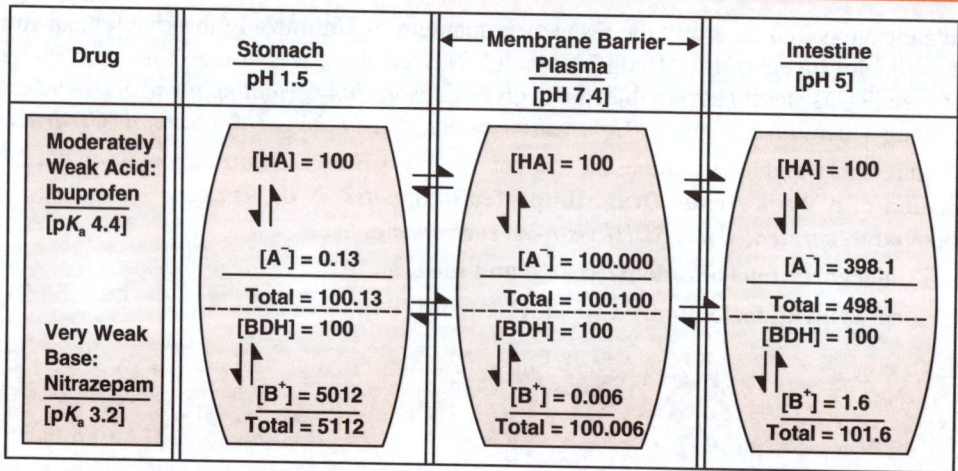

Fig. 2.32: The Critical Influence of pH Upon the Ionization of a Drug.

- [HA] and [BDH] designates the concentration of unionized acid and base and
- [H] and [B] represent the concentration of ionized acid and base.

Lipophilicity and Absorption of Drug: It has been established beyond any reasonable doubt that the '**pK of a Drug**' is solely responsible for *determining the degree of ionization at a specific pH level*. Besides, the **Unionized Drug** gets adequately absorbed into the systemic circulation provided the same shows *sufficient* **Lipoidal Solubility** profile. Thus, we may observe the following *typical situation* such as:

1. **Drug in Unionized State** may get absorbed rather slowly and sluggishly provided it has an inherent **poor lipid solubility (*i.e.*, Low $K_{o/w}$ value),** and

2. **Drug having Optimized Absorption** may exhibit enough aqueous solubility so as to get dissolved in the fluids at the absorption site besides exhibiting a **critical lipid solubility ($K_{o/w}$) high enough** to facilitate and augment the portioning to the '**Drug Substance**' right into the lipoidal membrane; and ultimately in the ensuing systemic circulation.

NOTE   In short, the excellent lipophilicity and drug absorption may be duly accomplished *via* a perfect hydrophilic-lipophilic balance (HLB) and it must be maintained by the crucial structure of the drug molecule having the optimum bioavailability.

Determination of Lipoidal Solubility of a Drug: It may be determined based on the **oil/water Partition Coefficient ($K_{o/w}$) Value of a Drug**. In a broader perspective, the $K_{o/w}$ **Value truly designates a measure of the degree of distribution of Drug prevailing between one of the several organic, water immiscible lipophilic solvents,** namely: **chloroform, *n*-heptane, *n*-octanol;** besides, **a hydrophilic phase,** *e.g.*, **water or an appropriate buffer solution.**

Example

An ideal oil/water system comprising **Octanol/pH 7.4 Buffer Partition Coefficient Value** ranging between 1 and 2 of a Drug is just enough for enabling the passive diffusion to commence very much across the lipoidal membranes.

Table 2.4 records the excellent comparisons between the **Intestinal Absorption of certain drug entities via the Intestine (animal model)** *vis-a-vis* $K_{o/w}$ **of the respective Ionized Form of the same drug (Schanker and Tacco, 1960)***

In conclusion it may be added that the **Bioavailability of a Drug** substance may be increased appreciably by *two* **known techniques**, namely:

- **Rate of Dissolution-invariably increased by changing the physical characteristic features,** *e.g.,* **crystalline structure, or particle size, and**
- **Rate of Permeability-usually promoted by critical and judicious modification of the drug's basic chemical structure by means of CADD****

2.7.4.6. *Limitations of pH-Partition Hypothesis*

There is no doubt that the scope and applicability of the **pH-Partition Hypothesis** have been exploited generously to decipher the so-called Intrigued and **Complicated Phenomenon of the Absorption of Drug**. Therefore, obviously it has its own *serious limitations as well as noticeable deviations from the aforesaid hypothesis,* namely:

- **specific presence of virtual membranes pH,**
- **critical absorption of ionized (polar) drugs,**
- **influence of GI surface area** *vis-a-vis* **residence time of drug substance, and**
- **crucial presence of aqueous unstirred diffusion layer.**

S. No.	Drugs	$K_{heptane/water}$	Absorbed Drug (%)
	Table 2.4. Comparison between Intestinal Absorption of Certain Drug Entities *via* Intestine (Rat Model) *vis-a-vis* $K_{o/w}$ of the Ionized State of the Same Drugs		
1	**Fast/rapid rate of absorption**		
	Phenylbutazone	100	54
	Thiopental	3.3	67
	Benzoic acid	0.19	54
	Salicylic acid	0.12	60
2	**Moderate rate of absorption**		
	Sulphanilamide	<0.002	24
	Theobromine	<0.002	22
	Theophylline	0.02	30
	Aspirin	0.03	21
3	**Slow rate of absorption**		
	Barbituric acid	<0.002	5
	Sulphaguanidine	<0.002	2

[*Adapted from*: Schanker LS. J. *Med. Pharm.*, 2, 343, 1960.]

* Schanker LS and Tacco DJ: *J. Pharmacol. Exp. Therp.*, **128**:115,1960
** **CADD**: Computer aided drug design.

The above *four* **vital and important aspects** will be discussed individually in the following sections:

(a) **Specific Presence of Virtual Membrane pH: It has been amply demonstrated that the pH-partition hypothesis duly proves** the **Critical Absorption of an Unionized Drug at a** *given* **GI-lumen pH exclusively;** In this manner, one may obtain a 'Sigmoid Curve' (*i.e.,* **an S-shaped curve) or the 'pH-Absorption Curve'** thereby representing the obvious **dissociation of a drug,** which may be obtained by **Plotting pH vs. Rate of Drug Absorption-as** depicted in Figure 2.33.

Explanation

The essential aspects are as follows:

1. **Salicylic Acid** clearly depicts the difference in the degree of absorption duly observed at a specific **GI-pH** *vis-a-vis* the values otherwise predicted by the respective **pH-Partition Hypothesis.**

2. **Experimental pH-Absorption Curves** are found to be much less steep and get *shifted towards LHS* (*i.e.,* **lower pH values**) as in the case of **Basic Drugs** (viz. **Guanethidine, Chloroquine, Morphines** etc); whereas, the curves remain *shifted towards RHS* (*i.e.,* **higher pH values**) as in the instance of **Acidic Drugs** (*viz.***Ibuprofen, Cloxacillin, Disodium Cromoglycate** etc).

3. **Virtual pH** (or **Microclimate pH**): The aforesaid logical findings and observations suggest strongly that a '**Virtual `pH'** (or **Microclimate pH**) *does exit predominantly at the surface of the membrane, which happens to be altogether different vis-à-vis the **Lumenal pH.***

In this manner, the presence of **Virtual Membrane pH,** in true sense, invariably and actually helps in the exact and precise determination of the degree of '**Drug Ionization'** and ultimately the '**Drug Absorption'.**

Critical Absorption of Ionized (Polar) Drugs: Importantly, the '**pH Partition Theory'** is heavily relied on the assumption that the unionized stated of a drug gets absorbed exclusively. Furthermore, the critical degree of permeation of the **Ionized State of a Drug** is found to be almost negligible due to the fact that its inherent rate of absorption stands at almost 3-4 folds less *vis-a-vis* the corresponding unionized state of the drug. these findings are indeed found to be quite realistic based upon the following *two* **critical observations,** *viz.,*

- **ionized drug substances exhibit low lipid solubility,** and
- **comparatively sluggish and slow permeability.**

Nevertheless, the '**pH-Absorption Curve'** (*see Figure 2.33*) indicating clear-cut shift, and vehemently supported the fact that the **Specific Ionized States of Certain Drug Substance** *do invariably undergo absorption to a significant extent perceptively.*

Interestingly, the important class of compounds called '**Morphinan Structural Analogies',** essentially having a *huge lipophillic moiety embedded in the structure,* **would get absorbed due to Passive Diffusion despite being ionized appreciably.**

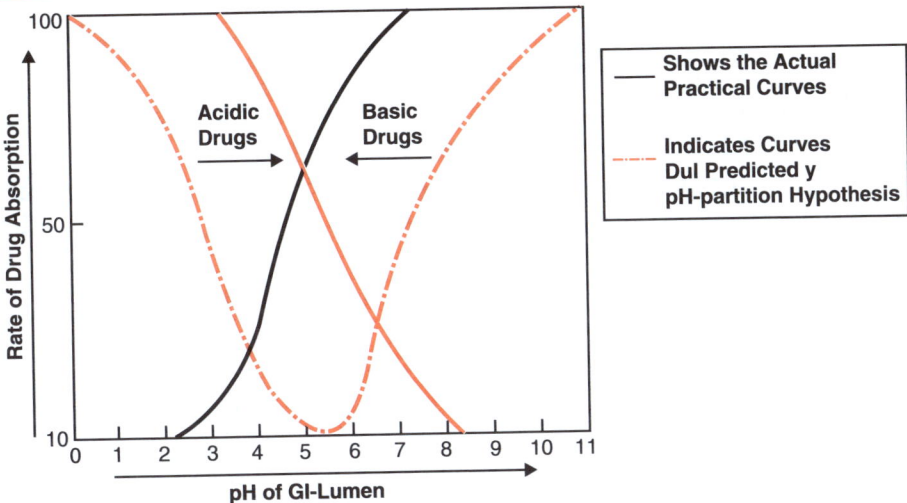

Fig. 2.33: A Sigmoid pH-Absorption Curve for Acidic and Basic Drug Substances.
[Acidic Drugs: Salicylic Acid; Basic Drugs Ephedrine]

NOTE   The critical and specific involvement of several other known mechanisms for the absorption of specific ionized drugs, *e.g.*, active transport, ion-pair transport and convective flow (as discussed elsewhere in this chapter).

Influence of GI Surface Area *vis-a-vis* **Residence Time of Drug Substance:** As per the **pH partition theory**, one may visualize the absorption of various types of drugs as indicated below:

- **Acidic Drugs:** They are usually absorbed to the optimum level from the stomach region (*due to acidic pH*)
- **Basic Drugs:** These are normally absorbed abundantly from the **intestinal canal** (*on account of alkaline pH*), wherein they remain eventually in an unionized state almost to a large extent.

Nevertheless, irrespective of the prevailing **gastrointestinal (GI) pH, together with the extent of ionization accomplished actually,** one may frequently take cognizance of the fact that both acidic as well as basic drugs rather get absorbed more profusely from the intestinal passage due to the following *two* **cardinal reasons,** namely:

- **first excessive huge surface area,** and
- **secondly, prolonged residence time of the drug in the intestinal canal.**

Crucial Presence of Aqueous Unstirred Diffusion Layer: The remarkable and efficient absorption of both acidic and basic drugs (*see Table 2.3*) is duly caused by the '**pH-shift**' which in turn comes into being by virtue of the fact that the usual '**bulk of the luminal fluid**' does not remain in direct contact with the biologic membrane, but instead comes into contact with a barrier invariably termed as the '**aqueous unstirred diffusion layer**' being interposed between them in a meticulous manner. Figure 2.34 illustrates a typical model showing vividly the critical presence of the aforesaid aqueous stirred diffusion layer located strategically upon the surface of the membrane.

Explanation

The various important aspects are as stated below:

1. The **'Aqueous Unstirred Diffusion Layer'** actually not only possess a definite thickness, but also serves a *potential barrier to the absorption of Drugs.*

2. The fundamental aspects of the **'pH Partition Theory'** relates predominantly the ensuing rate-limiting step to the respective absorption of drugs due to the **effective partitioning in the Lipid Barrier.**

3. The advent of the **'Aqueous Unstirred Diffusion Layer'** enables a drug to undergo critically:

   • *first* **diffuse *via* the aqueous barrier,** and

   • *secondly,* **diffuse *via* the lipodial barrier.**

4. Therefore, such drug substances with a prominently large partition coefficient may undergo fast and rapid penetration *via* the ensuing lipoidal membrane. However, the critically observed **'Rate-Limiting Step'** being their **effective absorption *via* the 'Aqueous Unstirred Diffusion Layer'** (see Figure 2.34)

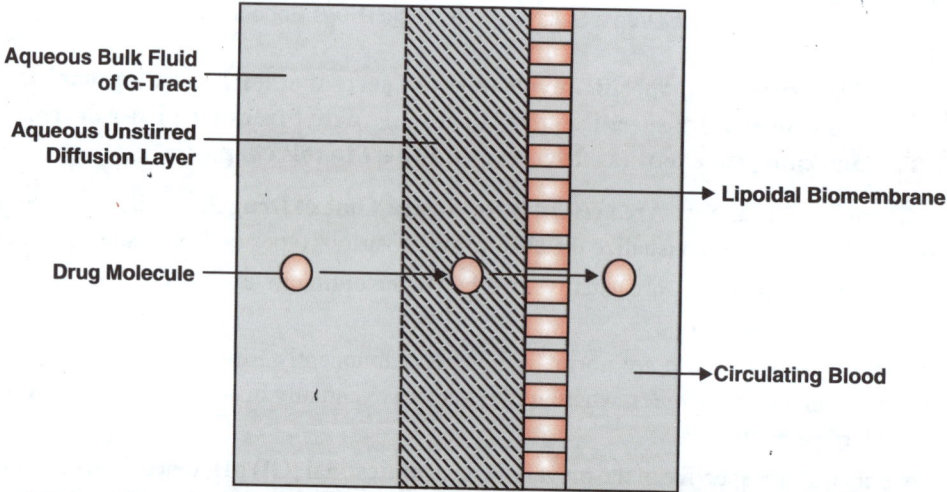

Fig. 2.34: Diagrammatic Representation of the Critical Presence of Aqueous Unstirred Diffusion Layer Located upon the Lipoidal Biomembrane Surface.

NOTE

1. **The above-cited phenomenon applies specifically to such substances having a high molecular weight, *e.g.*, bile acids, fatty acids etc.**

2. **Though the pH partition theory comprises several serious limitations, it still remains the most useful and effective means to have the fundamental concepts and ideas pertaining to the**

   • **phenomenon of absorption of drug and**

   • **critical movement of drug between different available body compartments.**

2.7.4.7. Deviations from the pH-Partition Hypothesis

A survey of literature has revealed that several attempts were made so as to rationalize the so-called **Experimental Deviation** from the *unmodified* **pH-Partition Hypothesis.** It is, however, worthwhile to state at this point in time that there exists absolutely no lack of concrete suggestions in this regard. Obviously, the following *two* **interesting factors** which may contribute to the aforesaid deviations are, namely:

- **microclimate,** and
- **a unifying hypothesis,**

which shall be discussed briefly in the following sections:

Microclimate pH: Microclimate pH is the most versatile factor which could be solely responsible for contributing to the **Deviation of the pH-Absorption Curves** (see Figure 2.33) from those duly predicted by the **Unmodified pH Partition Theory,** thereby causing a significant difference between the **Lumenal pH and the Microclimate pH*,** recurring at the cell membrane. It is, however, pertinent to state here that '**Microclimate pH Hypothesis**' is adequately supported by the glaring fact that H^+ ions are specifically secreted right inside the intestinal lumen.

Hogerle and Winne (1978)** researched meticulously to characterize the '**Microclimate**' almost directly by measuring the **pH** of the critical surface of the jejuna mucosa in *vivo*. It exists over a wide range between **4 and 10.8.**

Important Observations: They essentially include the following *three* **aspects,** *viz.,*

1. In most instances, the pH got shifted to the neutral point immediately after lowering the pH-electrode virtually down to the tips of the villi.
2. The microclimate pH was observed to be 5.4, when the luminal pH stood at 7.
3. Importantly, the microclimate pH varied negligibly with the corresponding changes in the lumenal pH that varied between 5.4 and 7.4 as observed over the entire range prevailing in the lumenal pH.

Hogerle and Winne** intelligently proposed the following relationship occurring between:

- **Microclimate pH,** and
- **Lumenal pH:**

$$\boxed{MpH = A + B\ (LpH{-}7) + C\ (LpH{-}7)^3}\qquad\text{(e)}$$

where,

MpH = Microclimate pH,
LpH = Lumenal pH,
A = 6.36,
B = 12.2×10^{-2} and
C = 10.3×10^{-3}.

A Unifying Hypothesis: Hogerle and Winne (1978)* duly extended their wonderful and remarkable researches, and finally developed a logical and acceptable '**Model**' applicable solely for the intestinal absorption which critically takes into account the above cited factual statements.

---

* It is also known as the '**Virtual pH**'
** Hogerle ML and Winne D: *Arch.Pharmacol.*, **322**:249, 1978.
*** Ibid, p 251.

Therefore, according to **Hogerle and Winne's Model,** the ensuing rate absorption of a drug substance may be expressed by the following equation:

$$\boxed{\text{Rate absorption} = \frac{C \times A}{(T/D + 1/P_u)f_u + f_i \times P_i/P_u)}}$$ (f)

where,

C = Drug concentration in the lumen,

A = Absorption surface area,

T = Thickness of unstirred layer,

D = Diffusion coefficient of the 'drug',

f_u = Unionized fraction of the 'drug',

f_i = Ionized fraction of the 'drug'

P_u = Permeability coefficient for unionized form of 'drugs' and

P_i = Permeability coefficient for ionized form of 'drug'. ,

It may be derived from the above that the degree of dissociation is duly designated by:

- **a critical function of the pK value of the 'Drug'**, and
- **the ensuing Microclimate pH**.

Nevertheless, one may calculate appropriately the 'f_u' and 'f_i' from the **Henderson-Hasselbalch Equation**. Thus, we may have:

For a '**Weak Acid**'

$$\boxed{pK_a - MpH = \log\left(\frac{f_u}{f_i}\right)}$$

For a '**Weak Base**'

$$\boxed{pK_a - MpH = \log\left(\frac{f_i}{f_u}\right)}$$

Importantly, as per Equation (e) the ensuing **Microclimate pH (MpH)** denotes a function of **Lumenal pH (LpH)**.

NOTE	The careful and cautions extension of the 'pH-Partition Hypothesis' to account for the judicious effects of the ensuing 'unstirred-layer' plus 'Microclimate pH' does cater for a rather more acceptable, logical and satisfactory rationalization of the derived experimental data.

2.7.5. Product Form (Dosage Form) Characteristics vis-à-vis Pharmaceutic Ingredients Affecting Drug Absorption

The intricacies and skillful manipulative phenomenon that are overwhelmingly associated with the '**drug absorption**' *in vivo* are meticulously modulated, guided and governed by an array of thoughtful novel concepts, ideas and technologies to produce ultimately a '**Better Drug for a Better World**'.

In order to accomplish the above aims and objectives, there is a strong and urgent need to explore the following *two* **important aspects**, namely:

- **product form characteristics**, and
- **pharmaceutic ingredients**,

which shall be discussed individually in the following sections:

2.7.5.1. *Product Form Characteristics*

The **product form characteristics** essentially comprise the following *six* **cardinal aspects**, such as:

- **formulation factors**,
- **disintegration time**,
- **processing variants**,
- **granulation variables**,
- **applied compression force**, and
- **packing of capsule contents**.

2.7.5.1.1. *Formulation Factors*

In general, the '**Excipients**' are mostly refered to as-'**non-therapeutic substance duly added to a drug product form so as to accomplish a suitable size or consistency**'.

From '**Pharmaceutic***' point of view, the '**Excipients**' are regarded as the '**pharmacodynamically inactive substances that may form an integral part of a 'formulation' to give rise to certain intended or desired functional characteristics features to the drug substance; and hence, the ultimate Dosage Form (or Product Form)**;

The '**Excipients**' are judiciously incorporated into the formulation of the tablet in order to achieve the following *five* **cardinal advantageous aims and objectives**, namely:

- **improving the compressibility of 'Active Drug'**,
- **modifying the stability of drug from undergoing degradation**,
- **minimizing the gastric irritation**,
- **modulate and control the rate of drug absorption from the absorption site**, and
- **enhance the drug availability**.

Table 2.5 (a) and (b) records certain frequently employed excipients in the '**Solid-Drug Products**' and '**Liquid-Drug Products**', respectively.

Salient Features of Excipients: These essentially comprise the following:

1. Excipients specifically for **Solid Oral Dosage Forms**, *viz*. **Compressed Tablets**, may essentially include the following integral components, namely:

   - **diluents**, *viz*. **lactose**   • **disintegrant**, *viz*. **starch**.

---

* **Pharmaceutics**: It refers to that branch of pharmacy involving the study of the chemical, physical and biological factors that critically influence **formulation, manufacturing, stability**, and **efficacy of the Dosage Form**

- lubricant, *viz.* **magnesium stearate**, and
- other ingredients, *viz.* **binding and stabilizing agents.**

2. **Alteration in Drug Bioavailability/Pharmacodynamic Activity Profile**: Improper and irrational usage of excipients critically in **Solid-Oral Dosage Formulations** may adversely affect these *two* **aspects**, namely:

- **drug bioavailability**, and
- **pharmacodynamic activity.**

Table 2.5(a). List of Commonly Used Excipients in Solid-Drug Products*

S. No.	Excipient	Property in Dosage Form
1	Cellulose acetate phthalate	Enteric coating
2	Dibasic calcium phosphate	Diluent
3	Hydroxypropyl methyl Cellulose (HPMC)	Tablet-coating
4	Hydrogenated vegetable oil	Lubricant
5	Lactose	Diluent
6	Magnesium stearate	Lubricant
7	Methylcellulose	Coating/granulating
8	Microcrystalline cellulose	Disintegrant/diluents
9	Polyvinylpyrrolidone (PVP)	Granulating agent
10	Starch	Disintegrant/diluents
11	Stearic acid	Lubricant
12	Sucrose (solution)	Granulating agent
13	Talc	Lubricant
14	Titanium dioxide	Combined with permissible dyes as coloured coating

Table 2.5(b). List of Frequently Employed Excipients in Oral Liquid Drug Products*

S. No.	Excipient	Property in Dosage Form
1	Alcohol	Solubilizing agent/preservative
2	Corn oil	As emulsion vehicle
3	Methyl propylparaben	Preservative
4	Polysorbates	Surfactant
5	Propylene glycol	Solubilizing agent
6	Sodium alginate	Suspending agent
7	Sodium carboxymethyl cellulose (sodium CMC)	Suspending agent
8	Sorbitol	Sweetner/vehicle
9	Sucrose	Sweetner
10	Sesame oil	As emulsion vehicle
11	Tragacanth gum	Suspending agent

| 12 | Veegum | Thixotropic/suspending agent |
| 13 | Xanthan gum | Thixotropic/ suspending agent |

[*Adapted From: Shargel L, Yu ABC. **Applied Biopharmaceutics and Pharmacokinetics,** 4th edn,: Mc Graw Hill Medical Publishing, New York, 1999.]

3. Excipients invariably influence and affect the profile of '**drug dissolution rate**' by changing critically the inherent medium by *two* **classical means**, namely:

- **Dissolution of the 'drug'**, and
- **Reaction with the 'drug' itself,**

Table 2.6 summarizes the overall and critical effect of some excipients upon the **Pharmacokinetic Parameters of Oral Drug Product** (or **Dosage Form**) thereby circumventing certain commonly encountered '**Manufacturing Problems**' which might affect both:

- **dissolution pattern of a 'drug'**, and
- **bioavailability of the 'drug product'**.

Table 2.6. Overall and Critical Effect of Some Excipients upon the Pharmacokinetics Parameters of Drug Product*

S. No.	Excipients	Exapmle(s)	K_a	t_{max}	AUC
1	**Coating agents**	Hydroxyprepylmethyl cellulose	–	–	–
2	**Disintegrants**	Avicel®, Explotab	↑	←	↑/–
3	**Enteric coat**	Cellulose acetate phthalate	←	↑	←/–
4	**Lubricant**	Hydrogenated vegetable oil, talc	←	↑	←/–
5	**Sustained-release agents**	Methyl cellulose, ethylcellulose	←	↑	←/–
6	**Sustained-release agent** (waxy agents)	Carbowax, Castrowax	←	↑	←/–
7	**Sustained-release agents** (gum/viscous agents)	Keltrol®, Veegum	←		←/–

* It may be caused due to *drug concentration* and drug dependence (drug concentration time curve) (K_a absorption rate constant t_{max}: time for peak-drug conc. In plasma; AUC: Area under the plasma.

(*Adapted From: Shargel* L,Yu ABC: **Applied Biopharmaceutics and Pharmacokinetics,** 4th ed.: McGraw Hill Medical Publishing, New York, 1999).

Specific Examples (Table 2.6): These include essentially the following aspects:

1. **Suspending Agents (e.g., Sodium Aginate, Sodium-CMC, Tragacanth):** They do enhance the viscosity of the drug vehicle; however, may lower the rate of drug dissolution from the ensuing suspension.

2. **Lubricants (e.g., Magnesium Stearate): Magnesium Stearate** being a *hydrophobic lubricants*, may in excessive quantity reduce the degree of:

- **critical drug dissolution,**
- **slow down the actual rate of drug absorption**, and
- **reduce the total quantum of drug absorbed.**

Remedial Measure: The above discrepancy may be abolished by any one of the following methods, such as:

      (a) **reduction in the level of lubricant,**

      (b) **replacing another selected lubricants,** and

      (c) **enhancing the quantum of disintegrant quite often may circumvent the retarding effect shown by the lubricants upon dissolution.**

3. **Disintegrants (*e.g.*, Starch, Microcrystalline Cellulose):** A suitable enhancement in the **Level of Disintegrant** to some poorly soluble drugs exhibit little or no effect pertaining to the **Drug Dissolution,** which is explained duly by the fact that the **fine-drug particulate matters never get wetted adequately and sufficiently.**

4. **Systemic Drug Absorption**: Excipients have a tendency to either **increase or decrease the rate and degree of systemic absorption of a drug entity**.

5. **Rate of Drug Dissolution and Absorption**: Such specific and critical **Excipients** that enhances the **rate of two major physical characteristics,** *viz.* **Dissolution** and **Absorption of a Drug,** also increase the '**Aqueous Solubility of the Drug**'.

Example

Sodium bicarbonate when used thoughtfully in a particular formulation may appreciably alter the pH of the surrounding medium of the '**Active Drug Substance**'.

In this manner '**Aspirin**' (a rather weak acidic drug, see Table 2.3), obviously in an Alkaline environment (due to $NaHCO_3$) shall be prone to form a water-soluble salt that enables the drug to undergo rapid dissolution phenomenon.

 NOTE   The aforesaid process of enabling a not-so-water-soluble drug to accomplish perfect solubility profile is invariably termed as 'dissolution in a reactive medium'.

6. **Formulation of Water-Soluble or Water-Insoluble Complex with a Drug: Excipients** may distinctly from either a water-insoluble complex with the drug substances present in the formulation.

Example

Calcium carbonate used in conjunction with **Tetracycline** (an '*antibiotic*') in a particular formulation would result into the formation of an **Insoluble Chelated-Complex of Calcium Tetracycline** that remarkably exhibits:

- **extremely slow rate of dissolution,** and
- **noticeably poor rate of absorption**.

7. **Excipients** show an obvious tendency to augment significantly the '**Actual Retention-Time**' of a drug substance present duly in the **GI-Tract**; and, therefore, possibly aid in the overall increment in the ultimate quantum of drug being used.

8. Lastly, **Excipients** may remarkably serves as **Carriers** so as to **increase the extent of drug diffusion very much across the intestinal wall.**

2.7.5.1.2. *Disintegration Time*

It may be observed that for immediate-release, the **Solid Oral Dosage Forms** (*e.g.*, **Tablets, Capsules, Dragees**), the **drug product** should have the ability to get disintegrated into small particulate matter and thereby help enormously in the **release of the Active Drug perceptively.**

USP (2004)* has promulgated an 'official disintegration test' so as to monitor a uniform and efficacious tablet disintegration profile.

Exempted Disintegration Tests for Certain Products: These **Solid Drug Products** have been exempted completely from the stipulated (**USP, 2004) Disintegration Tests,** such as:

- **tablets that are meant to be chewed,**
- **troches, and**
- **tablets that are intended for prolonged release or repeated action or sustained release.**

Importantly, the **'Disintegration Time (DT)'** is of specific and prime importance in such an event when one deals with either **'Tablets'** or **'Capsules'.**

NOTE	The stipulated *in vitro* 'DT' is certainly not a fool-proof 100% guarantee with regards to a drug's bioavailability, which is solely due to the fact that in case the so-called 'Disintegrated Drug Particles' do-not undergo actual dissolution, the absorption is not possible at all.

Nevertheless, in a particular situation when a solid dosage form fails to comply the stipulated DT, it usually **Foreshadows the Bioavailability Problems** significantly, since the immediate follow-up dissolution phenomenon may turn out to be:

- **much slower and sluggish, and**
- **extent of absorption remains insufficient**.

It is, however, pertinent to state here that the **'Sugar-Coated Tablets'** in particular remarkably process **longer DT**. Besides, the **Rapid Disintegration** is an absolute must in accomplishing the desired **'Therapeutic Success'** with respect to the **Solid-Dosage Form** under critical evaluation.

Interestingly, the **DT** of a **'Tablet'** shows a direct relationship between these *two* **aspects:**

- **quantity of binder present in the formulation, and**
- **compression force used in the making of a tablet.**

Thus, a **'Harder Tablet'** usually utilizes more amount of binder and process a *relatively longer DT.*

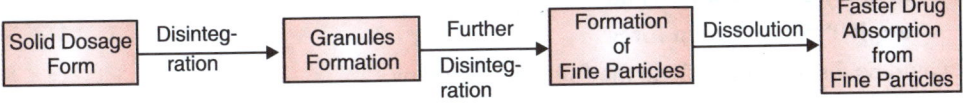

---

    * **The United States Pharmacopocia:** Published by United States Pharmacopocia Convention, Inc.Rockville MD (USA), 24th ed, 2004

The above flow chart shows explicitly the ultimately faster mode of drug absorption from fine particles duly obtained *via* the **Disintegration of** *Solid-Dosages Forms-Granules Formulation-Fine Particles Formulation* **in a sequential manner*.**

Incidentally, though the **DTs** do permit exact and precise measurement of the critical generation of **fragments-granules aggregates** adequately from **Solid Dosages Forms**-even then one may not obtain any useful or valuables information(s) from these aforesaid tests upon the rate of dissolution pertaining to the **'Active Drug Substance'**.

Amidon *et al.* **(1995)**** reported that the **Disintegration Test (DT)** proves to be some useful critical interest, whereas, the dissolution test is practically of no interest, essentially for the drug product that fulfill the various cardinal aspects of the **Biopharamceuticals Classification System (BCS)** specifically or

- **extremely soluble 'Drug Substances'** and
- **highly permeable 'Active Drug Entities'.**

NOTE	In short, *DT* caters a an useful integral component in the overall *'quality assurance'* in the *'Tablet Manufacturing Process'.*

2.7.5.1.3. *Processing Variants*

The **Processing Variants (or Manufacturing Variants) may be determined by the most effective single factor drug dissolution with respect to the absorption of drugs, particularly from the abundantly used conventional solid dosage forms,** *viz.* **Tablets, Capsules and Dragees.** However, the various recognized dosages from associated important criteria which predominantly influence the phenomenon of dissolution; and, therefore, the *respective absorption of a drug from such types of typical formulationsare as stated under:*

- **excipient used** and
- **manufacturing process variants employed**:

Importantly, the critical and important **Influence of the Excipients**, for instance: **Binders, Lubricants, Disintegrates etc., do exert their effective prominent role in the dissolution of an 'Active Drug' and discussed elsewhere.**

Following are **the** *two* **vital and importantly Manufacturing variables or Processing Variants that largely influence the Dissolution of Drug from the Solid Drug Form to the Solid-Dosage Forms.** The *two* **most important processes** that are employed most frequently in the manufacture of **'Tablets' are** *viz.,*

- **granulation variables**, and
- **applied compression force**.

that would be discussed briefly in the following sections.

2.7.5.1.4. *Granulation Variables*

Granulation may be defined as-**'a process of preparing finely divided to moderate-size**

---

*   That is, formulation ingredients apart from **'the active principles'** used.

** Amidon GL *et al.*: *Pharm. Res.*, **12**: 413-420, 1995

particles of varying shapes (mostly spheroid) to produce a definite degree of structure for easy flow and compressibility'.

Generally, the **granulation process** essentially involves the following *three* **major variants**, namely:

1. **Wet granulation method,**
2. **Precompression method** and
3. **Agglomerative Phase of Communication (APOC).**

        (a) **Wet Granulation Method:** The **wet granulation method** refers to the most conventional techniques that critically makes use of a granulating solution which is being employed so as to import adhesivness to the various ingredients in order that they may form first the '**granules**'; and secondly the 'firm tablets' when compressed duly.

It is a common practice to make use of a '**granulating solution**', since it is more effective in comparison to the same quantum of the '*dry powder binder*'.

Limitation of Wet Granulating Method: These mostly include the following:

1. The critical formation of a '**crystal bridge**' by the sheer presence of the liquid.
2. At times, the very presence of the liquid may serve as a potentially viable medium for carrying out certain '**chemical reactions**', *e.g.*, hydrolysis of esters (acetylsalicylic acid or 'aspirin').
3. The drying step involved in preparing '**dry granules**' may also help in the harmful degradation of certain highly thermolabile drugs.

Table 2.7 provides some of the more commonly and abundantly employed '*granulating agents*' in the **Wet Granulation Method:**

S. No	Granulation Agents	Granulating Fluid Added (%)
\multicolumn{3}{c}{**Table 2.7. Some Selected Granulation Agents Used in the Wet Granulation Method**}
1	Sugar	70-85
2	Glucose	25-50
3	Acacia	10-20
4	Gelatin	10-20
5	Cellulose Derivatives	5-10
6	Starch	5-10
6	Polyvinylpyrrolidone	3-15
7	Alcohol [95% *v/v*]	qs
8	Deionized Water	qs

In fact, the **wet granulation method** predominantly involves a plethora of steps each of which mostly influence such crucial and important functionalities, such as:

- **dissolution method,**
- **duration of blending,**
- **details of method selected,**
- **total times involved**, and
- **precise temperature of drying.**

(b) **Precompression Method**: In the **Precompression Method** frequently used to manufacturing compressed tables, one makes use of the 'dry formulated mass' duly compressed into a '**slightly oversized tablet or slug**', that is consequently ground to a uniform size for recompression into the finished tablet.

Necessity of Precompression Method

1. It is mostly suitable with such drugs which get decomposed rapidly because of exposure to moisture and heat.

2. Besides, the **Precompression Method** specially circumvents the disastrous effect of moisture and heat and, thus, enormously saves man hours and time factor because it completely avoids/ eliminates such operations as **wet mixing**, *drying* and *granulating*.

The following are the *three* typical advantages:

- **It enables the compression into a 'Single Tablet' of acids and bicarbonate, *e.g.*, effervescence tablet.**

- **The formulation must be designed to possess a reasonable degree of adhesiveness moderately dense and easy flow.**

- **The latest progressive advantages in the precompression method being the inclusion of 'Spray-Dried lactose', for such 'Active Drugs' with a small dose, as a specific diluents.**

2.7.5.1.5. *Applied Compression Force*

The term **Compression** refers to the –'process of rendering a discrete quantity of substance more dense or more compact, *e.g.*, solid-granules to 'tablets', and gases (LPG, CNG, Ammonia, N_2, O_2 etc.) to liquid states'.

It is, however, pertinent to state here that the specific and critical compression (or compaction) force duly used in the meticulous '**Tableting Process**' may predominantly influence such physical characteristic features of '**Tablets**':

- **density,**
- **porosity,**
- **hardness,**
- **disintegration time,** and
- **dissolution test.**

Figure 2.35 illustrates explicitly the precise influence of the applied compression force upon the ensuing **Dissolution Rate of Tablets.**

There are *four* different situations that may arise due to the application of varied **Compression Forces**, namely:

Situation 1: Application of higher compression force enhances the density and hardness of tablet thereby decreasing the porosity; and, therefore, gives rise to a number of changes in the status of a 'Tablet', such as:

- **reduces penetrability of solvent inside the body of the tablet,**
- **minimizes wettability by producing a firmer and rather more effective sealant layer by lubricant, and**

- **provides much tighter bonding created in between the particle crevices,**

which concertedly result in exhibiting the **Dissolution Rate of Tablets** as depicted in **Curve 'A'** (*Figure 2.35*).

Situation 2: Usage of *higher compression forces would cause deformation fractures, or even crushing of Drug Particles right into respective:*

- **smaller particulate matters,** and
- **help in the conversion of a spherical granule into a 'Disc-Shaped Particulate Matter' having a large enhanced surfaces area effectively.**

Ultimately, it gives rise to an increased dissolution rate of the **'Tablets'** as depicted in **Curve 'B'** (*see Figure 2.35*).

Situation 3 and 4: A logical, feasible and possible combination of **the** *two* **curves 'A' and 'B'** may also be accomplished as illustrated duly in **Curves 'C' and 'D' (Figure 2.35).**

NOTE	Conclusively, it may be pertinent to mention here that the specific and critical influence of the ensuing compression force upon the 'rate of dissolution' is invariably a difficult task to predict precisely. Perhaps, it could be achievable by carrying out a thorough investigative study particularly in each individual formulation so as to ensure overwhelmingly better dissolution and bioavailability of the 'tablet'.

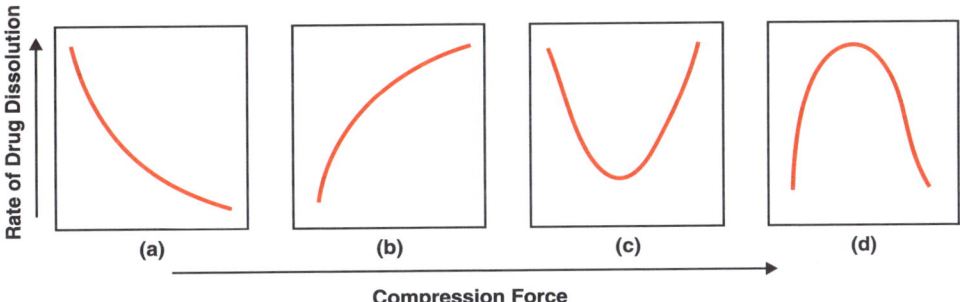

Fig. 2.35: Varied Influence of Compression Forces [A-> D] on the Dissolution Rate of Tablets.

2.7.5.1.6. *Packing of Capsule Contents*

Just similar to the **applied compression force** (see **Applied Compression Force** in this section) particularly applicable to only **'Tablets'**, the so-called **'Packing Density'** in the particular instance of the **'Capsules Dosage Form'** (or **'Capsules Product Form'**) may either inhibit or promote dissolution.

Critical Observations: These essentially comprise the following:

1. The actual diffusion of GI fluids into the tightly filled capsules prominently gives a high pressure very much within the capsule itself thereby causing:

   - **fast and rapid bursting,** and
   - **immediate dissolution of its contents.**

2. It has been amply proved and demonstrated that such capsules having excessively finer particles and intense packing do exhibit the following typical and characteristic features:

- **definite poor drug release profile,**
- **reduced dissolution rates on account of the appreciable decrease in the poor size of the compact,** and
- **distinctly poor permeability seen in the GI fluids.**

2.7.5.2. *Pharmaceutic Ingredients*

The **Pharmaceutic Ingredients** are also referred to in the literature as **'Pharmaceutic excipients;** or sometimes also as **'Formulation Factors'.**

In a broader perspective, an **'Active Drug'** is administered very rarely in its original form into a human system. The most commonly adopted means being the well known **conversion product form** (or **dosage form**) invariably administered via an **appropriate route,** *viz.* **Oral, IM, IV, SC, CSF** and the like.

Obviously, the **Orally Administered Solid-Dosage Form** does contain an array of **'Excipients',** also termed as the **'Non-Drug constituents of a Formulated Drug Product'.** The very purpose of incorporating the **'Excipients'** are as enumerated below:

- **accomplish and ascertain acceptability**,
- **ensure enough physiochemical stability in the course of extended shelf life of product,**
- **perfect uniformity of composition and dosage strength,** and
- **optimized biovavailability and functionability of the intended drug product.**

Characteristics of Excipients: The characteristics essentially consist of the following cardinal aspects:

1. In spite of the inert nature of excipients and their superb utilities in the formulated drug product, they may influence the **Normal Absorption of Drugs.**
2. One may usually encounter more complex problems with regard to **Absorption Pattern and Bioavailability Profile,** when more number of excipients are used in the **Dosage Form.**
3. The most commonly and extensively used **Excipients** in a variety of **'Drug Products'** are as given below:

- **diluents (fillers),**
- **binders and granulating agents,**
- **vehicles,**
- **lubricants**,
- **disintegrants**,
- **emulsions,**
- **coatings,**
- **surfactants,**
- **suspending agents,**
- **buffers,**
- **colorants,**

- **complexing agents,**
- **sweeteners,**
- **stabilizers,**
- **preservatives, and**
- **crystal-growth inhibitors.**

Some of the above-mentioned **Excipients** (or *Pharmaceutic Ingredients*) will now be discussed briefly in the following sections:

□ **Diluents (or Fillers) Diluents** may be defined as-'**any substance added to dilute or make less concentrated: solids, *e.g.*, Sucrose, lactose, Starch, Liquids, *e.g.*, Alcohol, Water, Glycerine; and Semi-liquid, *e.g.*, Liquid Glucose, Sorbitol'.**

In usual practice, the **Diluents** are incorporated invariably in **Tablet** and **Capsule Formulations** in such a situation when the required dosage regimen is not enough to produce the ultimate necessary required bulk. Moreover, the **Diluent could be either Organic or Inorganic in Nature.**

□ **Organic Diluents**: **Carbohydrates** occupy a very vital and important covert status as a **Diluents in Solid-Dosage Formulations**.

Examples

Carbohydrates designates the most important class of organic diluents which essentially comprise **Microcrystalline Cellulose, Starch and Lactose.**

Mechanism of Action: These **Carbohydrates** behave as *hydrophilic materials* and are found to be extremely useful in distinctly substantiating and promoting **specific dissolution of not only Hydrophobic Drugs, but also springly water soluble drugs, *e.g.*, Triamterene (a potent diuretic) and Spironolactone.**

1. **Steroidal diuretic/anti-hypertensive**: It predominantly forms a sufficient coat upon the hydrophobic surface of the drug particles, rending them hydrophilic in nature genuinely.

2. **Inorganic diluents**: **Dicalcium Phosphate (DCP)** represents one of the *most versatile and abundantly used Inorganic Diluents.*

Mechanism of Action: The most **Classical Drug-Diluent Interaction** that causes seriously poor bioavailability profile may be observed with **DCP** and **tetracycline** (*a potent broad-spectrum antibiotic*). It is due to the critical production of a '**Divalent Ca-Tetracycline Complex**', *which is found to be soluble sparingly;* **and, hence, poses an unobservable feature.**

□ **Binders and Granulating Agents: Binder** refers to- '**a substance being added to a formulation so as to cause particles to adhere (usually for 'granulation' and subsequent tablet compression)'.** It is also sometimes called as '**Adhesives**'.

In true sense, the **Binders** and **Granulating Agents** are used most frequently to **hold powders together to form granules** or to **afford and promote adequate 'Cohesive Compacts' specially for directly compressible materials, and also to render the 'Tablet' perfectly in an 'Intact State' after compression.**

Examples

Following are ***three* examples of commonly employed Binders and Granulating Agents;** *viz.,*

- **Naturals, synthetic and Semi-synthetic Polymeric Materials-** *e.g.*, acacia, cellulose derivatives, polyvinylpyrrolidne (PVP) and starch,
- **Hydrophilic (Aqueous Binders-usually display better Dissolution Profile with relatively sparingly Wettable Drugs by providing critically the desired Hydrophilic Characteristic features to the surface of granules,** and
- **Strong Binders-need to be used in the 'tablet formulation' with great care and caution, since their correct proportion in the formulation itself remains extremely critical and important.**

PEG-6000 proved to be a **'Deleterious Binder'** for the **'Active Drug'** phenobarbatone because it does *form a sparingly soluble complex with the drug itself.*

Besides, excessive quantum of these **'Binders'** invariably *enhance the hardness, minimize the Disintegration Rate,* and *reduce the Dissolution Rates of Tablets'.*

- **Non-Aqueous Binders**-also apparently lower the **Drug Dissolution** *to an* **appreciable extent,** *e.g.*, **Ethyl Cellulose.**
- ❑ **Vehicles: Vehicle** is referred to as – a **'Carrier or inert medium used as a solvent (or diluents) in which a medicinally active agent is duly formulated and/or administered'.**

In other words, **Vehicle** or **Solvent System** designates the major component of the particular **Class of Products** known as **'Orals and Parenterals'.** There are in all *three* different categories **of vehicles** that are used generally, such as:

1. **Aqueous vehicles,** *e.g.*, **syrup, water,**
2. **Non-aqueous water miscible vehicles,** *e.g.*, **sorbitol, glycerol and propylene glycol,** and
3. **Non-aqueous water immiscible vehicles,** *e.g.*, **edible vegetable (double refined) oils.**

Salient Features: These essentially include the following:

1. A **Drug's Bioavailability Profile** solely rests upon the ability of the **Vehicle** in exhibiting its *enormous degree of miscibility in the Biological fluids (viz., Blood, CSP)*
2. Both **'Aqueous' and Non-aqueous (water miscible) Vehicles'** are duly observed to be miscible with the body fluids; and the drugs are adequately absorbed from there in an efficient manner. Thus, it promotes overwhelmingly the **rapid absorption of the 'Active Drugs'.**
3. However, it may be observed quite frequently that an **'Active Drug'** which happens to be more soluble in **'Water Miscible Vehicles'** (*viz.* **propylene glycol-performing as a 'Co-solvent')** definitely displays much improved and better Bioavailability Profile.

NOTE	Importantly, careful and judicious dilutions of such vehicles along with the body fluids (*e.g.*, blood CSF, plasma) may result in the critical precipitation of the 'Active Drug' as fine particulate matters that would also undergo rapid dissolution phenomenon.

4. Potential **'Solubilizer'** *viz.* **Tween 80** is at times used invariably to augment and promote the desired solubility of an **'Active Drug'** in the aqueous vehicles.
5. Interestingly, one may take cognizance of the fact that in **Non-Aqueous Water Immiscible Vehicles,** the observed rate of drugs absorption depends almost exclusively upon its *due and effective partitioning taking place from the respective 'oil-phase' to the corresponding*

'*Aqueous Body Fluids*', *that may categorically turn out to be a* '*Rate-Limiting Factor*'.

6. The critical **Absorption of Drug Substances** is prominently modulated by the **Viscosity of the Vehicles'**. It, therefore, gives rise to a **diffusion process right into the bulk of GI Fluids, thereby rendering the critical absorption of an 'Active Drug'** from the core of a '**Viscous Vehicles' rather slower in pace.**

- ❑ **Lubricants (or Anti-frictional Agents): Lubricants** or **Anti-frictional Agents** are defined as-'**slippery, fine powder usually mixed with tablet granules to facilitate a uniform flow of drug granules into a tablet die, and to check and prevent the sticking problems usually encountered during compression'.**

In other words, the '**Lubricants**' judiciously and intelligently incorporated in '**Tablet Formulations'** do muster adequate and paramount support to the flow of granules, minimize ensuing **interparticle friction and adhesion** (*sticking*) of particles to the dies and punches in a **High-Speed PC-Based Tableting Machine.**

Examples

These essentially comprise the following:

1. **Metallic steatrates, saturated fatty acids** (*hydrogenated vegetables oils*), *e.g.,* **magnesium stearate, stearic acid, hydrogenated fatty acids**, which are known to cause distinct inhibition of wettability, sealing of moisture into tablet, and its respective disintegration and dissolution.

Mechanism: The **Lubricants** help in the effective coating of the added disintegrants when blended simultaneously in the formulation of a tablet. However, the **Lubricants** may be incorporated in the final stage, *i.e.,* just prior to the compression of the granules into a '**Tablet**'.

2. **Soluble Lubricants,** *e.g.,* **Carbowaxes** and **Sodium Lauryl Sulphate [SLS],** which are obviously the best alternative lubricants to prompt the dissolution of an '**Active Drug**' efficaciously.

- ❑ **Disintegrants (or Disintegrating Agents): Disintegrant** is defined as-'**a substance added to a tablet granulation during its preparation and after granulation to facilitate the breaking apart of the tablet into granules, and the splitting apart of the granules on being subjected to the fluids of the GI tract'.**

In true sense, these substances, *viz.,* **dried starch, microcrystalline starch,** critically overcome the cohesive strength of **Tablet,** and eventually break them up immediately on contact with water, which being a cardinal pre-requisite to the process of '**Tablet Dissolution'.**

Important points: These essentially include the following

1. **Most disintegrants are usually hydrophilic in nature.**

2. **Use of Lesser Disintegrant in a Tablet Formulation** may significantly lead to an obvious reduced bioavailability.

3. **Adsorbing disintegrants,** *e.g.,* **veegum, bentonite,** must be avoided particularly with **low-dosage active drugs,** such as: **potential alkaloids, steroids, digoxin,** as a relatively large quantum of dose gets absorbed permanently, whereas, only an extremely negligible fraction remains available for absorption ultimately.

NOTE	Importantly, it may be observed that 'microcrystalline cellulose' though serves as a highly effective disintegrant, nevertheless, at higher compression forces, it would effectively reduce the drug dissolution.

- ❑ **Coatings:** It has been duly observed on a broader perspective that the various coatings do exert a marked and pronounced harmful effect upon the ensuring drug dissolution from a tablet-dosage form follows the under-mentioned order:

Enteric Coat > Sugar Coat > Non-Enteric Film Coat

It is, however, pertinent to state here that the critical as well as specific **'Dissolution Characteristic Feature'** of certain typical coating materials do alter on ageing, such as: the so-called **'Shellac-Coated Tablets'** upon storage for a long period, invariably get dissolved more gradually in the intestinal passage. The above discrepancy may be easily circumvented by adding a small quantum of **PVP** in the **'Coating Formulation'** judiciously.

- ❑ **Surfactants:** It is indeed a common practice to make use of the **Surfactants** widely and abundantly in a variety of **'Tablet Formulations'** specifically as **Wetting Agents, Emulsifiers and Solubilizers.**

Mechanism: The exact and precise **Mechanism of Action of the Surfactant upon their influence on Drug Absorption profile** seems to be rather complex in nature. Importantly, the surfactants could either increase or decrease critically the **Rate of Drug Absorption accomplished by the following methods;** such as:

- interaction with the 'active drug',
- interaction with the 'membrane', and/or
- interaction with both 'drug and membrane'.

Nevertheless, the **Specific Mechanisms** that predominantly enhance only the **absorption of the 'drug' by using Surfactants** are as follows:

- **Specific augmentation in both wetting and dissolution of the 'active drug',**
- **Improved contact of drug with membrane for better absorption significantly,** and
- **Definite increased membrane permeability of the 'Active Drug'.**

NOTE	The advantageous beneficiary overall effect of the surfactants have been thoroughly investigated and evaluated specifically at the 'pre-critical micelle* concentration levels.

Physiological Surfactants: Interestingly, the **Physiological Surfactants**** do help in the much needed efforts to promote and substantiate the remarkable **Absorption of the Hydrophilic Drugs,** namely:

- **Steroidal drugs** (*viz*, **Testosterone, androsterone etc.**),
- **Fat-soluble vitamins** (*viz*.**vitamins A, D,K**), and
- **Griseofulvin,**

---

* **Micelle:** It refers to the agglomeration amphiphillic surfactant molecules in a dispersion medium (solvent) having a diameter of the order of **50 A or equivalent to 5 nm**

** **Physiological Surfactants**: Bile salts (anionic in nature), *e.g.*, alkali salts of bile: sodium glycochoclate, and **sodium taurochoclate; Lysolecithin (non-ionic in nature):** obtained duly from Lecithin *via* the action of an enzyme present in **Cobra Venom** by virtue of their **highly specific Micellar Solubilizing Characteristic Feature.**

Surfactants Causing Reduced Absorption of Active Drug(s): It has been proved beyond any reasonable doubt that one many definitely note a marked decrease in the absorption of active drug(s) b the critical presence of certain '**Surfactants**', which may be duly caused on account of:

- adequate creation of absolutely unabsorbable '**Drug-Micelle Complex**' at the critical surfactant concentration prevailing very much at a level just above the ensuing 'critical-micelle concentration; and

- excessive '**Surfactant Concentration**' is prone to cause definite laxative/purgative action.

- ❑ **Buffers**: A **Buffer** refers to- '**a system containing chemical constituents that eventually resist small changes in H ion and OH ions concentrations, designed to keep the pH relatively constant'.**

It may be observed that the **Buffers** do sometimes prove to be really beneficial creating the perfect congenial environment for accomplishing **Drug Dissolution**, *e.g.*, **Buffered-Aspirin Tablets**.

Nevertheless, contrarily there are certain **Specific Buffer Systems** comprising: K^+ ions *that critically inhibit the Absorption of the Drug, e.g.,* **Sulphanilamide, Viatmin B$_2$**.

Mechanism: The most **probable Mechanism** proposed for such an activity is the crucial up take of fluids of the intestinal epithelial cells by the virtue of which the following *two* **actions** come into play in a sequential manner:

- **reduction of the effective-drug concentration in the tissue**, and
- **substantial decrease in the rate of absorption the active drug.**

Interestingly, the observed inhibitory effect of certain viable and commonly used **Buffer Cations** upon the **Rate of Drug of Transfer is as given in the following order:**

$$K^+ > NH_4 > Li > Na^+ > TRIS^+$$

 NOTE   It is, therefore, an absolute necessity to have in a given 'buffer system' for a salt of an 'active drug' must contain the same cations as that of the drug salt, so as not to introduce any additional cations.

- ❑ **Colorants** It may be amply observed that even the actual presence of a very low concentration of a water-soluble dye could afford an '**inhibitory effect**' upon the critical rate of dissolution of quite a few crystalline active drugs.

Mechanism: This actually takes place due to the dye molecules being strategically adsorbed upon the '**Crystal Faces**', thereby giving rise to the ultimate inhibition of the **Drug Dissolution** appreciably.

Example

Brilliant-Blue (a dye) significantly reduces the dissolution of sulphathiazole.

NOTE   1. There are certain dyes that specially cause inhibition of the 'micellar solubilization effect' of the ensuing bile acids (*viz.* cholic, glycocholic and taurocholic acids) that may categorically impair the critical absorption of certain hydrophobic drugs, *e.g.*, steroids.

2. Importantly, some cationic dyes are found to be more reactive *vis-a-vis* the anionic dyes perhaps on account of their more prominent ability for absorption upon the primary particles.

❑ **Complexing Agtents:** It has been duly established that the extent of complex formation has exploited meticulously and advantageously to bring in certain effective changes in a 'Drug':

- **physiochemical characteristic features**, and
- **biopharmaceutical properties.**

Thus, a duly '**Complexed Drug Entity**' should posses the following typical characteristic features, namely:

- **changed stability,**
- **altered solubility,**
- **different molecular size,**
- **altered partition coefficient,** and
- **changed diffusion coefficient.**

Fundamentally, these aforesaid **complexed-drug molecules** are proved to be absolutely inert pharmacologically and, therefore, should have the ability to undergo critical dissociation either at the absorption site or eventually soon after absorption right into the systemic circulation system.

Examples

Following are some typical and vital examples wherein the '**complexation**' phenomenon has been exploited obviously to increase the extent of **drug bioavailability to an appreciable level**, such as:

1. **Increased GI absorption of 'Heparin'** (*an anti-coagulant*) due to increase membrane permeability in the critical presence of **EDTA** that specifically chelates the **Bivalent Cations,** *viz.* Ca^{2+} **and** Mg^{2+} **from the membranes.**

2. **Caffeine-PABA Complex:** It has been essentially an **enhanced lipophilicaly for much improved and better membrane permeability.**

3. **Ergotamine Tartrate-Caffeine Complex and Hydroquinone Dioxin Complex:** These *two* complexes do show an **increased degree of dissolution due to the formation of soluble complexes.**

   ❑ **Crystal Growth Inhibitors:** Besides maintaining and sustaining the primary physical characteristic features of an '**Active Drug**' duly present in a suspension, the very role of the so-called crystal-growth inhibitors, *e.g.*, **PVP** and **PEG**, do go a long way in affording the inhibition for the conversion of a 'high-energy metastable polymorph' right into:

- **less soluble,** and
- **fairly stable polymorph.**

2.7.6. *Drug Absorption vis-a-vis Patient-Related Factors*

It is, indeed, pertinent to mention in the very outset that before undertaking the discussion related to the specific patient-related factors which critically influence the **bioavailability** profile of a drug, one may have to understand vividly the anatomy and physiology of the **GI Tract** as illustrated in Figure 2.36.

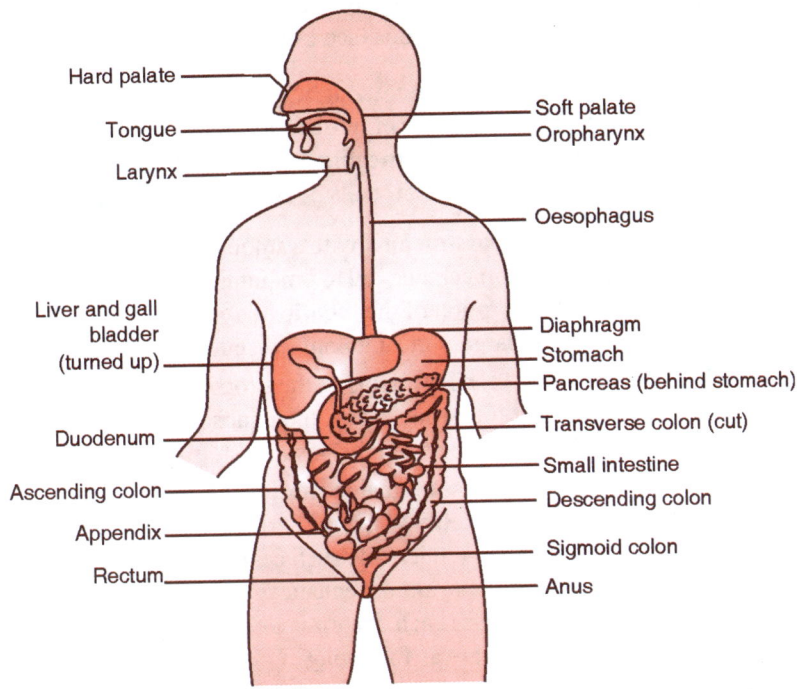

Fig. 2.36: A Schematic Representation of the GI Tract and Various Important Sites of Drug Absorption.

Mouth (pH 6.8): Lipophilic Basic and neutral drugs get absorbed directly into the systemic circulation.

Stomach (pH 1.3): **Lipophilic Acidic** and neutral drugs get absorbed but much lesser than that from intestine.

Small intestine (pH 5-7.5): Major site for the absorption of all types of drugs (*viz.* acidic/basic/neutral/lipophilic).

Large intestine (pH 7.5-8): All kinds of drugs get absorbed but only to a lesser degree.

Rectum (pH 7.5-8): All types of drugs get duly absorbed; almost half of the absorbed drug enters directly into the systemic circulation.

Liver: Designates a major site for drug metabolism, *e.g.*, first-pass metabolism.

Bile (pH 7.8-8.6): Helps in the critical absorption of lipophilic drugs; the actual route for 'active secretion' polar drugs/metabolites.

GI tract: It essentially consists of a plethora of vital components that modulate prominently such primary function as:

- **secretion,**
- **digestion**, and
- **absorption.**

However, the important functional components of the **GIT** (entire length: 450 cm) are namely: stomach, **small intestine (*comprising: duodenum, jejunum and ileum*)** and the **large intestine** (*also known a colon*), which distinctly and grossly differ from one another in terms of their individuals pH, anatomy, functions and secretions (see Figure 2.36).

NOTE	The complete length of the GI mucosa right from stomach to the large intestine is meticulously lined by a thin layer of 'mucopolysaccharides' (*viz.* mucus/mucin) that invariably serves as an impermeable barrier to the specialized particulate matters, for instance food particles, cells or microorganisms.

Stomach: It is more or less a 'sac-like structure' with a smooth mucosa and, of course, a small surface area. The acidic secretion in stomach due to HCI maintains a pH between 1 and 3, which predominately favours the critical absorption of the '**acidic drugs**', after getting duly solubilized gastric juice, because they do remain largely in an unionized state large degree in an acidic pH.

Besides, the **acidic gastric juice (pH 1-3)** helps in the proper dissolution of a host of basic drugs by virtue of their respective salt formation. Thus, their subsequent ionization renders them from being absorbed to a much lesser degree from the ensuing stomach.

Small Intestine: It actually represents the major site for the most preferred absorption of array of 'active drugs' based on the availability of a huge surface area. **The Folds of Kerckring**, as could be seen in the intestinal mucosa, renders the surface area to almost three times. Further more, '**Villi**', *i.e.*, the finger-like projections, almost enhances the exposed surface area to almost 30 folds. The resulting microvilli increases each absorptive cell lines up to **600 folds**. Thus, the overall dimensions of the small intestine are as following:

Length:~285 cm

Surface Area:~200 sq.m.

The observed blood flow in the small intestine ranges between 8 and **10 folds** than that of the stomach. Interestingly, the prevailing pH range between 5 and 7.5 proves to be most desirables and favourable for a good number of '**Active Drugs**' belonging to the therapeutic armamentarium, which remain unionized virtually.

In short, based on the above enormous advantageous plus points, the '**Intestine**' is proved to be the best available recognized acceptable site for the critical absorption of a host of drugs.

Large Intestine: Both the **length (110 cm)** and the **mucosal surface area (0.15 sq.m)** are smaller when compared to villi/ microvilli/ small intestine and, therefore, the ultimate absorption of drugs from 'colon' appears to be almost insignificant.

The **large intestine plays *two* major roles**, namely:

- **enormous absorption of water and electrotypes,** and
- **excessive residence time (6-8 hrs)-the 'colonic transit' may prove to be quite vital and important in the critical absorption of certain sparingly soluble drugs, and also some sustained release drug products (or dosage forms).**

The various patient-related factors have been discussed elsewhere in this chapter.

FURTHER SUGGESTED READINGS

Cadawallader DE. : **Biopharmaceutics and Drug Interactions**, 3rd ed. Raven Press, New York, 1983.

Gennaro AR. *Remington* : **The Science and Practice pf Pharmacy**, 20th ed., Vols. 1 and 2 Lippincott Williams and Wilkins, New York: 2004.

Gibaldi M, Perrier D : **Pharmacokinetics**, 2nd ed: Marcel Dekker Inc., New York., 1982.

Notari RE : **Biopharmaceutics and Clinical Pharmacokinetics**, 4th ed. Marcell Dekker Inc., New York 1987.

Rowald M Tozer TN : **Clinical Pharmacokinetics Concepts and Applications**, 3rd ed: Lea & Febiger New York., 1995.

Shargel L, Yu, ABC : **Applied Biopharmaceutics and Pharmacokinetics**, 4th ed: McGraw Hill Medical Publishing, New York, 1999.

Swarbick J (Ed.) : **Encyclopedia of Pharmaceutical Technology, Vol. 1** 3rd ed. : Informa Healthcare USA Inc., New York, 2007.

Chapter

3

PHARMACOKINETICS

3.1. INTRODUCTION

Pharmacokinetics is defined as–**'the study of the metabolism and action of drugs with particular emphasis on the time required for absorption, duration of action, distribution in the body, and method of excretion'.**

Alternatively, **Pharmacokinetics** relates to–**"the critical study of the quantitative relationships of the rates of the drug absorption, distribution, metabolism, and elimination (ADME) phenomenon: data used to establish dosage amount and frequency for the desired therapeutic response".**

Professor Dost (1953)*-first and foremost introduced the term '**Pharmacokinetics**' in the well-known text:

"Der Blutspiequelkinetic der Konzentration-Sablauffe in der Kreislanfflussiqkeit".

Though the concept of **Pharmacokinetics** and **Compartment Analysis** is certainly not a new one, yet the intrinsic level of interest and sophistication in this particular field has increased almost rapidly in the recent past. In 1920, the **Swedish scientists** first initiated the preliminary investigative studies related to the kinetics of drug elimination, and drug plasma concentration levels after administration of multiple doses. However, within a span of *two* **decades** the '**Compartmental Model'** was duly introduced followed by a comprehensive report pertaining to the kinetics of the distribution profile of drug substances *in vivo.*

Nelson (1961)** first and foremost presented a '**Review on Pharmacokinetics**' with regard to drug absorption, distribution, metabolism and excretion (**ADME**). **Notary (1980)***** established a logical correlation between **ADME** of drug substances and their inherent pharmacologic, therapeutic or toxic response in animals and humans. Importantly, the development of mathematical models is an absolute requirement to the interpretation of the typical prevailing kinetic phenomena.

The various **Important Aspects of Pharmacokinetics** shall be discussed in an elaborated manner using appropriate examples whenever necessary in the following sections.

---

*   Dost FH: *Drug Intell.Clin.Pharm.,* **11**: 747, 1953

**   Nelson *E: J. Pharm.Sci.,* **50**: 181, 1961

***   Notari RE: **Biopharmaceutics and Clinical Pharmacokinetics,** 3rd ed., Marcel Dekker Inc., New York, pp. 3, 46-47, 1988.

3.1.1. *Effects of Pharmacokinetics*

The various cardinal effects of **Pharmacokinetics** may be invariably explored and expatiated under the following sub-heads, namely:

- **Preformulation**,
- **Dissolution Testing,** and
- **Bioavailability and Bioequivalence,**

which shall now be discussed individually in the sections that follows:

3.1.1.1. *Preformulation*

Intensive and extensive investigative studies have revealed that '**Preformulation**' ascertains predominantly:

"the most prevalent and explicit effect that 'pharmacokinetics' has had upon the art and science of formulation".

However, it is rather quite difficult and cumbersome to determine with any definite certainty as and when the actual practice would turn out to be common.

Obviously, before 1960s- one may observe that the art and science of formulation was quite unusual; whereas, it almost became the essential and vital *'Norm'* in majority of the so-called:

'**Research-Based Pharmaceuticals companies by 1990s globally'.**

Remarks: Importantly, in certain Pharmaceutical Companies- the '**Preformulation**' episodes are being carried out by such qualified and intelligent personnels who are eventually involved in such glaring aspects as:

- **Design and evaluation of Drug-Delivery Systems (DDS),** and
- **Deal exclusively with Preformulation Task.**

Preformulation may also be defined as-

"a reconnaissance (to miss out) in depth to state precisely the characteristics features of a *Drug Molecule* most likely to affect the overall *design* and *performance* of the Drug Delivery System".

Highlights of Preformulation: These essentially include:

- *Preformulation Data* fail to convey precisely which path to follow in the on-going Formulation exercise; and thus, it quite often does inform us-'*which points are the Dead-Ends'*;
- *Preformulation Phenomenon* indeed implies a fairly '*good example'* of the so-called **successful philosophy** that-'**prevention is always better than cure';**
- At the very outset-*Preformulation* was vehemently associated with the underling fact which relates to: '**how the *possible incompatabilies* usually encountered between the *drugs* and *excipients* could ultimately affect the stability of *drug formulation*;** and
- There exists no **Standard Menu** (*Guideline*) that might be accepted by **All Pharmaceutical Companies** in the world for enabling them to follow:

'**the *activities* of a Preformulation Group'.**

However, the following *nine* **aspects summarizes perceptively** the various divergent areas of a detailed study common to several such groups, namely:

- **pK,**
- **Particle size spectrum,**
- **Aqueous solubility,**
- **pH solubility profile,**
- **Dissolution rate of pure drug substance,**
- **Distribution coefficient or some measure of drug membrane flux,**
- **Tests for polymorphism,**
- **Scan of incompatabilities with excipients,** and
- **Stability scan.**

*Prerequisites for Preformulation Study-*In fact, there are *two* **vital and important prerequisites** commonly observed in a critical **Preformulation Study** of a newly developed **Drug Product** or **Dosage Form**, such as:

- ➤ **Availability of Drug (Active Ingredient) in reasonable quantum**; and
- ➤ **Validated Assay Method.**

Points to Ponder: These essentially comprise:

1. A **significant ingenuity** (*showing originality*) has been shown by certain *Preformulation Groups* in performing the so-called:

"**miniaturizing preformulation tests perceptively**",

In order that the *actual demands for drug substance do got reduced appreciably.*

2. In addition, the critical and precise development of the intended-'**Stability-indicating Assays**' concerning various **drug substances** having actual *Molecular Weights (mw)* **less than 500 Daltons** (*i.e., micromolecules*) has virtually turn out to be almost routine practice in several **Pharmaceutical Companies** across the globe.

3. Importantly, such '*Drugs*' having either **Acidic or Basic Functional Moieties** – it would be an absolute must to determine their respective inherent '*pK*' **value**- that being a common *preformulation exercise* largely.

4. An accurate measurement of both '**Aqueous Solubility**' and '**pH Solubility Profile**'-does focus an:

"**Obvious relevance to the absorption phenomenon from the Gastrointestinal (GI) Tract predominantly**".

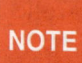

> **NOTE**   Nevertheless, it must be taken cognizance of the fact that these *equilibrium (Classic Thermodynamic) values* may be definitely of less importance *vis-a-vis* the critical determination of *Dissolution Rate (Kinetic Profile)* perceptively.

3.1.1.2. *Dissolution Testing*

Dissolution testing (Dissolution Test) refers to the means of measuring the *precise time* for the **Active Ingredients** of a '**Drug Product**' (*Dosage Form*) to undergo complete dissolution.*

---

* Refer to **USP, NF**-for the detailed procedures.

Another school of thought defines **Dissolution Testing as:**

'**definitely the so-called: Offspring of Pharmacokinetics**'.

Amazing, whether the '**parent**' (*i.e.*, **pharmacokinetic**) would remain comfortable in acknowledging the said relationship (between *father-son duo*) remains a *debatable factual episode*.

Remarks: In earlier discourse *i.e.*, before the advent of **Pharmacokinetics**- the various *Pharmacopocial Tests* (**IP, BP, USP, NF, Eur.P**, and **Intl P**) did provide *very little attention* to: "**Qualifying accurately the *Rate of Release* of Drug from the delivery systems perceptively**".

Consequently, the **Drug Product Data** duly published critically showed that:

"**for a good number of *Important Drug Substances*, the respective *Marketed Versions of the same Drug Product*, - though fully complied with the *Pharmacopocial Standards* but showed quite significant variation in the *Blood Concentration Profile*".**

Based on the aforesaid anomaly an attempt was made to adopt certain more '**Specific Tests**' so as to quantify the actual **drug release pattern** *in-vivo* with a thunderous zeal and gusto. **Scenario of Majority of Drugs Between 1960-1980:**

Interestingly, between the *two* **decades (1960-1980)** the various '*Drugs*' duly evolved by the *Pharmaceutical Scientists* were proved to be:

'**Weak-electrolyte Micromolecules**'.

Hence, it was reasonable to predict that:

"**dissolution was indeed the *Rate-determining* Step in the overall sequence of: Disintegration-Dissolution-Membrane Flux, and Intracorporeal transport to the general circulation in the human body**".

Inclusion of Dissolution Testing in Quality Assurance Test of Drug Products (Dosage Forms):

At this point in time there were great *hopes, belief*, and *expectations* that the practice of '**Dissolution Testing**' may prove to be a great asset in the following *two* **aspects**:

➢ **Utility as a viable and reliable Quality Assurance Test to monitor and regulate the** *batch-to-Batch variability;* and

➢ **Obviously prove to be predictive qualitatively of the *Blood Levels* which may be attributed by a given drug-delivery system perceptively.**

3.1.1.3. *Bioavailability and Bioequivalence*

Based on the scientific revelations and literature survey one may critically take cognizance of the fact that:

"**one of the most striking differences being observed predominantly between the so-called: *Pharmaceutical Formulation (Preparation)* in the 1990s and the prevailing practices in the 1960s lies in the gross overwhelming difference as-on-date given to the *in-vivo* performance of the *Drug-Delivery Systems*".**

Bioavailability [or *Bioequivalence Data*]- Following are some of the important and vital considerations pertaining to **Bioavailability [and/or Bioequivalence Data]**, namely:

1. They do have a major, *if not paramount*, status with respect to the aims and objectives of a host of so-called *Formulating Projects*.

2. Importantly, **US-FDA** and **other Regulatory Agencies** do predominantly and prevailing do essentially require either:

- **Bioavailability**, or
- **Bioequivalence Data,**

to be duly submitted to the competent **Drug Regulatory Agencies** together with either:

- **NDAs: New-Drug Applications**, or
- **ANDAs: Abbreviated New Drug Applications**.

3. In addition, the requisite relevant data pertaining to all such products intended to be *'Marketed'*, the **sponsor*** will invariably carry out other intimately concerned – *'Biostudies'* at various stages particularly in the course of:

' a Targeted Formulation Sequence'

4. In a broader sense, the critical **Bioavailability Studies** do play a pivotal role with regard to:

"**building a Bridge between a *'Formulation'* used extensively in the *Clinical Testing Episode;* and the one duly selected and intended to be used in the Final Market Product**".

> **NOTE**
> Importantly, the *Regulatory Agencies* (*viz*. US-FDA) may require vehemently that the *'Bioequivalence'* may be established meticulously between the *Formulation* upon which the so-called: Clinical justification for approval is based exclusively; and that will be marketed ultimately.

5. Perhaps one of the most encouraging development in the specific field of '**Bioavailability Tests'** largely relates to:

" the generous use of Neural Network Computing Techniques (NNCT)- that obviously seen to possess *very commendable potential* to enhance the- *statistical power of Biostudies* which essentially make use of a small number of subjects (*i.e.*, healthy-human volunteers)"******

> **NOTE**
> In case, these above mentioned hopes are fully realized-the so-called *'Formulators'* are most likely to accomplish a much more utilization of the *Bio studies*-as a critical segment of development they undertake at present.

3.2. CLINICAL SIGNIFICANCE OF PLASMA PROTEIN DRUG CONCENTRATION MEASUREMENT

It has been duly demonstrated that most **Drug Molecules** *in vivo* (*i.e.*, in a human body after administration of a drug) do invariably show a tendency to undergo critical interaction with several tissue constituents of which the *two* **major recognized categories are**-as given under:

- **plasma protein (available in circulating blood)** and
- **cardiovascular tissues.**

Importantly, an array of typical '**Macromolecules'**, *e.g.*, **deoxyribonucleic acid (DNA-a nucleic acid)**, plasma protein (obtained from human blood), and **Adipose Tissue (fat depots in a**

---

* **Sponsor**: The Agency who promotes (or launches) the product

** **Shimada T:** *J Physiol*, **392**:113, 1987

human body) are adequately formed by the **Interacting Molecules,** *i.e., the drug-protein binding.* Therefore, one may logically explain the '**protein-binding of drugs**' as caused by the unique process of **Complex Formation of Drugs and Proteins**. In reality, the different **Blood Proteins** to which the '**Drugs**' usually bind are:

- **human serum albumin**,
- α_1-**acid glycoprotein**, and
- **lipoproteins**

It is, however, important to state here that the respective '**Protein-Bound Drug**' entity due to its relatively large size fail to pass across the cell membranes. On the contrary, the corresponding '**unbound drug**' entity can pass through various cell membranes easily and conveniently. Therefore, in usual practice, based on the ease of detection, one may determine the drug concentration in plasma rather than the **assay of free-drug concentration**. Perhaps, for the same good logical explanation, the so-called '**Recommended Therapeutic Concentrations**' are frequently expressed in terms of the '**total drug concentration in plasma**'.

> **NOTE** **Methods employed for measuring free-drug concentration are found to be time consuming, tedious and expensive, and show lack of accuracy and precision in results; and therefore, are totally replaced by the assay for 'total drug concentration in plasma'.**

3.2.1. *Significance of Drug-Protein Binding Complex*

The vital significance of **Drug-Protein Binding Complex** is as enumerated below:

1. **Inert Pharmacokinetically**-These complexes are found to be quite pharmacokinetically.
2. **Inert Pharmadynamically**-These complexes strongly suggest that why a '**Protein-Bound Drug**' entity largely behaves as:

- **ineffective towards mobilization** *in vivo,*
- **non-excretable** *via* **the biological system,**
- **fails to exert any pharmacological activity** *in vivo.*
- **remains confined to a specific tissue for which it shows an enhanced affinity level and**
- **retards significantly the 'free membrane transport'; due to its huge bulk size, thereby increasing the biological half-cycle ($t_{1/2}$) appreciably.**

The critical and specific binding of drugs to the different tissue constituents *vis-a-vis* its concerted response to either meaningful disposition or anticipated clinical effect is as depicted in Figure 3.1.

Generally, the **drug-protein binding process** designates a reversible process. Nevertheless, a few typical drug substances may bind to proteins in an irreversible manner, *e.g.,* the specifically reactive intermediate metabolites of **Paracetamol** at higher dosage regimens that bind with liver proteins irreversibly; and thus, give rise to an **ultimate status of hepatotoxicity**.

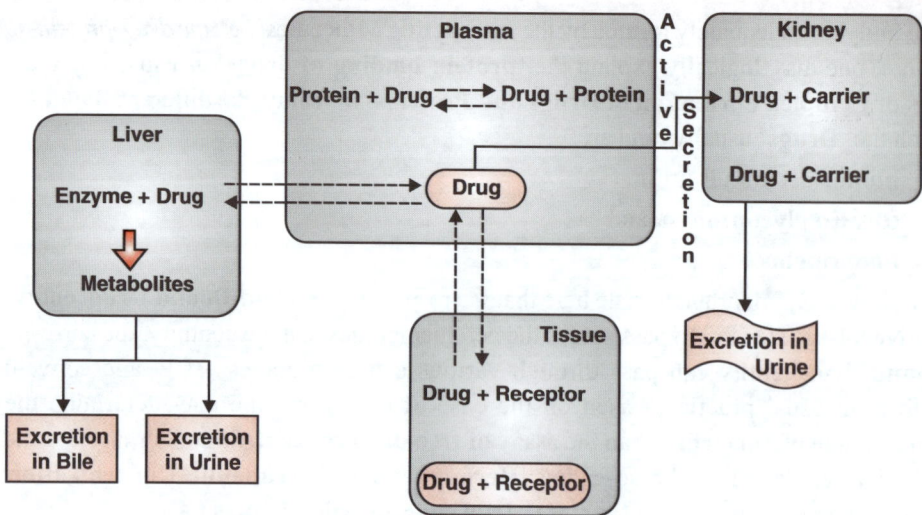

Fig. 3.1: Schematic Representation of the Effect of Reversible Drug-Protein Binding Interaction upon Drug Distribution-Metabolism-Excretion (*via* Kidney)-Therapeutic Effect.

How Does 'Binding of Drugs' Commence *in vivo*: On the basis of the copious volumes of extensive and intensive research outputs across the globe, one may rightly arrive at the following two important reasons concerned with the '**Binding of Drugs**':

1. **Blood constituents, *e.g.*, plasma or blood cells,** and
2. **Extracellular tissue proteins, *e.g.*, adipose tissues, bone marrow, cardiovascular tissues.**

Table 3.1 records explicitly the '**Blood Proteins**' that get bound to different '**Drug Substances**'. Importantly, the '**Binding of Drugs**' systematically takes place in a human body at various ports, namely:

- **serum albumin,**
- α_1**-acid glycoprotein (also known as α_1-AGP or AAG),**
- **lipoproteins,**
- **globulins**, and
- **erythrocytes [or red blood cells (RBCs)],**

which shall now be discussed individuall in the following sections:

Table 3.1. Different Blood Proteins to which Drugs Usually Bind

S. No	Blood Proteins	Molecular Weight (Da)	Concentration [%]	Drugs Binding to Protein
1	Human Serum Albumin	65,000-69,000	3.5-5	Broad spectrum of most drug substances
2	α_1-Acid Glycoprotein (Orosomucoid)	44,000	0.04-0.1	Imipramine lidocaine, quinidine (*i.e.*, basic drug substances)
3	Lipoproteins (*i.e.*, Macro-molecular	2,00,000- 3,400,000	Occurs in a variable range	Chlorpromazine (*i.e.*, basic lipophilic drug)

	complexes of Lipids and Proteins			
4	α-Globulin	59,000	0.003-0.007	Cyanocobalamine (vitamin B_{12}), thyroxine and corticosterone (a cortico-steroid)
5	α-Globulin	1,34,000	0.015-0.06	Fat soluble vitamins, *viz.* vitamins A,D,E and K; and Cu^{2+} (cupric ons)
6	Haemoglobin	64,500	11-16	Phenobarbital, phenytoin and phenothiazines

3.2.1.1. *Serum Albumin*

Obviously, **Serum Albumin** renders the most vital and prominent contribution to drug binding in the plasma that almost constitutes 50% of the total plasma proteins having a concentration ranging between 3.5% and 5%. In fact, the **Human Serum Albumin (HSA)** is largely synthesized b liver, and has a molecular weight varying between **65K and 69K Da**. The following are the *seven* important characteristics of HSA, namely:

- **HSA is usually present in plasma and extracellular fluid of different tissues.**
- **Nearly 120 g albumin is present in plasma for a man weighing 70 kg.**
- **Approximately 60% of total albumin in a human body is invariably found outside the plasma.**
- **Lower concentrations of serum albumin are usually found in pregnancy and some other disease conditions.**
- **HSA critically maintains the osmotic pressure of the blood.**
- **HSA takes care for the crucial *in vivo* transportation of**
  - ➤ **endogenous substances*.**
  - ➤ **exogenous materials.**
- **Albumin gets bound to a good number of weak acidic drugs and neutral drugs.**

Different Sites on HSA for Drug-Binding: In fact, there exist *four* different crucial sites strategically located on **HSA** which have been duly identified and recognized for drug binding, as illustrated in Figure 3.2.

Explanation

Following are the brief explanations with regard to the aforesaid four distinct drug binding sites:

Site 1: Warfarin (or Azapropazone) Binding Site- It mostly designates the specific region at which a large number of drug substances usuall get bound appropriately:

---

* **Endogenous Substances**: Albumin undergoes complexation with bilirubin, free-fatty acids (FFAs), tryptophan, and a number of hormones (*viz.* **Aldosterone, Cortisone, Thyroxine** etc.) to serve as a 'transport protein' for the endogenous substances.

Examples

NSAIDs, *viz.* **indomethacin, naproxen and phenylbutazone; Sulphonamides,** *viz.* **sulphamethizole, sulphadimethoxine; Phenytoi; Bilirubin: Sodium Valproate.**

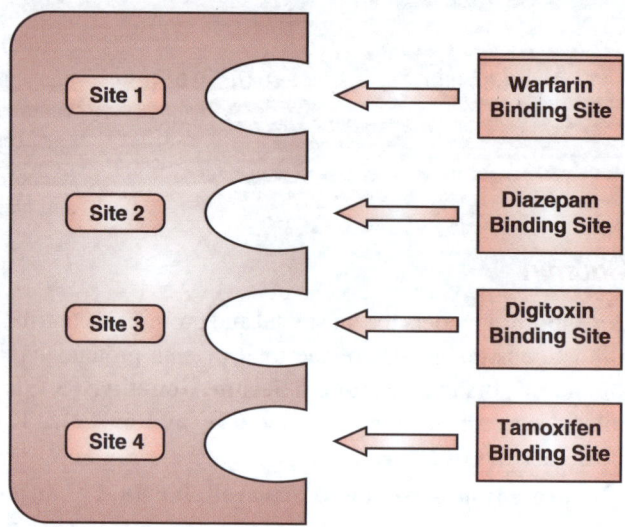

Fig. 3.2: Diagrammatic Representation of Four Major Drug Binding Sites on Human Serum Albumin (HSA).

Site 2: Diazepam Binding Site- it refers to such drug substances that particularly bind to this region and essentially comprise: **benzodiazepines, cloxacillin, ibuprofen, ketoprofen, medium chain fatty acids (MCFAs), probencid** and **tryptophan.**

> **NOTE**   It is worthwhile to state here that 'Site 1' and 'Site 2' are solely responsible for enabling the maximum quantum of drug-binding sites.

Site 3: Digitoxin Binding Site-Rarely a few drugs get bound to this site.

Site 4: Tamoxifen Binding Site-it also serves as a **'remote site for drug binding'**.

Salient Features for Binding Sites: There are quite a few salient features with particular reference to the available binding sites, namely:

1. A specific **'Drug'** may easily get bound to more than one site. In such a situation, one may call the main-binding site as the **'*primary site*'** while the less prominent binding site as the **'*secondary site*'**.

Example

Dicoumarol (a *natural anti-coagulant*) has the following *two* **distinct sites, namely**:
- **Site 1-refers to the 'primary site'** and
- **Site 2-designates the 'secondary site'**.

2. Certain groups of drugs that usually bind to the same are found to compete with each other for binding progressively.

Example

Sulphonamides for Site 1.

3. Some drugs which critically get bound to one site are found not to inhibit competitively the binding of drugs to other sites at all.

Example

Cloxacillin and **Ketoprofen** that usually bind to **Site 2** exclusively.

3.2.1.2. α_1-Acid Glycoprotein (or α_1-AGP or AAG)

It is also termed as the **Orosomucoid** which represents a **low molecular weight (~40,000 Da) protein** and is a 'Globulin'. Usually, the **average plasma concentration of α_1-acid glycoprotein per 100 mL ranges between 40 and 100 mg.**

Important Features: $\alpha1$-AGP (or AAG) has *two* important features, namely:

- **Its concentration in the plasma gets elevated in certain typical disease conditions,** *viz.*
  - ➤ **inflammation,**
  - ➤ **excessive physical/mental stress,** and
  - ➤ **several malignant disease states.**

Besides, one may critically observe a **marked decrease in plasma concentration of** *AAG in such disease condition as:*

  - ➤ **nephritic syndrome, and**
  - ➤ **hepatic disease.**

It primarily gets bound to a good number of basic drug entities, *e.g.,* **imipramine, lidocaine, propranolol** and **quinidine,**

In a broader perspective, one may obviously visualize the most vital aspects pertaining to protein binding duly found to be quite variable among the patients having altogether variant therapeutic status. Amazingly, several diseases may change perceptively the **Drug-Protein Bindings** by reducing significantly the quantum of proteins available readily for **Binding Phenomena**, as shown in Table 3.2.

Extent of Drug-Protein Binding: The actual extent of **drug-protein binding** *is expressed invariably as the ratio of bound drug to total drug concentration.*

The observed ratio usually ranges between **0 and 1**. The drugs having a ratio of more than 0.9 are regarded to be falling under the category of **'highly protein-bound drugs'**.

Importantly, the ability of **drug-protein binding** shall depend solely upon the molar concentrations of drug and protein specifically.

Consider a particular protein possessing a **Single-Binding Site,** we may have the following expression:

$$\boxed{\textbf{Drug + Protein} \xrightleftharpoons{K_1} \textbf{Drug – Protein Complex}} \qquad \textbf{(a)}$$

S. No.	Plasma Protein	Reduced Plasma Protein	Enhanced Plasma Protein
		Table 3.2. Plasma Protein Changing Conditionalities	
1	Albumin	Severe burns, chronic liver ailment chronic renal failure, pregnancy and trauma (sudden shock)	Hypothyroidism
2	α_1-Acid Glyco-protein (or α_1-AGP or AAG)	Nephrotic syndrome (*i.e.*, related to impaired kidney function)	Renal failure, celiac disease, Crohn's disease, myocardinal infarction, rheumatoid arthritis and trauma

where, K_1 = **Association constant** (*i.e.*, the ensuing affinity of the protein for a drug).

At this point in time, one may logically arrive at the following *two* **distinct analogies,** such as:

- **'high affinity' indicates that the prevailing equilibrium lies specifically to the far right,** and
- **higher the ensuing protein concentration for a given drug concentration, higher would be the ultimate bound drug concentration or** *vice-versa.*

Thus, **Equation (a)** may be expressed as

$$C_u + P \rightleftharpoons C_b d \qquad \text{(b)}$$

where,

C_u = Concentration of unbound drug,

P = Unoccupied protein and

$C_b d$ = Concentration of bound drug.

Now, based upon the '**Law of Mass Action**', **Equation (b)** may be expressed as stated below:

$$K_a = \frac{C_b d}{C_u \times P} \qquad \text{(c)}$$

Therefore, one may further extend the present on-going discussion a step forward by intelligently classifying the '**Drugs**' as acidic or basic, as given in Table 3.3.

Acidic Drugs-These invariably get bound to **plasma albumin**; and, therefore, the simultaneous administration of these drugs may clearly displace one another duly from their respective binding sites.

Basic Drugs-These usually get bound to either α_1-**acid glycoprotein or albumin.**

3.2.1.3. *Lipoproteins*

Lipoproteins represent the so-called **Macromolecular Complexes of Lipids and Proteins.** In general, they are duly classified based on their actual density. **Lipoproteins** are largely responsible for the transport of plasma lipids *in vivo*. In a situation when the **Binding Sites** on albumin get almost saturated, the **lipoproteins** may take eventually an active participation in the ensuing **drug-binding interactions**.

In a broader perspective, the critical binding of drugs to either **Human Serum Albumin (HSA)** or α_1-**Acid Glycoprotein (α_1-AGP)** involve **hydrophobic bonds**. As we know that the **lipophilic drugs** exclusively show their inherent ability to undergo specific **hydrophobic bonding,** the '**Lipoproteins'** may also get bound to such drug substances by virtue of their high-lipid content predominantly.

Table 3.3. Selective Representation of Acidic and Basic Drugs Exhibiting Greater than 90% Binding Potential to Plasma Proteins

S. No.	Range of Acidic Drugs	Range of Basic Drugs
1	Aspirin (Acetylsalicylic Acid)	Alfentanil
2	Cloxacillin	Amitriptyline
3	Naproxen	Desipramine
4	Penicillin	Diazepam
5	Phenylbutazone	Lidocaine
6	Phenytoin	Lorazepam
7	Probenecid	Nifedipine
8	Sulfinpyrazone	Propranolol
9	Tolbutamide	Quinidine
10	Warfarin	Verapamil

NOTE It is necessary to make it absolutely clear that the 'plasma concentration of lipoproteins' remains at a much lower level *vis-a-vis* HSA and α_1-AGP.

Modus Operandi: **Lipoproteins*** usually help a '**Drug**' to get bound by causing dissolution specifically in the **lipid-core of the protein**, which evidently suggests that their actual underlying capacity to bind solely depends upon its inherent lipid content.

Classification: Based upon the '**density of lipoproteins**', they are classified into four major categories, namely:

- **Chylomicrons,**
- **Very low density lipoproteins (VLDL),**
- **Low density lipoproteins (LDL)** and
- **High density lipoproteins (HDL).**

Important Points: These essentially comprise the following:

1. **Lipid core** of such macromolecules contains **cholesteryl esters** and **triglycerides.**
2. External layer of these macromolecules consists of **apoproteins (proteins and free cholesterol).**
3. VLDL serves as a rich source of **triglycerides**.
4. HDL represents a rich source of **apoproteins.**
5. **Essential binding of drugs to lipoproteins** is established to be non-competitive in nature.

---

* The molecular weight of **Lipoproteins** range between 2 and 34 lakhs depending on their actual chemical composition

** Found to be predominant in humans.

Examples

Following are certain typical examples of drug variants bound to lipoproteins:

- **Acidic Drugs**   : **Diclofenac**
- **Basic Drugs**   : **Chlorpromazine**
- **Neutral Drugs** : **Cyclosporin A.**

However, in the particular instance of the **Basic Lipophilic Drugs**, one may observe the following *two* **cardinal facts:**

- **They do exhibit comparatively much more affinity**, and
- **Lipoproteins binding process appears to be rather more appreciable in such instances of drug substances which get bound to them specifically when levels of HSA and in-α_1-AGP plasma are reduced significantly.**

3.2.1.4. *Globulins (α-, β-, γ-Globulins)*

Globulins refers to-'**a type of protein which is essentially round in structure, soluble in dilute salt solutions, insoluble in pure water and coagulable by heat'.**

Globulins are solely responsible for the transport of most **endogenous materials***; however, they do play a limited role of activity with regard to binding of a drug.

Examples

There are *two* **typical examples** of *drug-globulin binding* as given below:

1. **Corticosteroids Binding Globulin (CBG)**** is found to be highly specific to certain **Steroids,** *viz.* **Prednisolone.**
2. **Transcortin,** an *α-globulin* that binds and transports the biologically active, unconjugated cortisol in plasma. It also gets bound to **Vitamin B_{12} (Cyanocobalamine)** and **Thyroxine.**

α_1-**Globulins** designates the **Serum Globulins** having the *most rapid electrophoretic mobility*, which may be further subdivided into:

- α_1-**globulins- with faster mobility** and
- α_2-**globulins-with slower mobility.**

α-**Globulins** represent the **Globulins** present in plasma which, in neutral or alkaline solutions, do exhibit an electrophoretic mobility lying between those of the **α-and γ-Globulins**.

γ-**Globulins** are the **Serum Globulins** possessing the **least rapid electrophoretic mobility** and the fraction is composed almost entirely of **Immunoglobulins (IGs)**. They have negligible role in **drug-binding activity.**

3.2.1.5. *Erythrocytes [or Red Blood Cells (RBCs)]*

Erythrocytes (or **RBCs**) contain iron to transport oxygen throughout the entire body, which are duly manufactured in the bone marrow and removed critically by the **spleen** after nearly 5 days interval.

---

*   **Endogenous Materials**: such materials that arise either from within or biosynthesized by the body,

** **Corticosteroids**: Any of the steroids elaborated by the adrenal cortex or any synthetic equivalents, and **used clinically for hormonal replacement therapy.**

RBCs do get bound to both *endogenous* and *exogenous* compounds *in vivo*. Erythrocytes usually comprise nearly **45% of the total volume of the blood in a human body**.

It is worthwhile to mention at this point in time that the actual **'Drug Uptake'** by *Erythrocytes* is a crucial function of **Plasma-Protein Binding**. Nevertheless, one may evidently observe a distinct **'Linear Correlation'** between such *two* **entities**, namely:

- **erythrocyte/plasma concentration ratio**, and
- **free drug concentration of certain 'Drugs' in plasma**, *viz.* **Haloperidol, Pphenytoin, Propranolol and Quinidine.**

Salient Features: These essentially consist of the following *three* **cardinal aspects**, such as:

1. Absorption and penetration of drug into the **RBC** is dependent totally upon the free concentration of the ensuing drug in the plasma.

Examples

Evidently, an increased level of a **'free drug concentration present in the plasma'** causes a linear increment in the respective levels of **Acetazolamide and Phenytoin in the RBCs**.

2. Importantly, only the measurable quantum of the drug could be present in **RBCs for a longer duration***.

3. **RBC** essentially has a diameter almost 500 times *vis-a-vis* **Albumin**, *i.e.*, the **major plasma-protein binding constituent**.

In general, **RBC** specifically consists of *three* **major constituents** that eventually may get bound to drug substances, namely:

- **Haemoglobin**,
- **Carbonic anhydrase**, and
- **Cell membrane**,

which shall now be discussed briefly in the following sections:

1. **Haemoglobin:** Haemoglobin is referred to as the *oxygen-carrying pigment of RBCs*.

It has *four* **different identified variants**, namely:

- **Haemoglobin A_1:** It represents the **normal adult haemoglobin in a healthy normal human subject****

Haemoglobin A_1: essentially comprises α_2, β_2 (*i.e.*, *two* α-globin*** duly combined with two β-globins).

- **Haemoglobin A_1:** It designates the **glycosylated haemoglobin** usually employed to *determine blood glucose levels in diabetic patients*.

- **Haemoglobin A_2:** It refers to the **normal adult haemoglobin, which essentially comprises 5% of the haemoglobin in the normal human subject. Haemoglobin A_2 is composed of α_2, β_2** (*i.e.*, *two* α-globins duly combined with *two* δ-(delta) globins.

---

* It could only be possible in such a situation provided the bondage of the drug to the **RBCs** represents an 'irreversible phenomena'.

** Up to 95% of the **haemoglobin.**

*** **Globin:** it refers to the **protein portion of haemoglobin.**

- **Haemoglobin F (Foetal Haemoglobin)**: The predominant **Haemoglobin** of the foetus that normally disappears before birth. It also occurs in:
  - ➤ **certain anaemias**, and
  - ➤ **may even persist after birth of an infant**.

It is invariably composed of α_2, γ_2 (*i.e., two*-a-globins duly combined with two γ-globin).

2. **Carbonic Anhydrase (CA)**: It designates the **specific metabolic enzyme** that predominantly **catalyzes the combining of carbon dioxide (CO_2) and water (H_2O) to give rise to the formation of carbonic acid (H_2CO_3)*: in various body processes.**

Examples

Following are some typical examples of drugs which are known to get bound to the **Carbonic Anhydrases**: *viz.,*

- **Acetazolamide [Diamox®]**,
- **Methazolamide [Neptazane®]**,
- **Ethoxzolamide [Cardrase®]**,
- **Diclofenamide [Daranide®]**, and
- **Disulphamide [Diluen®]**.

Modus Operandi: The modus operandi of a few of these drugs are as follows:

Acetazolamide-It goes absorbed appreciably from **GI tract**, bound largely to the plasma proteins, and fails to undergo **Biotransformation.**

Ethoxzolamide-It exerts its action by **lowering the intraocular pressure** before surgery when used preoperatively in **acute angle closure glaucoma**.

Disulphamide-Its action resembles that of **Chlorothiazide (CTZ)** for the relief of **fluid retention in the body.**

3. **Cell Membrane**: It refers **to-'the membrane pertaining to any of the protoplasmic masses making up organized tissue, consisting of a nucleus surrounded by Cytoplasm enclosed in a Cell or Plasma Membrane'.**

Example

Imipramine and Chlorpromazine (CPZ) are found to bind with the RBC membrane particularly.

 NOTE   **The rate and degree of entrance right inside RBC is distinctly more for the lipophilic drugs, *viz*. Phenytoin; whereas, the hydrophilic drugs, *viz*. Ampicillin, fails to enter the RBCs.**

3. Pharmacokinetic Models

The fundamental basis of **Pharmacokinetics Modelling**** is to define the human body as:

---

*   **Carbonic Acid (H_2CO_3)**: It is highly unstable and breaks up to five a mole each of CO_2 and H_2O in vivo

**   Harvey SC and Withrow CD: **Remington's Pharmaceutical Sciuencies**, 17th ed., Easton, PY:Mack Publishing Co., 1979; Notari RE: **Biopharmaceutics and Pharmacokinetics**, 4th ed., Marcel Dekker Inc., New York 1987; O'Reilly NJ: *Can. J. Pharm. Sci.,* **7**: 66-72, 1972

- **a compartment**, or
- **a battery of compartments.**

Which are usually found to be interconnected by various rate processes regarded to be of **First-Order Kinetics**. In true sense, such a **Method of Rationalization and Generalization** of *generated data* helps to allow the reasonable perfect predictions on which to **Test New Data.** Therefore, this **Technique of Compartmental Analysis** represents the method most widely applied to the **Pharmacokinetics Data.** Though it is rather difficult to define a **'Compartment'** in precise *Anatomical Terms*; nevertheless, it may be defined largely upon its **Pharmacokinetic Parameters** exclusively.

In other words, the elaborated study of handling of drugs by a human body invariably designates a rather difficult task due to the **various intricate complexities of human anatomy and physiology**, respectively. In such a situation, the ensuing **'Pharmacokinetics Models'** do serve as a useful source of information in carrying out an elaborated study pertaining to the prevailing *'time-course throughout the entire human body'.*

Besides, in the **Pharmacokinetic Models,** one may assume the body to be composed of a number of compartments. It is indeed worthwhile to make it clear that these said **Compartments** do not represent either **Anatomic or Physiologic Compartments**, but are the *imaginary or virtual compartments*.

Central Compartment: In actual practice, the **'Central Compartment'** duly designates both *plasma* and *tissues*, which readily get equilibrated with drug substances. However, it is pertinent to observe *precise size* and *number of compartments* are usually determined by the following *two* aspects, namely:

- **Perfusion of the tissues and organs**, and
- **Physiochemical characteristic features of the drug.**

> **NOTE**   In Pharmacokinetics, a compartment usually refers to tissues or organs for which the rates of critical uptake and clearance of a drug remains almost identical.

Importance of Pharmacokinetic Models: Following are the *ten* **most important aspects of the Pharmacokinetic Models,** such as:

1. They specifically help in the **typical characterization of the behavioural pattern of drugs in human subjects.**
2. They precisely **predict the concentration of drug in various body fluids at any dose levels.**
3. They also aid largely in the exact prediction of the multiple-dose concentration curves derived from the so-called **single-dose experiments.**
4. **Pharmacokinetic models** help in the calculation of optimum dosage regimens.
5. Exact evaluation with regard to the **'risk of toxicity'** associated with some typical dosage regimens.
6. Establishing a candid correlation between the **plasma-drug concentration** and **pharmacological response.**
7. They do aid in evaluating the relationship prevailing between:
   - **Bioequivalence** and
   - **Bioinequivalence**

in various available '**formulation of the same drug substance**'.

8. They determine precisely the most portable accumulation in a human body of :
   - **Drug substances,** and/or
   - **Metabolite(s).**
9. **Pharmacokinetic Models** do exert a vivid influence upon the
   - **Disease condition,** and
   - **Altered physiology,**

   in a typical *drug* **Administration-Distribution-Metabolism-Excretion (ADME)** profile.
10. They also throw enough light in the different *drug-drug interactions in vivo* (**which cautions a physician enormously**).

3.3.1. *Pharmacokinetic Models vis-a-vis Mathematical Models*

In actual practice, several **Mathematical Models** may be developed intelligently so as to study and evaluate the **on-going rate phenomena of drug with regard to its ADME**. Generally, these **Mathematical Models** are found to be quite reliable, dependable and useful while establishing '*specific equations*' in order to elaborate the ensuing drug concentrations in vivo as a determinant function of time. Obviously, since the '**drug concentration**' are solely time dependent, therefore, the **resulting** *two* **variables**, namely:

- **drug concentration,** and
- **time,**

are invariably termed as '**dependent**' and '**independent variables**', respectively.

Data: **Data** usually refer to-'**the collective estimated experimental values duly obtained from a set of dependent and independent variables'.**

Nevertheless, these '**Data**' derived from a **Pharmacokinetics Model** goes a long way in accomplishing:

- **determination,** and
- **testing for validity**

of the *generated* **Pharmacokinetic Parameters**.

Preferred Model for Analysis of Data

The most preferred selected **Model for Analysis of the Data** is solely based upon *two* **aspects**, namely:

- **a hypothesis,** and
- **an array of assumptions,**

which eventually describe the **critical biological events in a proper mathematical form**.

It is, however, pertinent to state that adequate care and attention need to be taken while having confidence in the chosen **Pharmacokinetic Model** to predict drug action precisely.

Modus Operandi: The various steps essentially include the following:

1. **Data** are required to be analyzed using the **Simplest Pharmacokinetic Model.**

2. **Proper application of the statistical methods** to know exactly *how best the proposed Pharmacokinetic Model fits into the Data**.

 NOTE It may, however, be observed that the obtained 'Pharmacokinetic Data' should never be exchanged with the 'clinical observations' in the concerned subject.

3.3.2. *Classification of Pharmacokinetic Models*

The **Pharmacokinetic Models** have been judiciously classified into the following *four* **categories**, namely:

- **Compartment Models,**
- **Flow Models (or Physiologic-pharmacokinetic Models),**
- **Non-compartmental Pharmacokinetics,** and
- **Non-linear Pharmacokinetics.**

The aforesaid *four* **categories of the Pharmacokinetic Models** shall now be discussed individually in the following sections.

3.3.2.1. *Compartment Models*

The major cardinal problem usually encountered in approaching and establishing:

- **more precise dosage regimen**, and
- **more logical interpretation of biological response for a particular dose**,

is exclusively dependent on the extent of precise inaccessibility **of Drug Concentration at the Active Site**.

Therefore, in an attempt to circumvent a rational solution to such a glaring problem, one may make use of the **Novel Method of Compartmental Analysis** effectively. In usual practice, the following line of action is adopted largely:

- **'Data' duly obtained from blood concentration *vs.* time is fitted into a simple mathematical model where the perfect suitability of the model is measured by the application of statistical methods appropriately,** and
- **In an event when the accrued 'Data' fails to fit rightly into the *Simple Model* one may make use of a more *Complex Model* and tested subsequently till such time one comes across the so-called *Best Model* which explains explicitly the perfect relationship between:**

Drug Concentration (in Blood) *vs.* Time Factor.

 NOTE The 'Pharmacokinetic Analysis of Data' pertaining to a human body (*i.e.*, a living system) may, therefore, be assumed to comprise an array of interconnected compartments.

---

* In case the proposed **Pharmacokinetic Model** to fit accurately and squarely all the experimental observations, one may propose and test an altogether new and more **complex model** (*i.e.*, **hypothesis**).

Compartment: It designates a *separate division* or *section of the body**** wherein the circulating blood serves as one compartment and all other body tissues are regarded as the' **Central Compartment**.

In other words, a **Compartment** usually refers to –'**a group of tissues that more or less acts in a uniform fashion with regard to the movement of drug *in vivo*'**. Thus, one may come across several instances where upon each tissue may exhibit critically a **different concentration of drug substance**. However, they could be seen in an **Equilibrium State** in such a manner that the **observed change in the drug concentration in these tissues may be either linear or similar in nature**.

In a broader perspective, the human body is duly **Compartmentalized** based upon the following *two* **important properties**, namely:

- **Vascularity**** and
- **Distribution profile of a 'Drug Substance'**.

These essentially refer to the following different aspects:

1. **Blood-Serum-Plasma**- predominantly comprise
   - **Lean-tissue group** that are usually perfused extensively and consisting of such components as lungs, kidneys, glands, heart and hepatoportal system, and
   - **Specific tissues protected by specialized tissue membranes** that include spinal cord and brain.
2. **Scarcely Perfused Lean-tissue Group**- consists of skin and muscle.
3. **Fat Group**-largely comprises the adipose tissues and bone marrow.
4. **Rarely Perfused Tissue Group**-mostly consisting of bones, teeth, cartilage, tendons, ligaments and hair.

Number and Shape of Compartments: These may be established by means of such well-defined steps as

- **Number of Compartments**: They may be determined by
  - ➤ carrying out the **'Graphical Analysis'** of the *plasma concentration time data following an IV injection,* and
  - ➤ performing the **'Statistical Analysis'** of *plasma concentration time data.*
- **Shape of Compartment**: The **log concentration *vs.* time graph** depicts lines with various shapes of different compartments.

NOTE	**Several' Computer Programmes' are adequately available to tackle such problems quite swiftly and efficiently.**

On the basis of the critical characteristic feature whether the **'Compartments'** are found to be arranged

- **in parallel,** or
- **in a series,**

---

* As may be seen in a '*pharmacokinetic two-compartmental model*'

** **Vascularity** Indicative of copious blood supply

the **Resulting Compartment Models** are subdivided further into *two* **distinct categories**, namely:

- **Mammillary Model**, and
- **Caternary Model**.

which is described briefly in the following sections.

Mammillary Model: The 'Mammillary Model' is regarded to be one of the most commonly encountered compartment models ever used in **Pharmacokinetics**.

In fact, the model comprises either *one or more* **Peripheral Compartments connected critically to a Central Compartment** more or less very much akin to the joining of 'Satellites to a Planet'. Indeed, the central compartment essentially contains not only the plasma, but also the largely perfused tissues wherein the 'Drug Substance' gets distributed rapidly. The drug first gaining entry to a **Compartment approaches the Central Compartment** and from there gets distributed to all other **Adjoining Compartments** that are eventually connected to it. Ultimately, the 'Elimination of the Drug' commences from the **Central Compartment** itself because the major organs, *viz.* kidney and liver, duly engaged in **Drug Elimination Process** are located strategically in the **Central Compartment** perceptively.

Table: 3.4. records various Compantment Model Variants

Table 3.4. Depicts Different Compartment Model Variants	
• **Central compartment (or plasma compartments)**	Also known as '**Compartment 1**' that predominantly comprises plasma and highly perfused tissues, *e.g.*, lungs, liver, kidneys, that readily get equilibrated with the drug.
• **Peripheral compartments (or tissue compartments)**	Also referred to as '**Compartments 2, 3 and 4**', and essentially possess low vascularity and, therefore, apparent poor perfusion.

Conventionally, the ensuing **Pharmacokinetic Rate Constant** is designated by 'K'; whereas, the numerical number actually represents the prevailing **Direction of the Movement of Drug** between the aforesaid compartments.

Examples

K_{14} (*K*-one-four) designates in reality the **Pharmacokinetic Rate Constant (K)** with regard to the critical movement of the drug right from '**Compartment 1**' to '**Compartment 4**'; and hence, the **Reverse Phenomenon as K_{41} (*K*-four-one).**

Obviously, in Table 3.4, the observed movement of drug in between the compartments is duly governed by the '**First-Order Rate Constants**' (*K*), and the '**Subscript**' shows explicitly the actual direction pertaining to the drug movement taking place in various **Mammillary Compartment Models from Model 1 through Model 6,** as given in Figure 3.3.

Explanation

The various **Models from 1 through 6** may be explained as stated under:

1. **Model 1** depicts a **one-compartment open model after an IV administration of a 'drug substance'.**

2. **Model 2** shows a one-compartment open model after **an extravascular administration of a 'drug'** i.e., *either routed via rectal or oral following a First-Order Absorption pattern.*

3. **Model 3** illustrates a *Two*-**Compartmental Open Model** having the Pharmacokinetic **Rate Constant (K)** with directions of the drug movement from **Compartment 1 to Compartment 2** and *vice versa.* Furthermore, the drug moves from **Compartment 1 to Compartment 3.** Importantly, all the aforesaid movement of drugs comes into play only after the **administration of IV.**

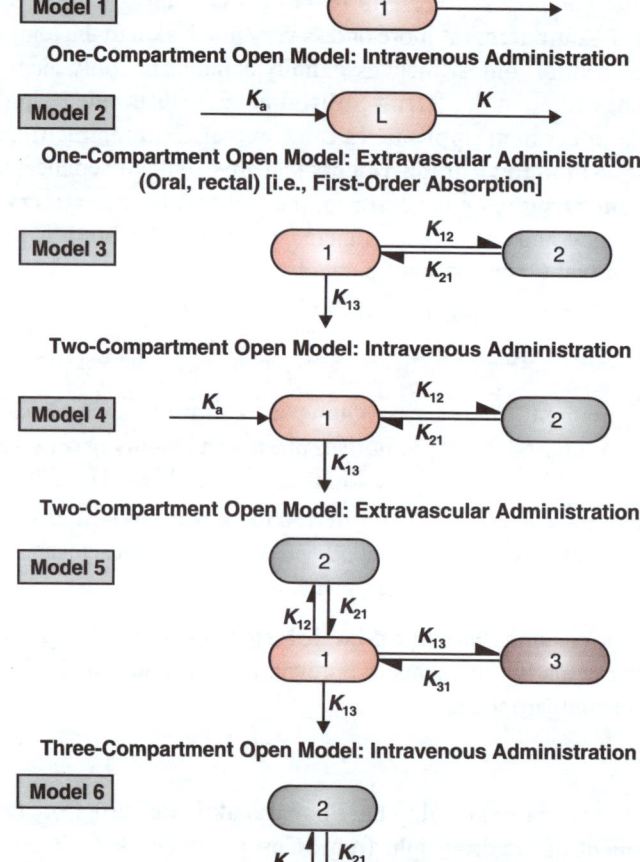

Fig. 3.3: Various Mammillary Compartment Models. (The Pharmacokinetic Rate Constant basically designates as 'K_a', i.e., the First-Order Absorption Rate Constant and the First-Order Elimination Rate Constant as 'K_e'.)

4. **Model 4** represents explicitly a *Two*-**Compartment Open Model** after the **extravascular administration of a drug.** In this specific instance, the **Pharmacokinetic Parameters**

essentially comprise the **Volume of Compartments 1 and 2**; whereas, the **Rate Constants**, *viz.* K_a, K_{13}, K_{12} and K_{21}, **in all constitutes six parameters.**

5. **Model 5** designates a *Three*-**Compartment Open Model** after an **IV administration of a drug.** in this particular instance, the respective **Pharmacokinetic Parameters** predominantly consist of the **Volume of Compartments 1, 2 and 3**; whereas, the **Rate Constants**, *viz.* K_{12}, K_{21}, K_{13}, K_{31} and K_{13}, in all gives rise to *eight* **parameters** perceptively.

6. **Model 6** shows vividly a *Three*-**Compartment Open Model** after an **extravascular administration of a drug substance.** Here, the various **Pharmacokinetic Parameters** that are intimately involved comprise the **Volume of Compartments 1, 2 and 3**; whereas, the **Rate Constants**, *viz.* K_a, K_{12}, K_{21}, K_{13}, K_{31} and K_{13}, **in totality constitutes nine parameters.**

In usual practice, the exact number of rate constants that may eventually appear in a **Specific Compartment Model** is designated by 'R'; and, therefore, we may have:

for IV administration: $R = 2n-1$, and

for EV administration: $R = 2n$

where, n = **Number of compartments.**

In general, looking closely at these different models, it is rather important to ascertain whether one may have an exact and precise access to the '**Drug Concentration Data**' obtained directly from each compartment separately. In Figure 3.3, the **Data Models 3 and 4** pertaining to **Compartment 2** may not be obtained so easily by virtue of the fact that the respective tissues do not usually:

- **get sampled frequently,** and
- **comprise a homogeneous concentration of 'drug'.**

Let us assume a typical situation whereby the exact quantum of drug substance being duly absorbed and eliminated per unit time is accomplished adequately by sampling **Compartment 1**, one may estimate suitably using various **Mathematical Models** the exact amount of the '**Drug**' present in the **tissue compartments (or peripheral compartments).**

 NOTE   **With the help of suitable 'Mathematical Equations' elaborating these typical models, it is a lot easier to determine and arrive at the different pharmacokinetic parameters being employed.**

Multi-Compartment Properties

It has been duly observed that by either:

- **IV Administration,** or
- **Bolus:* Administration.**

quite a few drug substances do acquire enough distribution *in vivo* rather slowly in order that a '**significant portion of the intended dose**' gets eliminated adequately before accomplishing the so-called **"Distribution Equilibrium" ****

---

*   **Bolus:** It refers to the rounded mass of a pharmaceutical preparation ready to swallow or such a mass passing through the GI tract

**   '**Distribution Equilibrium**': The equilibrium achieved due to the partitioning of drug to the various locations or compartments in the body or another heteroge system.

Thus, we may have *two* **different types of plots a Drug having Multi-Compartment Properties**, such as:

- semi-logarithmic plot of plasma-drug concentration *vs.* time after IV administration of drug, and
- semi-logarithmic plot of plasma-drug concentration *vs.* time after extravscular administration of drug.

The aforesaid *two* **aspects** shall now be treated separately along with their respective **plots** and appropriate explanations in the following sections:

Semi-logarithmic Plot of Plasma-Drug Concentration *vs.* Time After IV Administration of Drug: It is, however, pertinent to state here that in a specific instance when the drug is administered *via* **IV**, usually more than one exponential term may be needed critically to differentiate and characterize the perceptive changes in the ensuing **Plasma-Drug Concentration** with respect to time. In fact, the number of the prevailing **Exponential Terms** does signify the actual number of compartments involved. Therefore, for a *Two*-**Compartment Model** one may have both:

- **Central Compartments**, and
- **Peripheral Compartment**,

as illustrated explicitly in Figure 3.4.

COMPARTMENT IN SERIES

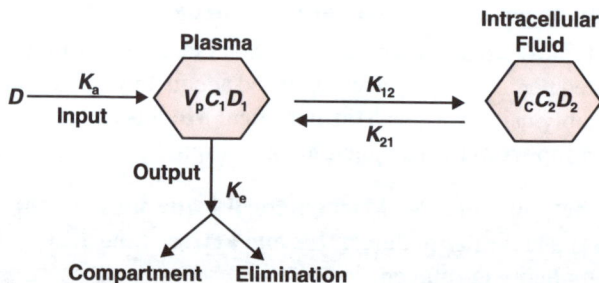

where,

K_a = Pharmacokinetic rate constant at input,

K_e = Pharmacokinetic rate constant at output,

V_p = Volume of 'Plasma'

V_c = Volume of 'intracellular fluid',

C_1 = Concentration in Compartment 1,

C_2 = Concentration in Compartment 2,

D = Drug used,

D_1 = Quantum of drug in Compartment 1,

D_2 = Quantum of drug in Compartment 2.

COMPARTMENT IN PARALLEL

Drugs adopting *Two*-**Compartmental Model:** There are a good number of drugs that predominantly adopt the *Two*-**Compartment Model.** Amazingly, **Vancomycin*** a **glycopeptides antibiotic**, represents a classical example, which follows specifically a *two*-**Compartment Model,** having a distribution phase extending for 1-2 hr.

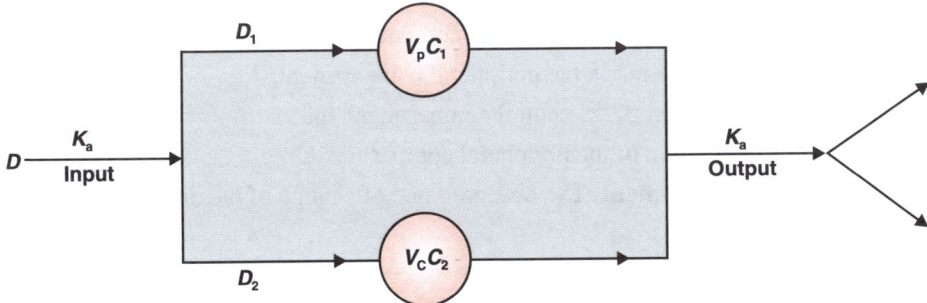

Fig. 3.4 Diagrammatic Illustrations of an Open Two-Compartment Pharmacokinetic Model.

Nevertheless, the observed distribution of drug taking place between the **central and peripheral compartments** invariably is guided by the **First-Order Kinetics.** Therefore, K_{12} and K_{21} (as seen in Figure 3.4) do represent the **First-Order Rate Constants.**

For Central Compartment- The observed change in the **drug concentration** may be expressed as:

$$\frac{dC_c}{dt} = K_{21} \cdot C_p - K_{12} \cdot C_c - K_e \cdot C_c \qquad \text{(d)}$$

where,

dC_c/dt = change in drug concentration in central compartment,

C_c = drug concentration in central compartment and

C_p = Drug concentration in peripheral compartment.

Remembering that:

$$X = V_d \cdot C$$

where,

X = Amount of drug in the body at time 't' after IV injection,

V_d = Volume of distribution** and

C = Amount of Drug in the body.

---

* **Vancomycin:** It is obtained from **Amycolatopsis orientalis** originally from the culture of an **Indonesian soil sample** and later on from **Indian soil.** In 1958, it was duly introduced as an antibiotic against certain *Gram +ve cocci, viz.* **streptococci, staphylococci,** and **pneumococci.**

** **Volume of Distribution:** It is referred to as an apparent biopharmaceutical terms expressing the perceived **Volume** (V_d) of the body in which a specific amount of the **unchanged drug** (A_b) is duly distributed based upon the ensuing **concentration** (C_b) of the drug in the blood. Thus, $V_d = A_b C_b$, a characteristic value for a specific drug, *i.e.*, an 'abstract volume' which is calculated from the ratio of the amount of drug in the body to its concentration in plasma once partitioning has been stabilized adequately (**at steady-state conditions**).

Therefore, one may now express **Equation (d)** as follows

$$\frac{dC_c}{dt} = \frac{K_{21} \cdot X_p}{V_p} - \frac{K_{12} \cdot X_c}{V_c} - \frac{K_E \cdot X_c}{V_c}$$ (e)

where

X_c = Amount of 'drug' present in the central compartment,

X_p = Amount of 'drug' present in the peripheral compartment,

V_c = Volume of distribution of the central compartment and

V_p = Volume of distribution of the peripheral compartment.

For Peripheral Compartment- The observed rate of change of the drug concentration may be duly expressed as follows:

$$\frac{dC_P}{dt} = K_{12} \cdot C_C - K_{21} \cdot C_P$$ (f)

However, **Equation (f)** can also be written in terms of the actual amount of drug present:

$$\frac{dC_P}{dt} = \frac{K_{12} \cdot X_C}{V_C} - \frac{K_{21} \cdot X_P}{V_P}$$ (g)

Several other equally important drugs that critically follow either a *two* or **even more Compartment Model** are as stated below:

- **Amphetamine,**
- **Chlordiazeperoxide,**
- **Digoxin,**
- **Epinephrine,**
- **Gentamycin,**
- **Lidocaine,**
- **Methicilline,**
- **Oxacillin,**
- **Sulphisoxazole,**
- **Theophylline**, and
- **Warfarin**.

Importantly, for an **IV Injection of a Drug** showing glaring *two*-**Compartmental Models**, one would invariably come across *two* **distinct phases of definite alteration in the 'Plasma-Drug Concentration'**; with regard to 'Time'. Thus, we may have in the respective:

Central Compartment: *Firstly*, a marked reduction in the drug concentration shall be rather fast and rapid (*i.e.*, **distribution phase**); and *secondly*, it would be sluggish (*i.e.*, **elimination phase or post-distributive phase**).

Peripheral Compartment: *Firstly,* there would be a sharp increase in the drug concentration which will be followed by a peak (*i.e.,* **distribution phase**); and *secondly,* it will distinctly exhibit an apparent decline in the ensuing **drug concentration** (*i.e.,* **elimination phase or post-distribution phase**).

Obviously, the distribution of a drug substance usually taking place between the **Central Compartment** and the **Peripheral Compartment** is being governed by the **First-Order Kinetics**. Figure 3.5 depicts the plot between the **log plasma drug concentration of a drug substance** *versus* **the time profile after the IV administration which clearly exhibits a *Two*-Compartment Model. Hence, it will give rise to *two* phases of change occurring in the plasma drug concentration with regard to time profile.**

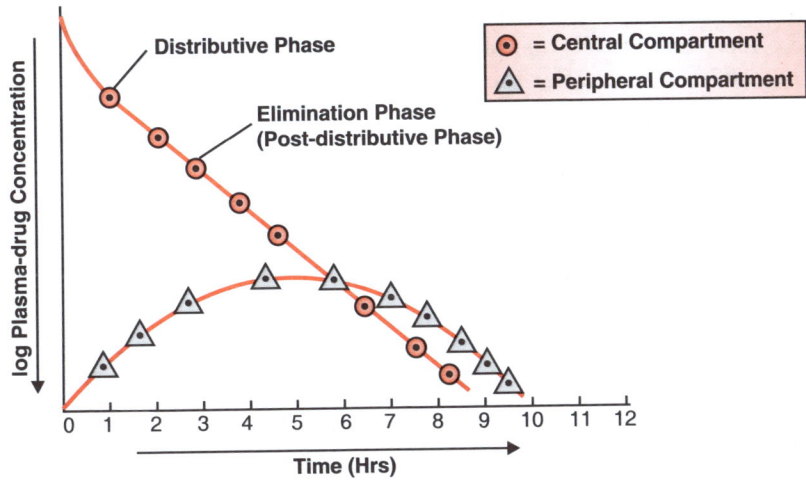

Fig. 3.5: Plasma Drug Concentration *vs.* Time Profile after the IV Administration of a Drug.

Therefore, one may virtually estimate the ensuing drug concentration present in **both Central and Peripheral Compartment** at any point in time by *integrating* Equation (*e*) and (*g*):

Thus, we may Have:

$$C_c = \frac{X_0}{V_c}\left[\left\{\frac{K_{21}-\alpha}{\beta-\alpha}\right\}\cdot e^{-\alpha\cdot t} + \left\{\frac{K_{21}-\beta}{\alpha-\beta}\right\}\cdot e^{-\beta\cdot t}\right] \qquad (h)$$

$$C_p = \frac{X_0}{V_p}\left[\left\{\frac{K_{12}}{\beta-\alpha}\right\}\cdot e^{-\alpha\cdot t} + \left\{\frac{K_{12}}{\alpha-\beta}\right\}\cdot e^{-\beta\cdot t}\right] \qquad (i)$$

where

C_c = Drug concentration in the central compartment,

C_p = Drug concentration in the peripheral compartment,

X_0 = Dose of the drug in IV administration,

α = First-order kinetic constant for rapid distributive phase and

β = First-order kinetic constant for slow distributive phase.

NOTE	It is worthwhile to state here that both a and b depend slowly upon K_{12}, K_{21}, and K_g.

It has been duly established that when a drug is administered via the **IV route**, it explicitly depicts a **plasma-drug concentration *vs.* time curve** of the drug that essentially follows a *Two-Compartment System*. Thus, it may be duly expressed by means of the '**Biexponential Equation**' as given below:

$$C = A \cdot e^{-\alpha \cdot t} + B \cdot e^{-\beta \cdot t}$$

(*j*)

where *A* and *B* represent the corresponding zero time intercepts.

It has been duly ascertained that **Equation (*j*)** may be eventually resolved into its respective components by adopting the **Method of Residuals***

Figure 3.6 represents vividly the plot between the **Two Components**, *viz.* **plasma-drug concentration profile *vs.* time after the IV administration of a drug.**

Example

It may be observed in Figure 3.6 that the initial decline duly caused by virtue of the '**distribution of drug**' appears to be much more rapid in comparison to the later phase *i.e.*, **elimination phase (or post-distributive phase).**

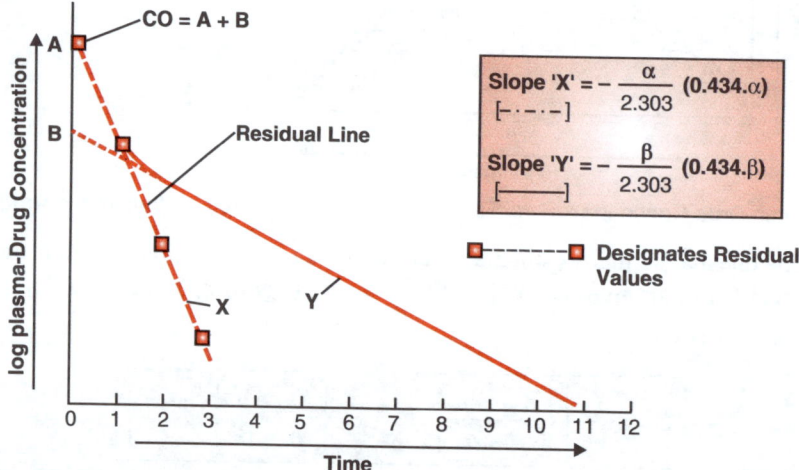

Fig. 3.6 Diagrammatic Representation of Plasma-Drug Concentration Profile *vs.* Time After IV Administration of a Drug.

In other words, α, *i.e.*, the **First-Order Kinetic Constant** for the *rapid distributive phase*, happens to be much **larger than** β *i.e.*, the **corresponding First-Order Constant** for the corresponding *slow elimination* phase. Therefore, one may critically take cognizance of the fact *A.* $e^{-\alpha t}$ (*i.e.*, **the zero time intercepts** of the **First-Order Constant for rapid Distribution Phase**) shall approach 'zero' rather more rapidly *vis-à-vis* **B.** $e^{-\beta t}$ (*i.e.*, the **zero time intercepts of the First-Order constant for slow elimination phase**). If this is the situation, **Equation (*j*)** may become

---

* '**Method of Residuals**': It refers to the determination of absorption and elimination rate constants having fairly comparable values.

$$C' = B \cdot e^{-\beta \cdot t} \qquad \text{(k)}$$

Thus, taking the *logarithm* we have

$$\log C' = \log B - \frac{\beta \cdot t}{2.303} \qquad \text{(l)}$$

Besides, the ensuing **Semi-Log Plot of Plasma-Drug Concentration** *vs.* time shall evidently give rise to a **linear terminal phase** having the *ultimate slope equivalent to* s–β. t 2. 303ˢ (or = **0.434β)**, that on being subjected to **extrapolation** to 'zero' produces an **intercept of log B.**
Hence, the **plasma half-life ($t_{1/2}$)** for **the elimination phase comes out to be**

$$t_{1/2} = \frac{0.693}{\beta} \qquad \text{(m)}$$

Furthermore, the subsequent *subtraction of the concentration time values* shall yield a series of **residual drug concentration time values (C_γ)** that may be given as:

$$C_\gamma = C - C' \qquad \text{(n)}$$

where
C = **Amount of 'drug' injected in the body,** and
C' = **Amount of plasma-drug concentration (after the distribution/elimination phases).**
Now, based upon the **Equation (*j*) and (*k*)** we have:

$$C_\gamma = A \cdot e^{-\alpha \cdot t} \qquad \text{(o)}$$

Again, taking the **Logarithm of Equation (o)** we have

$$\log C_\gamma = \log A - \frac{\alpha \cdot t}{2.303} \qquad \text{(p)}$$

Therefore, a **semi-log plot** of the **Residual-Drug Concentration ($C\gamma$)** *vs.* **Time** shall virtually give rise to a **'Straight Line'** having:

- $\boxed{\textbf{Slope} = -\dfrac{\alpha}{2.303} \textbf{ and}}$
- **a zero time intercept upon Y-axis of log A.**

At this point in time, it is absolutely necessary to point out that due to the **Method of Residuals in Equation (*j*)** all the parameters may be duly calculated with great case and fervor. Perhaps it would certainly help to determine the various parameters of **a *Two*-Compartment Model,** *viz.* K_{12}, K_{21}, V_d.

Semi-logarithmic Plot of Plasma-Drug Concentration *vs.* Time After Extravascular Administration of Drug: It has been duly observed that after the **extravascular administration of a 'Drug'** particularly in a *Two*-Compartment Model, one may come across *three* processes being involved simultaneously, such as: **absorption-distribution-elimination.** Importantly, the aforesaid **First-Order Absorption Phenomenon in an extravsacular administration** may be expressed as follows:

$$C = A \cdot e^{-\alpha \cdot t} + B \cdot e^{-\beta \cdot t} - C_p^{0-ka \cdot t}$$

(q)

where

A and B designates the corresponding zero time intercepts (as described earlier), C°_p is the Y-axis intercept of the absorption residual line, and theoretically equals A + B. Nevertheless, the above **multi-exponential components** may be suitably resolved by the help of the 'Method of Residuals' as already discussed earlier:

Figure 3.7 depicts the **Semi-Logarithmic Plot of the Plasma-Drug Concentration** *vs.* **Time after the extravascular administration of a Drug.**

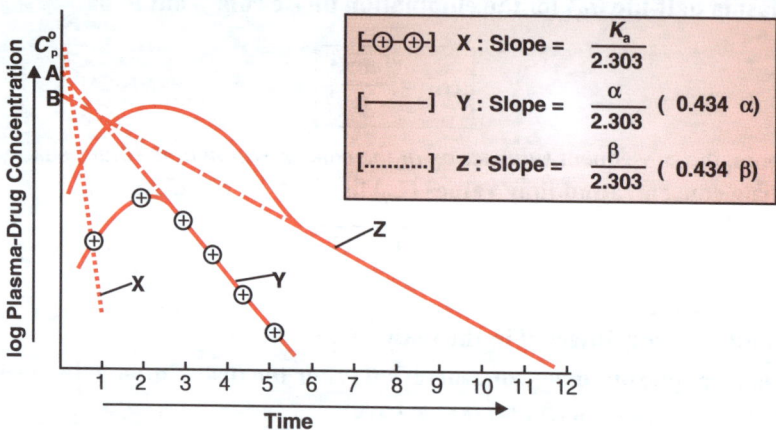

Fig. 3.7: Semi-logarithmic Plot of the Plasma-Drug Concentration *vs.* Time for a *Two*-Compartment Model: After Extravsacular Administration of a Drug.

Explanation

The various steps essentially comprise the following:

1. The pioneer step being the actual subtraction of the **'Line of Elimination'** (*see Figure 3.7 the 'solid line' with slope Z*) from the curve.

2. It will eventually result into the formation of a *two*-**Compartment Residual Plot.**

3. Importantly, the aforesaid *two*-**Compartment Residual Plot bears** essentially a critical **Post Absorptive Linear Segment** (see in Figure 3.7 the slope Y shown by ®–®)

4. In case, the residuals are subtracted carefully from this plot, one may obtain a plot having the **Slope X** as depicted by '…' *in Figure 3.7.*

5. The *two* observed intercepts , namely 'A' and 'B' remain the same as described earlier.

6. C°_p designates **the Y-axis intercept of the respective absorption residual line**; and, therefore, **equals to A + B theoretically.**

Caternary Model: In the **Caternary Model**, the various compartments are specifically joined to one another in a row very much similar to the compartments of a train, as shown in Figure 3.8.

It essentially has the following *three* important features, namely:

- Quite contrarily, the **Mammalian Model** comprises either one or more compartments around a **Central Compartment very much akin to satellites.**

- The **Caternary Model** can be noticeable neither anatomically or physiologically since the different organs are linked almost directly to the **blood compartments.**

- Because most of the so-called '**Functional Organs of the Body**' are associated directly to the **Plasma, Caternary Model** *finds its remote usage in a human body.*

Merits and Demerits of Compartment Modelling Approach: The various **merit and demerits of the Compartment Modelling Approach** have been enumerated in *Table 3.5*:

3.3.2.2. *Flow Models (or Physiologic-Pharmacokinetic Models)*

In general, these models are also known as:

- **Blood-flow Rate-limited Models**, and
- **Perfusion Rate-limited Models.**

As the name suggests, the **Physiologic-Pharmacokinetic Models** are duly based upon the known values of both **physiologic and anatomic data**; and, therefore, signifies a rather *more realistic and true picture of the drug disposition in different tissues and organs in a human body.*

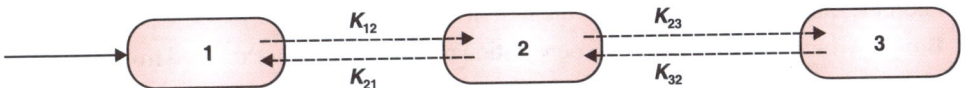

Fig. 3.8: The Caternary Model Using Three Compartments.

S. No.	Merits of Compartment Modelling
\multicolumn{2}{c}{Table 3.5. Merits and Demerits of Compartment Modeling}

S. No.	Merits of Compartment Modelling
1	Provide an explicit visual representation of rate process variants intimately involved in **drug disposition.**
2	Determines the precise number of rate constants that are absolutely necessary to describe these process vividly.
3	The **Pharmacokinetic experts** are duly empowered to derive the various '**differential equations**' pertaining to each of the rate phenomenon so as to elaborate drug concentration changes occurring in each compartment.
4	Extremely important aspects with regard to the development of the dosage regimens.
5	Perceptively useful in predicting the relationship between the drug concentration and time profile in • **Normal physiologic**, and • **Pathologic conditions**.

S. No.	Demerits of compartment Modelling

1	There exists no relationship between
	    • **physiologic functions**, and
	    • **anatomic structure of species.**

Hence, there is a dire need to have several assumptions so as to facilitate the data interpretation.

2	Exhaustive efforts are needed to develop a befitting '**Model**' which would predict and designate suitably the **ADME of a typical 'drug'**.
3	**Compartment Model** is solely based upon curve fitting of plasma concentration to the resulting complex multi-exponential mathematic equations.
4	Model may invariably exhibit variance very much within a study population.
5	Applicability only confined to a particular drug under investigation.
6	**Drug profile** within the body may fit into various compartmental models pertaining to the route of administration.
7	**Complexities** may arise when comparing results using both human and animal experiments.

In fact, the said models do describe kinetically the data with critical consideration of the fact that the blood flow is exclusively responsible in the proper distribution of a drug substance to various segments of a human body. Besides, the actual uptake of a drug into various organs is estimated ultimately due to the obvious binding of a drug in these tissues.

Salient Features: Following *four* **Salient Features**, such as:

1. The **actual number of compartments** that are involved in these models solely depends upon the disposition properties of the individual drug substance.
2. **Bones*** which have absolutely no penetration of drug are totally excluded from such models.
3. Since there exists a good number of **tissue organs present in a human body**, it becomes quite necessary and important that the **Tissue Volume** should be determined; and hence, its ensuing **Drug Concentration (g mL^{-1} or mcg mL^{-1}) specified appropriately**.
4. However, most of the **Valid Information** which is required essentially for proper description of a **Physiological Pharacokinetic Model Experimentally is difficult to achieve** ordinarily.

NOTE	Contrary to the serious limitations, the physiologic pharmacokinetics model fails miserably to give a much better insight of how the ensuing physiologic factors would cause a definite change in the drug-distribution profile from a particular animal species to another.

Figure 3.9 illustrates explicitly a **Physiological Pharmacokinetic Model** (or **Flow Model**) where the various **Compartments** are duly arranged in a series in a *descriptive* **Flow Diagram**.

1. The **IV administration of drug** carries it to the lungs, and from there right into the arterial blood.

Description: The various aspects in Figure 3.9 may be described as below:

2. From the **arterial blood, the drug passes into the following** segments (organs) of human body:
   - **heart,**
   - **gut and liver-in a sequential manner- and gets away via the hepatic elimination (K_m),**
   - **kidney and gets away through the urinary excretion (K_e),**

---

* **Bones**: They refer to the hard, rigid form of connective tissue constituting most of the skeleton of vertebrates, composed chiefly of calcium salts.

- venous blood after passing via the highly perfused tissues (HPT), and
- venous blood after entering through the poorly perfused tissues (PPT).

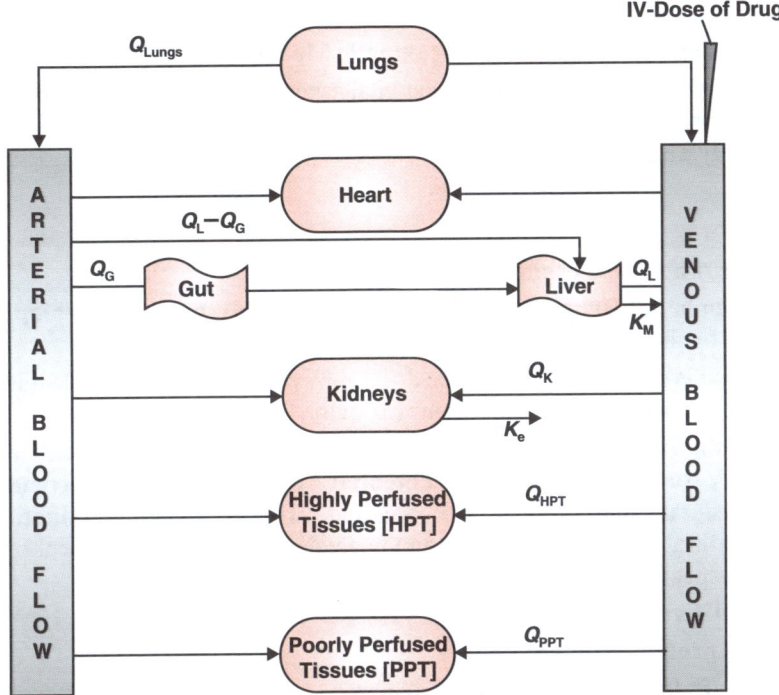

Q Designates Blood Flow Rate to a Body Region

K_m is the Rate Constant for Hepatic Elimination

K_e is the First-order Rate Constant for Urinary Excretion

Q_{HPT} Designates Blood Flow Rate in Highly Perfused Tissues

Q_{PPT} Represents Blood Flow Rate in Poorly Perfused Tissues

Fig. 3.9: The Schematic Representation of a Physiologic Pharmacokinetic Model of Drug Perfusion.

3. Thus, one may explicitly observe the *'drug' administered through IV passing across the venous blood to the arterial blood by means of an array of physiologic **Pharmacokinetic Modes**.*

Three Major Differences: There are in all *three* **major differences** with regard to the **Physiologic Pharmacokinetic Models**, namely:

1. Devoid of Data-Fitment in Perfusion Model: The **Perfusion Model** is devoid of any sort of **Data-Fitment Demand**. Consequently, the requisite **Drug Concentrations in different tissues are predicted precisely by such critical requirements:**

- **organ tissue-size,**
- **ensuing blood-flow,** and
- **drug-tissue-*blood ratio** estimated experimentally.**

---

* That is, **partition of the drug between the tissue and blood**

2. Observed Variance in Blood-Flow/Tissue-Size/Drug-Tissue-Blood Ratios: One may apparently observe a **significant variance in Blood-Flow, Tissue-Size,** and **Drug-Tissue-Blood Ratios** necessarily caused by virtue of certain **Pathophysiologic Status***: Therefore, it is a almost mandatory to take into consideration the overall effects of these variants upon the **Drug Distribution** specifically in Profile **Physiologic Pharmacokinetic Models.**

3. Possibility of Extrapolation: The most vital aspect of all **Physiologic Pharmacokinetic Models** may be applicable to many species and certain critical **Drug-Human Data may be extrapolated easily and conveniently.**

Examples

Following are *two* **typical examples,** such as:

- A good number of **Drugs,** *viz.* **Digoxin, Lidocaine, Methotrexate, Thiopental,** can be described by the aid of the **Perfusion Models** exclusively.
- **Tissue Levels** of quite a few of these drugs may not be predicted as accurately as can be accomplished with the **Compartment Models.**

Importantly, the *real significance of a* **Physiologic-Pharmacokinetic Model of Drug Perfusion** is solely based upon the ensuing **Potential Application of this Particular Model** in the viable and accurate prediction of the so-called '**Human Pharmacokinetics'** from the accomplished '**Animal Data'.** However, one may achieve the following critical information in humans and other species, such as:

- **mass of different body organs or tissues,**
- **degree of protein-binding,**
- **capacity of 'drug metabolism',** and
- **blood flow.**

Interestingly, the aforesaid **anatomical and physiological parameters** may be employed explicitly to:

- **predict the ensuing effects of drug substances in humans,** and
- **their consequent effects upon the animal models in all such instances whereby the 'Human Experimentation' becomes rather difficult to accomplish.**

Merits of Physiologic-Pharmacokinetic Models: The **Physiologic-Pharmacokinetic Model** essentially has *certain glaring merits,* namely:

1. The **Mathematical Treatment** is mostly of a *straight-forward nature.*
2. Obviously, here the '**Fitment of Data'** is hardly necessarily. Besides, one may gainfully predict the actual drug concentrations duly present in various regions of the body based upon such factors as:
   - **tissue or organ volume,**
   - **rate of perfusion** and
   - **tissue to plasma 'Partition Coefficient' estimated experimentally.**
3. It does provide a precise description of the prevailing **Drug-Concentration Time Profile** present duly in any specific organ or tissue; and, therefore, it may provide a much **better picture of the ensuing Drug-Distribution Features in a human body.**

---

* **Pathophysiologic Status**: It refers to the physiology of disordered function.

4. It is quite possible to record the influence of an altogether **changed pathology or physiology** upon the *disposition of drug*, which may be predicted both easily and conveniently based upon the changes taking place in **Different Pharmacokinetic Parameters**.

> **NOTE**   These 'Pharmacokinetic Parameters' predominantly are related to the actual anatomic and physiologic values.

5. Logical and judicious correlation of data in many **animal models is evidently possible. Even certain drug substances may be carefully extrapolated to humans**.

Important Note: The one and only major demerit of such **Comprehensive Models** is retaining meaningful **Experimental Data** that certainly proves to be a *Herculean and Exhaustive Task.*

3.3.2.3. *Non-Compartmental Pharmacokinetics*

Due to the well-know fact there exist numerous, disadvantages along with several difficulties invariably encountered with the '**Classical Compartment Models**', gave birth to many '**Newer Approaches**' to carry out an elaborated study confined to the time-course of drug substances in a human body. It is usually termed as the **Non-Compartmental Pharmacokinetic Model**.

However, it is also-known as the '**Independent Model Method**';. Besides, it may be applicable to any available **Compartment Model** only in such condition where:

- **the drug substances**, and
- **their respective metabolites**,

strictly adhere to the '**Linear Kinetics Exclusively**'.

Statistical Moments Theory :The **Non-Compartmental Pharmacokinetic Models** normally employed for the *calculation of absorption, distribution, and elimination parameters* **are solely based upon the Statistical Moments Theory**.

It essentially involves the meticulous collection of various **Experimental Data obtained duly from the Single-Administration of a 'Drug'**. Now, considering the **time-course of a drug concentration duly present in plasma representing specifically the 'Statistical Distribution Curve', we may have the** following expression:

$$\boxed{\text{MRT} = \frac{\text{AUMC}}{\text{AUC}}} \qquad \text{(r)}$$

where,
MRT* = Mean residence time,
AUC = Area under 'zero-moment curve' and
AUMC = Area under 'first-moment curve'.
Importantly, one may obtain **AUMC easily from a plot:**

- **product of plasma-drug concentration (at time '*t*'. *i.e.*, '*C*'ₜ), and**
- **time '*t*' (from o→α),**

---

*   **MRT:** It may be defined as 'the average amount of time consumed by a drug in the body before being eliminated'. Evidently, it refers to the statistical moment analogy of plasma half-life ($t_{1/2}$). In true sense, MRT designates the actual time taken for ~63.2% of the IV bolus dose to be eliminated. Obviously, the MRT values shall always be greater in a situation when the drug is being administered via a route other than the IV bolus.

as illustrated in Figure 3.10

Hence, **AUMC may be expressed mathematically by the following expression:**

$$AUMC = \int_0^\alpha C_t dt \qquad \qquad (s)$$

In the same manner, **AUC** may be arrived at from a plot of the ensuing plasma-drug concentration *vs.* time duly extending from o→α. Therefore, **AUC** may be expressed mathematically by the following expression:

$$AUC = \int_0^\alpha C dt \qquad \qquad (t)$$

Explanation

The various vital aspects of Figure 3.10 may be expatiated as follows:

Both '**Area Under First-Moment Curve' (AUMC)** and Area Under Zero-Moment Curve may be calculated based on the respective *graphs* (or *plots*) duly obtained by the '**Trapezoidal Rule'**. In other words, the entire curve is duly divided into a series of vertical lines (*see Figure 3.10*) into an array of **Trapezoids**. Subsequently, the specific area of each **Trapezoid is calculated individually, and then they are added up together finally.**

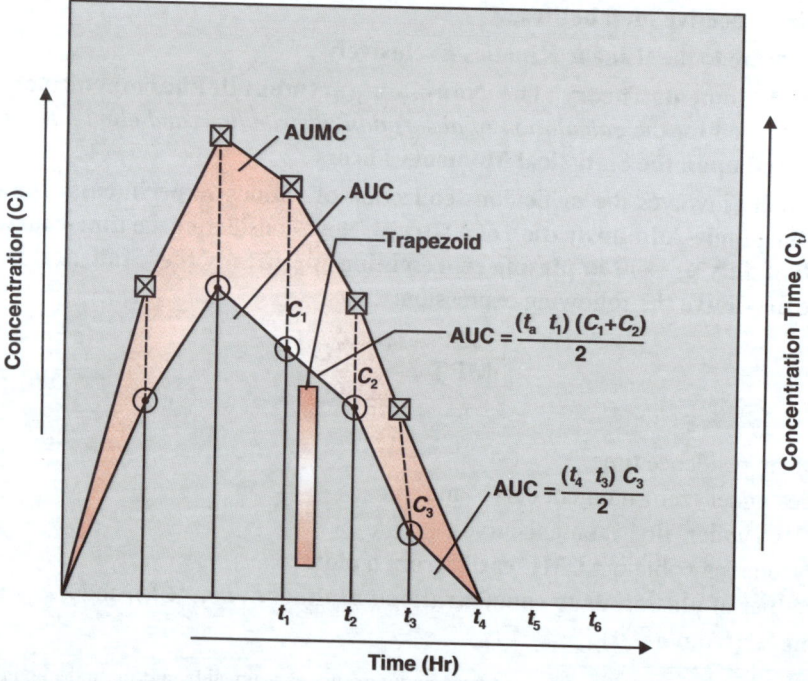

[*Trapezoidal Rule: It refers to the method for estimating integrals (*i.e.*, areas under absorption curves) by adding the areas of discrete trapezoids. It is frequently used for estimating several other pharmacokinetic integrals to determine either quantity and/or extent of occurrence of a process.]

Fig. 3.10: Diagrammatic Representations of AUMC and AUC Plots.

Important Applications: The important applications of the **Non-Compartmental Pharmacokinetic Model** are concerned with the determination of various **Pharmacokinetic aspects,** namely:

- **Bioavailability,**
- **Clearance,**
- **Volume of distribution (V_d),**
- **Plasma half-life ($t_{1/2}$),**
- **Rate of absorption,** and
- **'First-Order' absorption rate of the drug substance.**

Merits of Non-Compartmental Pharmacokinetics: These essentially comprise the following:

1. The **Pharmacokinetics Parameters** may be derived quite easily by using **Simple Agebraic Equations.**

2. Importantly, one may make use of *similar* **Mathematical Treatment** to practically any sort of :

- **drug substance,** or
- **metabolite,**

only if they rigidly follow the **'First-Order' kinetics.**

3. The necessary of an elaborated description of the **drug disposition characteristic feature is ruled out completely.**

NOTE	**The only major disadvantage of this technique being the scanty provision of absolute restricted information pertaining to the critical *Plasma-Drug Concentration-Time Profile.***

3.3.2.4. *Non-Linear Pharmacokinetics*

The **Pharmacokinetics Models** discussed so far have been duly constructed on the assumption that the ensuing **Pharmacokinetics Pathways** are invariably described by these *two* **vital factors,** namely:

- **linear differential equations,** and
- **'first-order' rate constants.**

In a broader perspective, these models need not be true and is quite important to state here that these are the typical instances wherein both the **Non-ideal and Non-Linear Behavioural Pattern** may take place effectively.

Evidently, the determination of a host of **Pharmacokinetic Parameters,** for instance,

- **absorption rate constant,**
- **elimination rate constant,** and
- **plasma clearance factor,**

are entirely based upon the assumption that all these **conditionalities** (*i.e., parameters*) actually fails to bring about either a significant alteration on the administration of a drug at different dose levels or in a situation when the multiple doses of a drug are duly administered.

Example

It has been duly observed that either the increased doses of certain drugs or the chronic medication may ultimately give rise to the apparent deviations with respect to the **ensuing Linear-Pharmacokinetics Profile** as shown with single-low doses of the same drug.

Furthermore, the **Non-Linear Pharmacokinetics** behavioural pattern is usually termed as the **'Dose Dependent Pharmacokinetics'**. It has been discussed more elaborately under *Section 3(7)*.

Time-Dependent Pharmacokinetics: When the actual time of the administration of a drug substance particularly influences the **Pharmacokinetics Parameters** of the drug, the overall phenomenon is known as the **Time-Dependent Pharmacokinetics**.

However, it is pertinent to state at this point in time that the **aforesaid Non-Linear Pharmacokinetics** may be the result of a typical pathologic alteration with regard to the respective **Drug Absorption-Distribution-Elimination (DADE)**.

The **Non-Linear Pharmacokinetics** shall be treated in details, under *Section 3(7)*.

3.4. Pharmacokinetics of Drug Absorption

The **'Orders of Processes'** related to the **Pharmacokinetics of drug absorption** could be **'Zero Order'**, **First Order'** or **'Second Order.** In true sense, the **'order'** solely depends upon the number of variables that ultimately determine the **'Rate of Reaction'**. However, in the domain of **Pharmacokinetics**, the **Zero Order and First Order** do play an extremely important role; and, therefore, shall be discussed in the following sections.

3.4.1. *Zero-Order Absorption Rate Constant*

The **Zero- Order Absorption** is prominently characterized by a **Constant Rate of Absorption**. Importantly, it is found to be absolutely independent of:

- **actual amount remaining to be absorbed (ARA),** and
- **regular ARA *vs*. t plot appears to be linear with respect to 'slope' that is equivalent to the rate of absorption; whereas, the 'Semi-Log Plot' is duly shown by an increasing-gradient with time (*t*), as illustrated in Figure 3.11.**

Contrarily, the **First- Order Absorption Rate Constant** determining phenomenon is markedly distinguished by means of a visible decline in the **Constant Rate of Absorption with ARA*** Thus, the actual **'Cartesian Plot'**** appears as a **Curvilinear Type; while the Semi-Log Plot'** comes out as a **'Straight Line'** *having the desired absorption rate constant designated duly by its 'Slope' (Figure 3.11).*

It has been duly established beyond any reasonable doubt that soon after the **Extravascular Administration (EV) of a Drug**, the observed **Rate of Change** in the actual quantum of the same in the body, **dx/d*t***, shows the prevailing difference between the **Rate of Input** (*i.e.*, **absorption**) given by **dx$_{EV}$/d*t***, and the **Rate of Input** [*i.e.*, **Elimination (*E*)**] given by **dxE/d*t***. Thus, we may have the following expression:

$$\frac{dx}{dt} = \frac{dx_{EV}}{dt} - \frac{dx_E}{dt}$$

---

* That is, the rate of absorption is solely dependent upon **ARA**.

** Also known as a **'Regular Plot'**

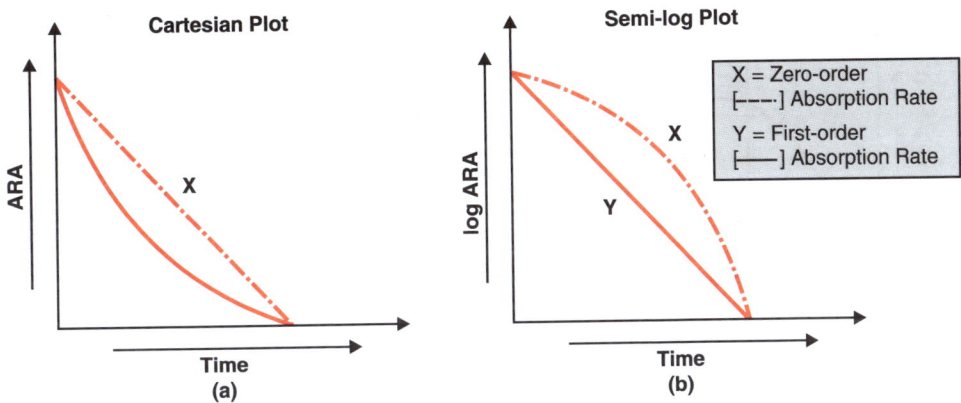

Fig. 3.11: An Explicit Distinction Between Zero-Order and First-Order Absorption Phenomenon (a) Cartesian Plot and (b) Semi-Log Plot.

3.4.1.1. *Plasma Drug Level-Time Curve for a Drug Administered in Single Oral Dose*

In a real perspective, it may be understood thoughtfully that the **critical rate of an on-going phenomenon exclusively depends upon the actual quantum of the drug duly available for such a phenomenon to accomplish at given time; and, therefore, is equivalent to the ultimate product of:**

- **rate constant**, and
- **quantum of drug at a given time.**

Obviously, one may conclude generously that the '**Rate of a Phenomenon**' undergoes a definite charge with respect to time since the ensuing quantum of '**Drug Substance**' alters with time.

Figure 3.12 records evidently the **Plasma Drug Level-Time Curve** duly accomplish following a '**Single-Oral Dose of a Drug Substance**'. Thus, the resulting '**Curve**' may be further subdivided into different zones genuinely based upon the following *two* **major factors**: *viz.*,

- **relative magnitudes of rate of absorption,** and
- **rate of elimination at different time points.**

Explanation

The following *four* **different phases of the plasma drug level-time curve obtained from a single oral dose of a drug substance** are as given below:

- **absorption phase,**
- **plateau phase,**
- **post-absorption phase,** and
- **elimination phase**

as shown by A, B, C and D in **Figure 3.12**, which will now be treated briefly in the following section.

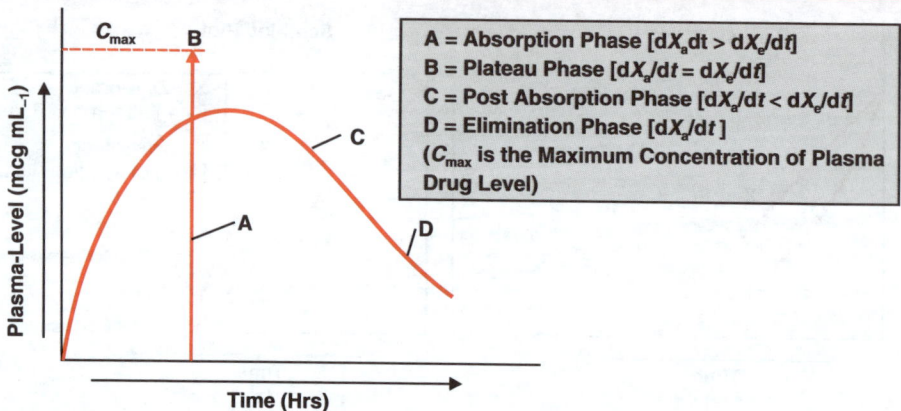

Fig. 3.12: Different Phases of a Plasma Level-Time Curve for a Drug Administered *via* a Single Oral Dose.

Absorption Phase (A): Immediately after the *oral administration of a particular Drug Substance,* almost the entire dose of the same is duly available for commencing the **Absorption Phase at zero time**. Thus, the quantum of the drug substance prevailing critically at the **Absorption site** starts declining as a **Function of Time (t)**. Therefore, one may obviously observe during the absorption phase pertaining to a **Plasma Level-Time Curve**, the **attained Rate of Drug Absorption appears to be markedly greater** *vis-a-vis* **the Rate of Drug Elimination.**

$$\frac{dX_a}{dt} > \frac{dX_e}{dt} \qquad \text{(u)}$$

Plateau Phase (B): It refers to the **Absorption of Drug Substance** into the systemic circulation rather slowly, which **enhances the Plasma Level of the Drug Substance till such time the Rate of Absorption Remains obviously greater in comparison to the Rate of Elimination.** In this manner, the slow and steady enhancement of the evening drug-level in plasma helps to increase the rate of elimination of the drug substance, dX_e/dt, as a function of time. It obviously suggests that the **rate of absorption of a drug substance decreases with time (t)**; whereas, the resulting **rate of elimination** of the same shall almost render to be **'equal'**.

Importantly, the critical **'time'** at which the aforesaid **'equality'** is accomplished is usually termed as the **'Time of Peak-Drug concentration (t)'** in plasma; and hence, the attained concentration of the drug substance is invariably called as the **'maximum plasma drug concentration (C_{max})'**, that may be duly accomplished soon after a single oral dose of the drug is administered. Evidently, one may observe that at 't_p':

Rate of absorption = Rate of elimination

$$\frac{dX_a}{dt} = \frac{dX_e}{dt} \qquad \text{(v)}$$

Post-Absorption Phase (C): Soon after the completion of the **'Plateau Phase (B)'**, the observed rate of elimination of a drug substance appears to be faster *vis-a-vis* rate of absorption, as designated explivitly by the distinct 'Post-absorption Phase (C)' (*see Figure 3.12*). interestingly, in the course of this particular phase, one may observe predominantly that there exists a **definite decline in the evening 'drug levels' because the on-going absorption of the drug substance remains still in active progress.**

Thus, we have the following expression:

$$\frac{dX_a}{dt} = \frac{dX_e}{dt} \tag{w}$$

Elimination Phase (D): It represents vividly a typical situation when the drug substance strategically located at the absorption site gets depleted overwhelmingly; and, therefore, the **Rate of drug Absorption** critically attains the 'zero level', *i.e.*, $dX_a/dt = 0$. Thus, the **Elimination Phase [D]** of the plasma level-time curve eventually represents the overall elimination of the drug substance from the body exclusively, and that happens to be a **first-order phenomenon.** It follows from the above stated facts that the actual rate of charge observed in the quantum of the drug substance present duly in the human body specifically in the aforesaid '**Elimination Phase**' is frequently expressed by the **first-order phenomenon, as given below:**

$$\frac{dX_e}{dt} = -KX \tag{x}$$

where,

K = Overall elimination rate constant and

X = Quantum of drug substance present in the human body at any time.

3.4.2. First-Order Absorption Rate Constant

The **First-Order Absorption Rate Constant** usually designates the **Oral-Administration of a Drug Substance** *i.e., the critical presence of the unchanged drug substance in blood/plasma.*

Therefore, for a specific drug substance which gains entry into the body by means of a **First-Order Absorption phenomenon** finally gets distributed throughout the human body *via* a **One-Compartment Kinetics.** Consequently, it is duly eliminated by the help of **First-Order phenomena;** and hence, the said model may be expressed as follows:

Where,

X_0 = Oral dose of a drug substance administered,

X = Amount of drug present in blood and body tissues at any time (t) (*i.e.*, equivalent to the product of the volume of distribution (Vd) of the drug and the plasma drug concentration),

K_a = First-Order Rate Constant of the drug absorption, K_e = First-Order Rate Constant of the elimination phenomena.

We have seen earlier that:

$$dX/dt = \text{Rate of absorption} - \text{Rate of elimination}$$

and the differential form of the above equation is given by the following expression:

$$\frac{dX}{dt} = K_a X_a - K_E X \tag{y}$$

where,

K_a = First-Order Rate Absorption Constant, and

X_a = Amount of drug substance present at the '**absorption site remaining to be absorbed (ARA)**'.

Integrating Equation (y) we may have:

$$X = \frac{K_a F X_0}{(K_a - K_E)} [e^{-K_E t} - e^{-K_a t}] \tag{z}$$

where, F = Fraction of the drug substance being absorbed systematically soon after an extravascular administration.

Now, transforming **Equation (z)** in terms of the concentrations, we may obtain the following expression:

$$C = \frac{K_a F X_0}{V_d (K_a - K_E)} [e^{-K_E t} - e^{-K_a t}] \tag{aa}$$

where,

V_d = Volume of Distribution (*i.e.*, $X = V_d XC$).

NOTE   Figure 3.12 illustrates a typical concentration-time profile of a drug substance administratered duly *via* the extravascular route.

Nevertheless, **Equation (aa)** elaborates explicitly the **Duration of Time of the Drug-Concentration in Plasma (C)** soon after the *Oral Route of Administration*. It has been amply demonstrated and proven that for majority of drug substances that are usually given in readily available dosage forms, one may observe the ensuing **Absorption Rate Constant [K_a] being appreciably greater than the Elimination Rate Constant [K_E]**.

Important Observations: In a situation, when the **First-Order Absorption Rate Constant** (K_a) turns out to be appreciably larger in comparison to be corresponding **Elimination Rate Constant (K_E)** * the **second exponential (e^{-K_a})** in Equation (aa) shall usually tend to approach 'zero' rather more swiftly that the **first exponential ($e^{-K_E t}$)**.

Furthermore, at larger values of **time 't'**, the **Equation (aa)** shall get reduced to the following expression:

$$C = \frac{K_a F X_0}{V_d (K_a - K_E)} \cdot e^{-K_t} \tag{ab}$$

Ultimately, **Equation (ab)** expatiates the critical **Elimination Phase**** of the following **Plasma Drug Concentration-Time Curve** as depicted in *Figure 3.13*.

---

*   That is, a '**good rule**' suggests that it must at least five folds larger (or K $_a$= 5K$_E$)

**   That is, the particular time when the ensuing '**absorption**' no longer comes into play

Equation (ab) may be expressed in the form of **common logarithms** as follows:

$$\log C = \log \left[\frac{K_a F X_0}{V_d(K_a - K_E)} \right] - \frac{K_t}{2.303} \qquad \text{(ac)}$$

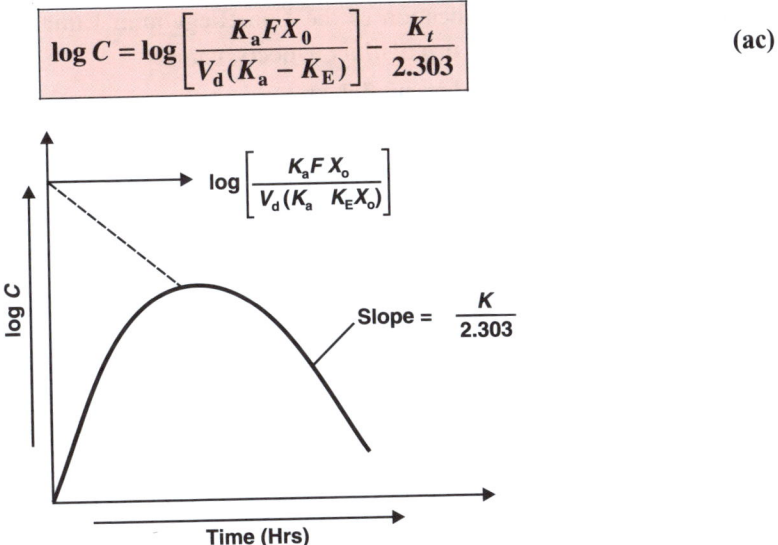

Fig. 3.13: Logarithm of Plasma Drug Concentration-Time Curve for a Single Oral Dose of a Drug Substance.

Explanation

Figure 3.13 clearly depicts a plot of the **'log' of Plasma Drug Concentration-Time(t)** which gives rise to a typical **'Bioexponential Curve'** at very initial stage; and eventually tends to be **'Linear'** in the course of the ensuing elimination phase (as duly described by **Equation (ac)** above). Obviously, the **'slope'** of the terminal end of the linear segment of the **Plasma-Drug Concentration-Time Graph** which is almost equal to $K/2.303$; whereas, the intercept is equivalent to **Log $[K_a FX/V_0(K_a-K_E)]$**.

Therefore, one may easily obtain the following *two* values from **Figure 3.13** as given below:

- **elimination rate constant (K) from the slope of the terminal linear segment**, and
- **elimination of the plasma half-life ($t_{½}$) of the drug substance as given by 0.693/K.**

3.4.3. The Loo-Riegelman and Wagner-Nelson Equations

In fact, both **Loo-Riegelman** and **Wagner-Nelson equations** do help in calculating the *actual percentage of a drug substance*, *i.e.*, **amount remaining to be absorbed (ARA) at any time.** Importantly, the resulting percentage is exclusively based upon the critical absorbable fraction of the dose particularly in the instance of an **Incomplete Absorption** (Notari et al., 1972)*

Nevertheless, a suitable plot (which could be either **Zero-Order or First-Order**) duly obtained from these data allows the logical calculation of the respective **Absorption Rate Constants, K or K.**

** Notari R E et al.: *J.Pharm, Sci.,* **61**:135, 1972.

3.4.3.1. *Loo-Riegelman Equation*

The usual effective application of the **Loo-Riegelman Equation** to a drug-substance is described **explicitly** by these *two* **distinct aspects,** namely:

- **two-compartment open model,** and
- **absorption via a first-order rate process.**

Vaughan and Dennis (1980)* and Wagner (1983)** have demonstrated adequately that the **Loo-Riegelman equation,** through based upon the **Model of Equation (ac)** below as given in *Figure 3.4* yet is reasonably applicable even the **Model of Equation (ii) oe Equation (iii) is in effect.**

$$\longleftarrow \quad ① \rightleftharpoons ② \tag{i}$$

$$① \rightleftharpoons ② \longrightarrow \tag{ii}$$

$$\longleftarrow \quad ① \rightleftharpoons ② \longrightarrow \tag{iii}$$

Based on the above facts, the **Loo-Riegelman equation** is found to be **Model Independent** as long as the '**input**' is confined to **Compartment 1** exclusively.

We may use the following equation:

$$\left(\frac{A_b}{V_C}\right)_{t_n} = C_{t_n} + K_{10}\ \text{AUC}(0 - t_n) + T_{t_n} \tag{ad}$$

where,

A/V_c = Total amount of drug absorbed,

V_c = Volume of the central compartment,

C and T = Concentration of drug in plasma and tissue and

T_n = Time of absorption.

Example

A proper explanation of **Equation (ad)** and its application is obtained through a typical example. A '**drug substance**' exhibits a biexponential disposition soon after an IV injection. The calculated values for the *Two*-**Compartmental Model Rate Constants, are** found to be $K_{12} = 0.30$; $K_{21} = 0.40$ and $K_{10} = 0.25$ (**per hr**). The same drug was given orally, and the data thus obtained are provided in *Table 3.6.* The aforesaid information shall be utilized to calculate the *two* **unknown, quantities given** in **Eqaution (ad),** namely: **AUC** $(0-t_n)$; and (A_b/V_c)***.

---

*   Vaughan DP and Dennis MJ: *J Pharmcokinet. Biopharm.,* **8**: 83, 1980

**   Wagner JG: **Fundamentals of Clinical Pharmacokinetics;** 2nd ed., Hamilton, IL: Drug Intelligence, p.196 1983,

*** Adapted from: Notari R E: **Biopharmaceutics and Clinical Pharmacokinetics,** 4th ed., Marcel Dekker Inc., New York:1987.

Table 3.6. Observed Plasma Levels of a Drug Substance Soon After the Oral Administration of 490 mg

S. No.	Time (hr)	Concentration (mg%)
1	0.5	3.2
2	1.0	4.8
3	1.5	5.5
4	2.0	5.7
5	2.5	5.7
6	3.0	5.4
7	4.0	4.8
8	5.0	4.1
9	7.0	3.1
10	9.0	2.2
11	11.0	1.8
12	13.0	1.4

Solution

The results are duly calculated in the following three steps in a sequential manner and subsequently recorded in *Table 3.7*.

Step 1: It essentially involves the calculation of the tissue concentrations as a function of time. The following equation has been employed:

$$T_{tn} = T_{tn-1} e^{-K_{21}Dt} + C_{tn-1} (1 - e^{-K_{21}Dt}) \frac{K_{12}}{K_{21}} + \frac{1}{2} K_{12} DCDt \qquad \text{(ae)}$$

Table 3.7. Answers Duly Recorded From Stepwise Calculations for the Loo-Riegelman Equation

		Step (1)			Step (2)			Step (3)		
(1)	(2)	(3)	(4)	(5)	(6)	(7)	(8)	(9)	(10)	(11)
t_n	Δt	C	ΔC	T_n	Area t_{n-1} to t_n	Area t_o to t_o	K_{10} X col.7	A_a/V_c= 3+5+8	Percent A_b/V_c	100%⁻ col.10
0.5	0.5	3.2	3.2	0.240	0.80	0.80	0.20	3.64	26.8	73.2
1.0	0.5	4.8	1.6	0.752	2.00	2.80	0.70	6.25	46.0	54.0
1.5	0.5	5.5	0.7	1.32	2.58	5.38	1.35	8.17	60.1	39.9
2.0	0.5	5.7	0.2	1.84	2.80	8.18	2.04	9.58	70.4	29.6
2.5	0.5	5.7	0.0	2.28	2.85	11.03	2.76	10.7	78.7	21.3
3.0	0.5	5.4	-0.3	2.62	2.78	13.81	3.45	11.5	84.6	15.4
4.0	1.0	4.8	-0.6	3.00	5.10	18.91	4.73	12.5	91.9	8.1
5.0	1.0	4.1	-0.7	3.09	4.45	23.36	5.84	13.0	95.6	4.4
7.0	2.0	3.1	-1.0	2.78	7.20	30.56	7.65	13.5	99.3	0.7
9.0	2.0	2.2	-0.9	2.26	5.30	35.86	8.96	13.4	98.5	1.5
11.0	2.0	1.8	-0.4	1.80	4.00	39.86	9.96	13.6	100.0	0.0
13.0	2.0	1.4	-0.4	1.43	3.20	43.06	10.8	13.6	100.0	0.0

Now, **Equation (ae)** shall be solved appropriately for **each data point**. In the above example, let us consider the **first-set of points**, *i.e.*, **0.5 hr at concentration 3.2 mg%**. Hence, we may have these data:

$$\Delta t = 0.5; \quad \Delta C = 3.5 \quad \text{and} \quad t_{n-1} = 0$$

In this manner, the concentrations of a drug in plasma and tissue at time (t_{n-1}) obtained are also 'zero' as there is absolutely 'no drug' present in the body at time 'zero'. Thus, the first entry in Table 3.7 under the Step 1 is carefully calculated from the following expression:

$$T_{0.5} = 0 + 0 + \tfrac{1}{2}(0.3)\,(3.2)\,(0.5)$$
$$= 0.24$$

(af)

and likewise, the second entry from the following equation:

$$T_{1.0} = 0.24e^{-0.20} + (1 - e^{-0.2})\,\frac{3.2 \times 0.3}{0.4} + \frac{1}{2}[0.3\,(1.6)\,0.5]$$
$$= 0.751$$

(ag)

and so on so forth. **All the entries of T is recorded in Table 3.7.**

Step 2: This particular step takes care of the calculation of elimination as a **function of time** (t_n). so far, we have duly calculated the values for T_t. as we have proceed the **data for C** (*i.e.*, **concentration of drug in plasma at time** t_n), there remains only one segment of **Equation (ad)** that need to be calculated, which being **[AUC(0–t)]** designating the '**area under the plasma time-concentration curve**' extending from time '**0**' to time '**t_n**'.

Wagner (1983)* suggested emphatically that the much needed precision and accuracy may be enhanced by incorporating the **interpolated points**** Furthermore, by making use of the **logarithmic Trapezoidal Rule***** during the terminal **Log Linear Segment****** and the critical extension of the aforesaid **Trapezoidal Rule right up the Peak Level.**

Needless to add that in this '**Specific Example**', it may be carried out very easily and conveniently by employing the '**Trapezoidal Rule**'. Hence, one should be able to draw the 'curve' for C *vs. t*, and subsequently, the respective '**individual areas**' duly calculated for each trapezoidal (or triangle) as elaborated by the various data points.

The answers thus obtained are provided in Table 3.7, column (6), which represent the areas of the different '**Trapezoids**'. Therefore, it is absolutely necessary to sum up each and every area up to including tn so as to get the '**total value**' of the **AUC (0-t_n)** in Equation (ad), as illustrated duly in Table 3.7, column (7). At the end, each of these values is multiplied by the so-called '**Elimination constant K_{10} = 0.25**' in order to obtain the values in the respective column (8) of Table 3.7.

---

   *   Wagner JG: *J. Pharm. Sci.*, **72**: 838, 1983

  **   That is, derived data from that which precedes and follows it.

***   **Trapezoidal Rule:** It is a method for estimating integrals (areas under absorption curves) by adding the respective areas of discrete trapezoids

****   Chiou WI: *J. Pharmacokinet. Biopharm.*, **6**:539, 1978

Step 3: Calculation of A_b/V_c in Equation (ad): The *three* major component segments of Equation (ad) are now supposed to be calculated individually, *e.g.*, **columns 3, 4 and 8 in Table 3.7,** which are ultimately summed up to get at the respective values contained in column 9. Now, a critical examination of the entries in column 9, as a function of time, shall reveal that A_b/V_c thus, accomplished are duly converted to a percentage of the aforesaid **'Maximum value'** of approximately **13.6**. Consequently, the values of A_b/V_c thus, accomplished are duly converted to a percentage of the aforesaid **'Maximum Value'**, as per the following expression:

$$\% \; \frac{A_b}{V_c} = \frac{100 \, A_b}{13.6 \, V_c} \qquad\qquad \text{(ah)}$$

and the accrued results are duly posted in column 10 of Table 3.7.

The percentage of **'Drug Unabsorbed'**, as a function of time, is represented in column 11, and this is calculated by subtracting column 10 from 100%. Therefore, the **First-Order Plot of the percent unabsorbed vs. time yields a value of 0.60 hr^{-1} for K.**

Curve-Fitting Technique: The well-known method for the determination of K_a, *i.e.*, **First-Order Absorption Rate Constant** designates a **Curve-Fitting Technique**. Importantly, this method is found to be most suitable for such drug substances which essentially possess the following characteristic features:

- **get absorbed rapidly,**
- **undergo complete absorption**, and
- **rigidly follow the one-compartment kinetics even when administered *via* the IV route.**

Nevertheless, in such instances when the particular drug substance undergoes the following *three* **modes of absorption**, namely:

- **gastrointestinal (GI) motility retardation,**
- **enzymatic degradation**, and
- **exhibits typical 'multi-component characteristic features' second IV administration,**

Eventually one may arrive at the K_a **value (duly computed by the Curve-Fitting Technique),** which proves to be **'incorrect'** even though the drugs were actually absorbed by the **First-Order Kinetics.**

Obviously, under such circumstances, the **value of K_a** so obtained probably at its best may provide a reasonable estimate with regard to the **First-Order Disappearance of the specific drug substance from the GI tract instead of the First-Order Appearance in the normal systemic circulation.**

3.4.3.2. *Wagner-Nelson Equation*

The **Wagner-Nelson Equation** serves as not only a **better estimation of K_a**, but also a **qualified alternative method** to the **'Curve-Fitting Technique'**. Interestingly, the **Wagner-Nelson Method** predominantly involves

- **critical estimation of K_a based upon the percent (%) unabsorbed-time plots,** and
- **independent of the assumption of both zero-order and first-order absorptions.**

Oral Administration of a Single Dose of a Drug Substance: It may be observed that soon after the oral administration of a single dose of a drug at any material time, the actual quantum of drug being absorbed right into the ensuing **systemic circulation (X_0), is given by the sum of quantum of drug present in the body (A_{un}), and the quantum of drug eliminated from the body (A_{un})** (*i.e.*, **amount unabsorbed**).

Thus, we may have the following expression:

$$X_0 = A + A_{un} \qquad \text{(ai)}$$

Therefore, the quantum of the drug absorbed (A) at any time (t) is equivalent to the sum of the quantum of the drug present in the body (X), and also the precise quantum of the drug duly eliminated from the body at any material time (X_E). We have the following expression:

$$A = X + X_E \qquad \text{(aj)}$$

Derivation of **Equation (aj)** gives

$$\frac{dA}{dt} = \frac{dX}{dt} + \frac{dX_E}{dt} \qquad \text{(ak)}$$

As we know that $X = V_d XC$, hence we may have the following version of **Equation (ak)**:

$$\frac{dX}{dt} = V_d \cdot \frac{dC}{dt} \qquad \text{(al)}$$

Besides, $\dfrac{dX_E}{dt} = KX$, but $X = V_d \cdot C$

Therefore, we have

$$\frac{dX_E}{dt} = K \cdot V_d \cdot C \qquad \text{(am)}$$

Putting the values of **Equations (al)** and **(am)** in **Equation (ak)** we have:

$$\frac{dA}{dt} = V_d \cdot \frac{dC}{dt} + KV_d C \qquad \text{(an)}$$

or

$$dA = V_d \cdot dC + KV_d C dt \qquad \text{(ao)}$$

Now, integrating **Equation (ao)** between the limits $t = 0$ to $t = t$ gives the following expression:

$$\int_0^t dA = V_d \int_0^t dC + KV_d \int_0^t C \cdot dt$$

or

$$A_t - A_0 = V_d (C_1 - C_0) + KV_d \int_0^t C \cdot dt \qquad \text{(ap)}$$

Evidently, A_o is equal to the quantum of a drug absorbed at $t = 0$ is also equivalent to '0'; besides, the actual ensuing concentration of the drug in the human body at $t = 0$ also becomes equal to '0'. Hence, **Equation (ap)** gets simplified to the following expression:

$$A_t = V_d \cdot C_1 + KV_d \int_0^t C \cdot dt \qquad \text{(aq)}$$

Equation (aq) may be suitably rearranged to

$$\frac{A_t}{V_d} = C_t + KV_d \int_0^t C \cdot dt \qquad \text{(ar)}$$

where,

A_t/V_d = Amount of drug absorbed at time 't' divided by the '**volume of distribution**',

C_t = Plasma (serum/blood) concentration at time 't' and

$\int_0^t C \cdot dt$ = Area under the plasma concentration vs. time curve up to time 't'.

Again, integrating **Equation (ao)** but now between the **limits $t = 0$ to $t = \alpha$**, and subsequently rearranging the respective **equation**, we may obtain the following expression:

$$\int_0^\alpha dA = V_d \int_0^\alpha dC + KV_d \int_0^\alpha C \cdot dt$$

or

$$A_\alpha = V_d (C_\alpha - C_0) + KV_d \int_0^\alpha C \cdot dt$$

Now, we know that $C_0 = 0$ and $C_a = 0$, hence the above expression may be represented as follows:

$$A_\alpha = KV_d \int_0^\alpha C \cdot dt \qquad \text{(as)}$$

Equation (as) may be suitably rearranged as below:

$$\frac{A_\alpha}{V_d} = K \int_0^\alpha C \cdot dt \qquad \text{(at)}$$

where,

A_α/V_d = Total quantum of drug absorbed from the dosage form up to an infinite time ($t = \alpha$) divided by the '**Volume of Distribution**', and

$$\int_0^\alpha C \cdot dt = \text{Area under the } \textbf{total plasma (serum/blood)} \text{ concentration } \textit{vs.} \text{ time curve.}$$

Fraction of the drug substance being critically absorbed at 'any time' is obtained realistically by dividing **Equation (ar)** with **Equation (at):**

$$\frac{A_t/V_d}{A_\alpha/V_d} = \frac{\left(C_t + K \int_0^t C \cdot dt\right)}{K \int_0^\alpha C \cdot dt} \tag{au}$$

or

$$\frac{A_t}{A_\alpha} = \frac{\left(C_t + K \int_0^t C \cdot dt\right)}{K \int_0^t C \cdot dt} \tag{av}$$

However, the 'Unabsorbed Fraction' at any 't' is usually given by the following expression:

$$\left[1 - \frac{A_t}{A_\alpha}\right] = \left[1 - \frac{\left(C_t + K \int_0^t C \cdot dt\right)}{K \int_0^\alpha C \cdot dt}\right] \tag{aw}$$

or

$$100\left[1 - \frac{A_t}{A_\alpha}\right] = 100\left[1 - \frac{\left(C_t + K \int_0^t C \cdot dt\right)}{K \int_0^\alpha C \cdot dt}\right] \tag{ax}$$

Based on **Equation (ax)** one may easily calculate the actual percentage of the unabsorbed drug substance at any time 't'. in this way, we may usually come across the following two commonly encountered situations:

1. **Percent-Unabsorbed drug** *vs.* **Time:** It gives a straight-line thereby showing that the absorption phenomenon follows a **Zero-Order Kinetics** (*see Figure 3.14*).

2. **Logarithm of Percent-Unabsorbed Drug** *vs.* **Time:** It also yields a straight line which shows that the absorption phenomenon is said to follow **First-Order Kinetics** (*see Figure 3.15*).

Remarks: In short, it may be added that the **Wagner-Nelson Equation** particularly helps one to have a clear vision, concept and understanding with respect to the critical '**Absorption kinetics**' without making any sort of assumptions whatsoever. Importantly, the methodology appears to be very much useful and efficacious for enabling an in-depth investigative study for deciphering the actual in-built mechanism for the specific release profile of drug substances from the dosage forms (or drug products) *in vivo*. Besides, the **inherent absorption phenomenon** itself invariably accounts for the **First-Order kinetics;** whereas, the subsequent on-going **dissolution of capsules, Tablets, more emphatically the meticulously designed sustained release drug products, should usually be elaborated by relatively more Complex Kinetic Mechanisms.**

The **Wagner-Nelson Method** essentially needs the collection of '**blood samples**' soon after a single-oral dose at regular intervals of time till such time the entire quantum of the drug substance gets duly eliminated from the body. Thus, K_E is usually derived from '**log C' vs. 't' plot, and a semi-log plot of percent unabsorbed (*viz*. percent ARA) *vs.* 't' gives a straight line whose slope is $-K_2.303$ (see Figure 3.15). In case a regular plot of the same happens to be a straight line, one may conclude that the absorption process is of the Zero-Order Kinetics.**

The major *disadvantage* of the **Wagner-Nelson Method** is its being applicable exclusively to such drug substances having **One-Compartment characteristic features**. The real problem gets triggered in a particular situation when a drug which obeys the **One-Compartment Model** after an **extravascular administration** typically exhibits the characteristic features of a **Multi-Component Model after an IV administration.**

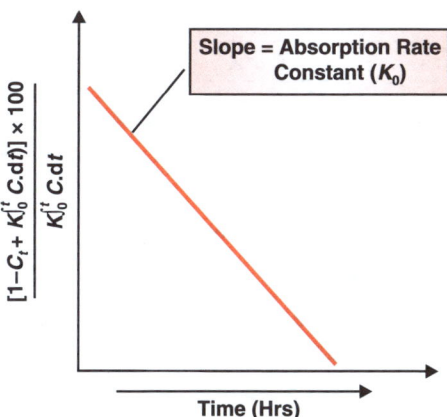

Fig. 3.14: Plot between Percent of Unabsorbed Drug *vs.* Time for a Single Oral Dose of a Drug Exhibiting a Zero-Order Absorption Phenomenon.

3.4.3.3. *Estimation of C_{max} and t_{max}*

The **maximum plasma concentration of a drug substance, C_{max}** as observed after the administration of a *single-oral dose* of the same usually takes place at the plateau of the ensuing plasma concentration time curve. Thus, the actual time essentially required to attain the maximum concentration is termed as the **Peak Time, t_{max}.** Furthermore, the time actually required to approach C_{max} is found to be quite independent of the '**dose of the drug**'. Instead, it solely dependent upon the **Rate Constants for the absorption (K), and also the elimination (K_E).**

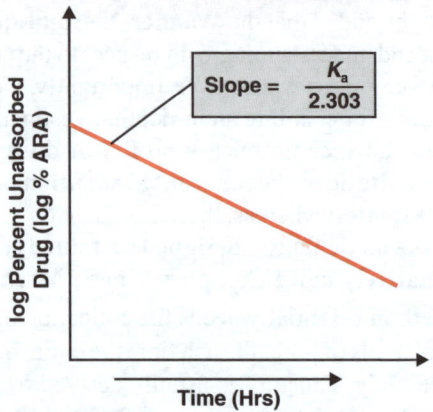

Fig. 3.15: Plot between Percent of Unabsorbed Drug (ARA) *vs.* Time '*t*' Showing the First-Order Absorption Process (*i.e.*, according to Wagner-Nelson Method).

However, it has been observed that the *maximum level of concentration of the drug*, invariably known also as the '**Peak Concentration**', the **Rate of Drug Absorption appears to be almost equal to the rate of the Drug Elimination**, which ultimately renders the ensuing **Rate of Concentration** change profile *dc/dt,* to become equivalent to '**zero**'.

Now, the **Rate of Concentration Change** observed may be accomplished by differentiating the following equation:

$$\frac{X}{V_d} = C = \frac{K_a F X_0}{V_d(K_a - K_E)}[e^{-K_n} - e^{-K_{at}}] \qquad \text{(ay)}$$

and above equation on being differentiated with respect to time gives the following expression:

$$\frac{dc}{dt} = -\frac{K K_a F X_0}{V_d(K_a - K_E)}e^{-K_{Et}} + \frac{K_a^2 F X_0}{V_d(K_a - K_E)}e^{-K_{at}} \qquad \text{(az)}$$

Since, the **Plasma Drug Concentration** reaches C_{max} **at time** t_{max}, then ultimately dc/dt becomes '**zero**'; and, therefore, we may have

$$\frac{K_E K_a F X_0}{V_d(K_a - K_E)}e^{-Kt_{max}} = \frac{K_a^2 F X_0}{V_d(K_a - E_E)}e^{-K_a t_{max}}$$

and the above expression may be easily simplified to

$$K_E e^{-Kt_{max}} = K_a e^{-K_a t_{max}} \qquad \text{(ba)}$$

or

$$\frac{K_a}{K_E} = \frac{e^{-Kt_{max}}}{e^{-K_a t_{max}}}$$

By applying common logarithms on either sides of the above equation

$$\log \frac{K_a}{K_E} = \frac{-K_E t_{max}}{2.303} + \frac{-K_a t_{max}}{2.303}$$

or

$$t_{max} = \frac{2.303}{(K_a - K_E)} \log \frac{K_a}{K_E} \qquad \text{(bb)}$$

As it has been expatiated earlier that 't_{max}' is solely dependent upon both the **rate constants** K_a and K_E, the observed maximum concentration of the drug substance in plasma concentration takes place at t_{max} predominantly. Therefore, by substituting 't_{max}' for 't' in **Equation (ay)** we obtain:

$$C_{max} = \frac{K_a F X_0}{V_d (K_a - K_E)} [e^{-K_E t_{max}} - e^{-K_a t_{max}}] \qquad \text{(bc)}$$

Nevertheless, one may judiciously obtain a rather much simpler expression based on Equation (bc) above, by affecting the substitution $e^{-K_E t_{max}}$ **equivalent to** $K_E/K_a \, e^{-K_E t_{max}}$ as per Equation (ba):

$$\therefore \qquad \begin{aligned} C_{max} &= \frac{K_a F X_0}{V_d (K_a - K_E)} \left[e^{-K t_{max}} - \frac{K_a}{K_E} e^{-K_E t_{max}} \right] \\ &= \frac{K_a F X_0 \cdot e^{-K_E t_{max}}}{V_d (K_a - K_E)} \left(1 - \frac{K_a}{K_E} \right) \\ &= \frac{K_a F X_0}{V_d} \cdot \frac{(K_a - K_E)}{K_a} \cdot e^{-K_E t_{max}} \end{aligned} \qquad \text{(bd)}$$

or

$$C_{max} = \frac{F X_0}{V_d} \cdot e^{-K_E t_p} \qquad \text{(be)}$$

Conclusion: In conclusion, it may be observed that the estimate C_{max} immediately after the **First-Order Input** represents prominently a definite function of the resulting fraction of the dose (of the drug) entering the human body systematically:

- apparent 'volume of distribution (V_d),
- apparent 'first-order absorption', and
- determined 'elimination rate constants (K_E).

3.4.3.4. Influence of Ka and K_E upon C_{max}, t_{max} and AUC

The various articulated influence caused specifically due to the changes in K_a **at constant** K_E, and that of K_E **at constant** K_a upon the *three* **cardinal components** C_{max}, **tmax and AUC of a drug substance when administered via the extravascular (EV) route is recorded explicitly in Table 3.8.**

Table 3.8. Critical Observed Influence of K_a and K_E upon C_{max}, t_{max} and AUC

S. No.	Grossly Affected Parameters	Observed influence when K_E Remains constant		Observed influence when K_a Remains Constant	
		Lesser K_a	More K_a	Lesser K_a	More K_E
1	C_{max}	-		-	
2	t_{max}	Long	Short	Long	Short
3	AUC	No change	No change	-	

[- : shows an increase; and : shows a decrease]

3.5. Volume of Distribution and Distribution Coefficient

First and foremost, let us understand the meaning of certain terminologies, such as **Distribution** and **Distribution Coefficient.**

Distribution: It refers to the portioning of a drug to the several locations or compartments in the body or another **Heterogeneous System.**

Distribution Coefficient: The **Distribution Coefficient** designates the ratio of the *solubility* (or concentration) of a substance in an organic immiscible system to the solubility (or concentration) of the same substance in water when observed in the same system under the specified conditions st equilibrium.

3.5.1. *Volume of Distribution (V_d)*

The **Volume of Distribution (V_d)** is a **Biopharmaceutical Terminology** which specifically expresses the perceived volume of the body wherein a certain quantum of an **unchanged drug** (A_b) gets properly distributed depending on the ensuing **concentration (C_b)** of the drug present in the circulating blood. Importantly, $V_d = A_b/C_b$ designates a characteristic value for a particular drug-substance. Besides, 'V_d', represents an altogether **abstract volume** which may be easily *calculated from the ratio of the quantum of drug present duly in a human body to its actual concentration in plasma only when the partitioning has been stabilized adequately (i.e., at steady-state parameters achieved).*

In other words, the **Volume of Distribution** or perhaps more logically '**Apparent Volume of Distribution**' of a drug is neither literally nor actually a '**volume**'; and, therefore, it must not be regarded as a specific **physiological volume/space** present very much within the body. Thus, truly speaking, the apparent volume of distribution vividly designates the apparent volume into which a drug substance gets evenly distributed in the human body at equilibrium. Hence, in a broader perspective (apparent), **Volume of Distribution, V_d,** represents the **Volume of Plasma* at a drug concentration (C), needed essentially to account for the total quantum of drug present in the body (X).**

Thus, we have the following expression:

$$V_d = \frac{X}{C}$$ (bf)

---

* This is usually measured as plasma rather than blood.

$$\boxed{\text{Apparent volume of distribution} = \frac{\text{Amount present in body}}{\text{Plasma drug concentration}}} \tag{bg}$$

Advantages of V_d: There are *two* major advantages of Volume of Distribution (V_d), namely:

➢ Determination of the plasma concentration in a situation when a known quantum of a drug substance is duly present in the body, and

➢ Estimation of the critically required 'dose' so as to attain a given (or targeted) plasma concentration at time '*t*', *i.e.*, after a certain duration.

3.5.2. *Presence of a Fraction of Drug Both Inside and Outside Plasma*

From **Equation (bf)**, the amount of drug present in the **body** (X) is given by the **product of** V_d **and** C.

hence,

$$\boxed{\text{Amount of drug in plasma} = V_p \cdot C}$$

where,

V_p = Volume of plasma and

C = Plasma drug concentration.

$$\text{Fraction of 'drug' inside body plasma} = \frac{V_p \cdot C}{V_d \cdot C}$$

or

$$\boxed{= \frac{V_p}{V_d}} \tag{bh}$$

Likewise, fraction of 'drug' outside body plasma $= \dfrac{(V_d - V_p)}{V_d}$ (bi)

Remarks: Equation (bh) explains clearly that Greater the Volume of Distribution (V_d), the Lesser would be the Fraction of Drug Present in the Body Plasma.

3.5.3. *Determination of Plasma Volume*

There are *two* **chemical substances** (or *reagents*), *viz.* **Evan's Blue** and **Indocyanine Green**, both of which are *high-molecular-weight compounds*, which possess a unique characteristic feature of remaining essentially confined to the **circulating plasma in the human body on being administered** *via* **the IV route.**

Evan's Blue

Indocyanine Green

These *two* **reagents** are invariably employed to determine the **Plasma Volume** and **Blood Volume** accurately in a situation after the estimation of '**Hematocrit**'* Besides, the *anions, viz.* Cl- and Br- that readily and evenly get distributed throughout the **extracellular fluid but fail to cross over the cell-membranes rapidly may be employed justifiably to determine the following** *two* **values:**

- **extracellular water volume,** and   • **extracellular fluid volume.**

3.5.4. *Volume of Total Body Water (or Fluid)*

It can be determined with reasonably good accuracy by making use of:

- **heavy water or deuterated water (D_2O),** or
- **certain specific 'lipid-soluble compounds',** *e.g.*, '**Antipyrine**',

that gets distributed swiftly in the entire '**Total Body Water Fluid**'.

Table 3.9 provides the approximately percentage or volumes for various body compartments.

3.5.5. *Volume of Distribution (V_d) vs. Protein/Tissue Binding of Drugs*

It has been amply proved and established that the duly estimated '**Apparent Volume of Distribution**' for each of the tracers, *viz.* **plasma, extracellular fluid, intercellular fluid, vascular fluid** *etc.*, as expatiated above almost turns out to be very much similar to its '**True Volume of Distribution**', based on the glaring fact that are virtually negligible.

S. No.	Table 3.9. Components in Body Fluid Water		
	Components in Body	**Percentage (%) Approx**	**Volume (L) Approx.**
	Fluid Water		
1	**Plasma**	5	3
2	**Extracellular Fluid**	20	12
3	**Intercellular Fluid**	-	24
4	Vascular Fluid **(or Blood)**	-	6
5	**Total Body Water**	70	42
•	**plasma-protein binding,** and		
•	**tissue-protein binding.**		

---

* **Hematocrit**: It refers to the percentage of erythrocytes in a specified volume of whole blood. It desig- nates the ration of RBCs to plasma.

Salient Features: The various *salient features* are as follows:

1. A majority of **drug substances** are appreciably bound to
   - **vascular components,**
   - **extravascular components,** or
   - **both components.**

2. The **drug substances** that are bound significantly to the respective '**Plasma Proteins**' do exhibit '**Apparent Volumes of Distribution (AVD),** which are indeed lesser than the '**True Volume of Distribution**'. Besides, 'V_d' of this kind of drug substances actually ranges between the *two* components, namely: **Blood Volume** and **Total Body Water Volume,** *i.e.,* **6-42 L.**

Example

Warfarin has V_d~7L.

3. Such drug substances which have a tendency to get bound intimately and extensively to the *EV* **tissues** do exhibit the '**Apparent Volume of Distribution**' that appear to be larger in comparison to their **Actual Distribution Space.**

Example

Amitriptyline has V_d~1,400 L, which shows explicitly that the quantum of drug present in plasma happens to be very meager and small *vis-a-vis* the quantum present in the *EV* **compartments**, thereby suggesting broadly that the tissue concentrations of rug are definitely very high.

NOTE   In general, the '**apparent volume of distribution**' (V_d) implies that it is the most prominent characteristic feature of a drug and hence, may vary from 0.04 to more than 20 L kg^{-1}.

3.6. Organ-Specific Clearance

Clearance may be explained as a phenomenon that removes the **Chemical Compound (Drug)** completely by the kidneys or liver specifically from **a requisite volume of blood* per unit of time.**

Total Clearance: In general, the '**Total Clearance**' of a drug substance from the body almost invariably encompasses more than one organ of elimination. The *human body*, **the God-gifted anatomy,** is created in a manner such that the ensuing observed clearance from the composite clearing organs critically takes place in parallel; and, therefore, proves to be of an '**Additive Nature**'.

Example

In a situation when a drug substances gets duly eliminated either by renal and hepatic elimination, the '**Total Clearance**', designed as **CL$_T$,** of the drug substance may be expressed as

---

*   **Blood:** It refers to the fluid tissue that circulates via the heart, arteries, veins and capillaries, carrying oxygen and nutrients throughout the body

$$CL_T = CL_R + CL_H \qquad \text{(bj)}$$

where,

CL_R = Renal clearance, and

CL_H = Hepatic clearance.

3.6.1. Concept of Organ-Specific Clearance

It is indeed possible and a lot easier to have the **Concept of Organ Specific Clearance** duly visualized with the help of Figure 3.16.

Explanation

Figure 3.16 may be expatiated with the aid of the following sequential steps:

1. The '**drug substance**' is carefully introduced as a single dose into **Compartment 1** (*in beaker*), and from which it further gets portioned into **Compartment 2** (*in beaker*).

2. The '**drug solution**' is now circulated almost at a constant rate '**Q**' *via* **Compartment 3**, wherein the effective removal of the '**drug substance**' right from the solution designates **elimination.**

> **NOTE**   **At this stage, the aforesaid** 'extraction of the drug substance' **may or may not be complete at all.**

3. Importantly, the extent to which the effective extraction takes place is critically reflected by the actual difference observed between the following *two* components, namely:

   • C_{in}, *i.e.*, **concentration of the solution gaming entry into the 'Extracting Compartments',** and

   • **Cout, *i.e.*, concentration of the solution leaving the 'Extracting Compartment'.**

4. In a situation when the drug gets extracted almost completely, one would expect **Cout = 0;** and when none is extracted, one may have $C_{out} = C_{in}$.

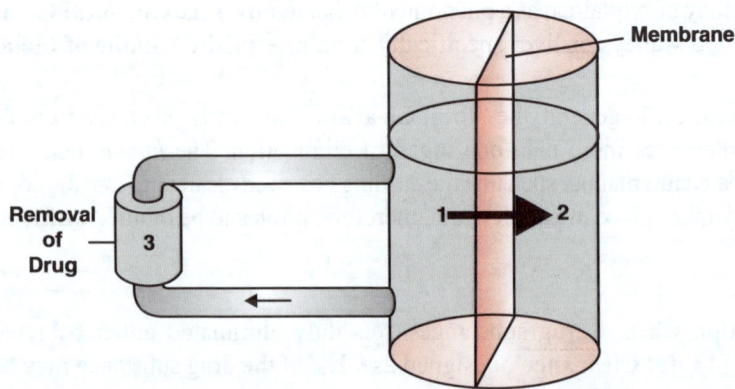

Fig. 3.16: Illustration of Organ-Specific Clearance Whereby Introduction of the Drug into Compartment I, from Which Drug Gets Distributed into Compartment 1. The solution being Circulated at a Constant Rate 'q' via Compartment 3 wherein Drug Undergoes Critical Removal from a Fixed Volume per unit time.

5. Ultimately, the prevailing limits for the critical concentration that leave Compartment 3 are as follows:

$$0 \le C_{out} \le C_{in}$$

Alternatively, the *three* terminologies, *viz.* **clearance, systemic clearance**, and **normalized systemic clearance**, may be explained as following:

Clearance [CL] is usually calculated soon after the IV administration (*i.e.*, 100% bioavailability) and may be expressed as

$$CL = \frac{D_{IV}}{AUC}$$

where,

D_{IV} = Amount of drug administered via IV route and

AUC = Area under the curve.

Systemic Clearance relates to **a single oral dose administration of a drug substance** (*with <100% bioavailability*) and is usually based upon **AUC ranging within time 0 → t (i.e., AUC)** Hence, the resulting **Trapezoid Calculation** is invariably given by the following expression:

$$CL = \frac{F \cdot D}{AUC_{0-t}}$$

where,

F = Fraction of the drug (dose) absorbed and

D = Dose of the drug administered.

Normalized Systemic Clearance refers to the body weight of a patient and may be suitably calculated with the help of the following expression:

$$CL_{Normalized} = \frac{CL}{Body\ weight\ (kg)}$$

3.6.2. Renal Clearance

Renal Clearance may be defined as **'removal by the kidney of a solute (or other substance) from a specific volume of blood per unit of time'.**

In other words, **Renal Clearance** refers to the ratio of the **Product of Urine Concentration of the Solute; and the Rate of urine Flow to the Plasma Concentration of the Solute.**

Fundamental Basis: A survey of literature reveals that the physiologists carried out an exhaustive study with regard to the renal clearance of both:

• **endogenous chemical entities,** and

• **exogenous chemical substances.**

much before the **recognition of the application(s) of the Clearance Concepts in Pharmacokinetics.** In fact, the wonderful revelations proclaimed by the renal physiologists, almost stretched over a few decades, paved the way for a better understanding pertaining to the **Clearance of Drug in Pharmacokinetics.**

It is important to state here that there exists *three* **most vital primary phenomena**, namely:

- **filtration,**
- **secretion,** and
- **reabsorption.**

Indeed metabolism designates actually a minor on-going phenomena. Interestingly, each of the aforesaid major phenomena is affected predominantly by several known **decisive factors.** Thus, the **Rate of Filtration (RF)** by the kidney for a drug substance is usually given by the following expression:

$$\text{Rate of filtration (RF)} = \frac{\text{GFR}}{C_U} \qquad \text{(bk)}$$

where,

$\qquad$ **GFR** = Glomerular filtration rate,

$\qquad C_U$ = Free-drug concentration.

Now, the observed clearance due to filtration is given by the '**quotient of the rate of filtration at a given concentration;** and, therefore, the renal clearance, CLR, of a particular drug substance caused due to filtration is given by the expression:

$$\text{CL}_R = (\text{GFR})\,(f_u) \qquad \text{(bl)}$$

where,

$\qquad f_u$ = Free-Fraction of drug.

From **Equation (bi)** one may obtain the renal clearance of a drug substance which gets eliminated only due to filtration and can be determined provided the following *two* **components** are known:

- **secretion,** and **glomerular filtration rate (GFR),** and
- **free-fraction of the drug substance.**

3.6.2.1. *Two Substance Used to Determine GFR*

Following *two* **substances** are commonly used to determine the **GFR** precisely, such as:

1. **Creatinine** *i.e.,* **an endogenous by product of muscle metabolism,** and
2. **Inulin** *i.e.,* **a polysaccharide substance.**

Importantly, it has been observed that both creatinine and inulin are essentially 100% eliminated in the urine due to filtration *via* the kidneys; and, therefore, the respective **CL values** of these *two* **aforesaid constituents** may be judiciously as the **reasonable acceptable estimates for the GFR.**

3.6.2.2. *Active Tubular Secretion (ATS)*

The **Active Tubular Secretion (ATS)** serves as another primary process closely involved in the renal elimination of drugs. In fact, there are quite a few active-transport systems prevailing in the proximal renal tubule which are solely responsible for the critical excretion of the drugs from the circulating blood into the urine. Interestingly, one may come across a *multiplying of systems for the ATS of both cations and anions.* There should always be a net tubular secretion together with the clearance by filtration in situation when the prevailing **Renal Clearance (CL$_R$)** comes out to be greater than:

- **product of GFR,** and
- **free fraction (f_u).**

Hence, the **Renal Clearance** due to **ATS (CL$_{ATS}$)** may be expressed by the following equation:

$$CL_{ATS} = \frac{(Q_{RP})(f_u CL_{u,s,int})}{(Q_{RP} + f_u\ CL_{u,s,int})} \qquad \textbf{(bm)}$$

where,

Q_{RP} = Effective renal plasma flow and

$CL_{u,s,int}$ = Unbound intrinsic secretary clearance.

Importantly, for such drugs which undergo both 'filtration' and '**Active Tubular Secretion (ATS)**', the actual **Renal Clearance (CL$_R$)** is given by the simple sum total of:

- **clearance due to 'filtration',** and
- **clearance due to 'secretion',**

which may be given as:

$$CL_R = (GFR)(f_u) + CL_{ATS} \qquad \textbf{(bn)}$$

3.6.2.3. *Kinetics of Urinary Excretion*

In a broader perspective, it is possible to obtain useful information(s) based upon the **urinary data pertaining to the elimination kinetics of a drug substance,** particularly in the absence of available plasma level time data. Therefore, the **kinetics of urinary excretion has several glaring advantages in the analysis of an established Pharmacokinetic System**. These essentially comprise the following:

1. It serves as a useful technique to determine precise concentration of drugs in plasma in the absence of a sensitive accurate procedure.

2. The present methodology is definitely a non-invasive procedure; and, hence, proves to be more patient (subject) friendly and improved patient compliance.

3. It is a lot convenient to collect '**urine samples**' at regular intervals in comparison to drawing blood samples periodically.

4. For estimating the '**urine-drug concentrations**' one may require a less sensitive method *vis-a-vis* the '**plasma-drug concentrations**'.

NOTE   In case, the urine-drug concentrations are found to be in a much lower range, assaying of 'Larger Sample Volumes' need to be carried out.

5. These generated data may help to determine in the effective computation of such vital factors:

- **First-Order Elimination,**
- **Excretion and Absorption Rate Constants,** and
- **Drug-fraction Excreted Unchanged.**

6. Besides, the **First-Order Metabolism** and/or **Extrarenal Excretion Rate Constant** may also be duly calculated accordingly from the difference:

$$\boxed{(K_E - K_C) = K_m}$$

where,

K_E = First-Order Constant of the elimination phenomenon, (or overall elimination rate constant).

K_C = Constant for the drug concentration and

K_m = Rate Constant for 'Hepatic Elimination' (*see Figure 3.8*).

7. Both **absolute and relative Bioavailability** can be measured directly; and this is quite possible without the necessity of the fitment of data into a known **Mathematical; Model.**

8. In association with the **Plasma Level-Time Data,** one may make use of the **Urinary Excretory Data** (or **Pharmacokinetics of Urinary Excretion**) in order to **estimate precisely the renal clearance of the unchanged drug,** as per the following expression:

$$\boxed{CL_R = \frac{\text{Total quantum of 'drug' unchanged}}{\text{Area under the plasma-level-time curve}}}$$

Computation of Volume of Distribution (V_d) and Renal Clearance (CL_R) from Pharmacokinetics of Urinary Excretion Data: It has been observed that if V_d is known, one may calculate the following *two* values easily:

- **total systemic clearance,** and
- **non-renal clearance.**

In actual practice, it may not be possible to compute the V_d and CL_R from the **Urine Data** exclusively. Nevertheless, the estimate **Renal Clearance (CL_R)** from **Pharmacokinetics of Urinary Excretion Data** may not be an **'Accurate Equivalent Substitute'** for the **Plasma Concentration-Level Data.** Therefore, the data obtained could be utilized judiciously as a more or less representation of a **Rough Estimate of the Pharmacokinetic Parameters'.** At this point in time, *two* **typical situations** may arise, namely:

- **Dosage Form:** showing an extremely **slow and sluggish drug-release pattern,** and
- **Drug Product:** exhibiting a very **prolonged biological half-life ($t_{1/2}$).**

Consequently, the ultimate **low-level of urinary drug concentration may** be too dilute for enabling a **precise determination of the 'drug' released.**

Importantly, in the second instance, *viz.* for such drug substances having a **Long Biological Half-Life ($t_{1/2}$),** one is required to collect urine output for several days at a stretch in order to determine the total drug excreted.

Factors for Generating Valid Renal Clearance (CL_R) from Pharmacokinetics (or Urinary Excretion Data Profile) Following are the 10 most important and critical factors that are invariably required for generating valid **Renal Clearance (CL_R)** based on the **Pharmacokinetic Evaluation Studies:**

1. Excretion of an appreciable quantum of drug in an unchanged form in the urine up to a level of at least 10%.

2. The selected '**Analytical Procedure**' for the assay of unchanged drug should be highly, and also it must not indulge in any sort of interference with the **ensuing metabolites.**

3. **Water-Loading:** The **Water-Loading** must be carried out by taking 400 mL of water soon after the overnight fasting so as to:

   - **Cause diuresis,** and
   - **Enable sufficient collection of required 'Urine Samples'.**

4. The underlying procedure needs to adopted rigidly:

   (a) **Before the actual administration of a drug, the urinary bladder should be emptied completely as far as possible, *i.e.*, up to a duration of 60 minute from water-loading.**

   (b) **The 'Urine Sample' obtained in (a) above is to be taken as the 'blank sample'.**

   (c) **'Drug' is now administered with 200 mL of water.**

   (d) **Ingestion of water may be followed by 200 mL at every hour on the hour, for the next 4 hr.**

5. **Healthy Volunteers** should be adequately instructed to empty their urinary bladders as completely as possible while collecting the respective '**Urine Samples**'.

6. More '**Frequent Sampling of Urine**' must be carried out so as to accomplish a reasonably '**Good Curve**'.

7. Precise time (duration) and volume (mL) of '**Urine Sample**' excreted must be noted carefully in the course of the sampling procedure.

8. Care should be taken that an '**Individual Collection Period Profile**' must not exceed one **biological half-life ($t_{1/2}$)** of the '**Drug Substance**' under investigation. It should be ideally much less.

9. Usually the urine samples should always be collected at least up to seven **Biological Half-Lives ($t_{1/2}$)** so as to ensure complete collection (**> 99.5%**) with respect to the excreted drug.

10. Ultimately, any change incurred in:

    - **pH of the urine,** and
    - **volume of urine collected,**

    may alter directly or indirectly the '**Urinary Excretion Rate**;.

Table 3.10 records the '**Urinary Excretion Data**; immediately followed by an IV bolus of 100 mg of a drug substance that essentially consist of *two* **separate criteria**, *viz.* **observation and treatment of data**. Thus, the various aspects of observations include:

- **number of samples collected,**
- **time (hr) of urine collection (*t*),**
- **volume of urine sample collected (mL), and**
- **concentration (mcg mL^{-1}) of unchanged drug in urine sample.**

Likewise, the various components of the treatment of data include perceptively:
- **urine collectioninterval (d*t* or Δ*t*),**
- **mid-point of urine collection (*t**),**
- **quantum of drug excreted in time interval ΔX_u,**
- **excretion rate (mg hr^{-1}) (or dX_u/d*t*),**
- **cumulative quantum of drug excreted (mg) X^t_u, and**
- **quantum of drug remains to be excreted ($X_u^\alpha - X_u^t$).**

NOTE	The various data duly calculated and recorded in Table 3.10 are processed in a systematic manner to arrive at an array of further valuable information.

Estimation of Elimination Rate Constant (KE) from Urinary Excretion Data:
In fact, the **First-Order Elimination (and/or Excretion) Rate Constant (KE)** may be easily computed from the urinary excretion data by either of the following *two* **methodologies**, namely:
- **excretion rate method,** and
- **Sigma minus method,**

which shall now be discussed briefly in the following sections.

Excretion Rate Method It refers to their *actual* **Rate of Urinary Drug Excretion, d*X*/d*t*,** which is proportional to the **quantum of drug '*X*' present in the human body,** and may be expressed as:

$$\frac{dX_u}{dt} = K_e X \tag{bo}$$

were,

K_e = **First-Order Urinary Excretion Rate Constant.**

Hence, according to the **First-Order Pharmacokinetics,** *i.e.,*

$$X = X_0 \cdot e^{-K_E t} \tag{bp}$$

where,

where K_E is the **Elimination Rate Constant.**

substituting **Equation (bp)** in **Equation (bo),** we may have

$$\frac{dX_u}{dt} = K_e \cdot X_0 \cdot e^{-K_E \cdot t} \tag{bq}$$

where,

X_0 = Dose of drug administered (*via* **IV bolus**).

Transforming **Equation (bq)** into the corresponding '**log**' form, we have:

$$\log \frac{dX_u}{dt} = \log K_e \cdot X_0 - \frac{K_E t}{2.303} \tag{br}$$

Table 3.10 Urinary Date Immediately Followed by IV Bolus of 100 mg of a 'Drug Substance'.

No. of Samples	Time of Urine Collection (hr)	Volume of Urine Sample Collected (mL)	Concentration of Unchanged Drug in Urine (mcg mL^{-1})	Urine Collection Interval dt or Δt	Midpoint of Urine Collection (t^*)	Quantum of Drug Excreted in time Interval (ΔX^t_u)	Excretion Rate (mg hr) dX_u/dt	Cumulative Quantum of Drug Excreted (mg) (X_u)	Quantum of drug Remains to be Excreted $[X^a_u-X^t_u]$
0	0	-	-	-	-	--	0	67.5	32.5
1	0-2	150	250	2	1	35	17.5	35	32.5
2	2-4	160	100	2	3	15	7.5	50	17.5
3	4-6	100	80	2	5	7.4	3.7	58.7	8.8
4	6-8	210	20	2	7	4	2	61.2	6.3
5	8-12	320	10	4	10	3.2	0.8	64.3	3.2
6	12-14	610	04	12	18	2.3	0.2	67.5	-

$$\downarrow$$
$$X^a_u$$

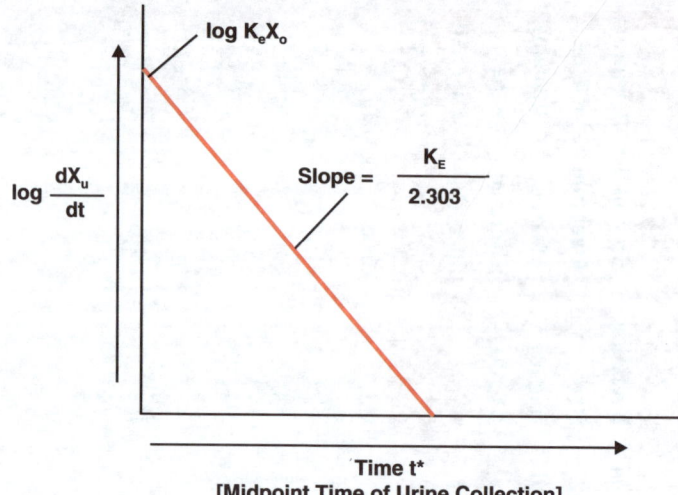

Fig. 3.17: Semi-Log Plot Rate of Excretion vs. Midpoint Time of Urine Collection Duration (t^*) for Computing the Elimination Rate Constant (K_E) after IV Bolus Administration of a Drug.

Obviously, the **Equation (br)** clearly states that the respective **Semi-Log Plot of the Rate of Excretion vs. Time Plot** shall give rise to a **straight line** having a **slope-K_E/2.303** as depicted clearly in Figure 3.17.

Explanation

Various aspects of *Figure 3.17* are expatiated as follows:

1. It should be considered that the **'slope'** duly obtained from a **Semi-Log Plot of an excretion Rate vs. Time Plot** is invariably related to:
   - **elimination rate constant K_E,** and
   - **certainly not to excretion rate constant K_a.**
2. However, one may duly obtain the **Excretion Rate Constant (K_E)** from the **Intercept on the Y-axis given by log $K_e X_o$.**
3. Thus, both K_E and K_e values may be judiciously employed to compute the following *two* **determinations effectively.**
   - **elimination half-life,** and
   - **non-renal elimination rate constant.**

Advantages of Excretion Rate Method: It has the following advantages, namely:

1. Drug substances with long inherent **Biological Half-Lives ($t_{1/2}$)**, the urine samples should be collected up to 3-4 half-lives only.
2. There is absolutely no necessity to collect **'all urine samples'** because the subsequent collection of **'any two consecutive urine samples'** usually gives rise to such valid points upon the excretion rate plot from which one may **easily construct a straight line (see Figure 3.17).**

Sigma-Minus Method It is possible to estimate the exact 'Cumulative Quantum' of the unchanged drug substance duly excreted in the urine sample up to anytime by integrating the following equation:

$$\frac{dX_u}{dt} = \frac{K_e K_a F X_0}{(K_a - K)} (e^{-Kt} - e^{-K_a t}) \qquad \text{(bs)}$$

where,

K_a = First-Order Rate Constant for drug absorption,

F = Fraction of the drug absorbed, and

K = First-Order Rate Constant for drug elimination.

Integrating **Equation (bs)** between the limits of 't' ranging between '0' and 't', we have the following expression:

$$\int_0^t dX_u = \int_0^t \left[\frac{K_e K_a F X_0}{K_a - K} \right] (e^{-Kt} - e^{-K_a \cdot t}) \, dt$$

or

$$X_u^t - X_u^0 = \frac{K_E K_a F X_0}{(K_a - K)} \left[\frac{e^{-Kt}}{-K} + \frac{1}{K} - \left(\frac{-e^{-K_a \cdot t}}{-K_a} + \frac{1}{K_a} \right) \right] \qquad \text{(bt)}$$

where,

X_u^0 = Cumulative quantum of drug substance duly excreted in urine at $t = 0$ equals 'zero'. Therefore, by simplifying **Equation (bt)**, we may have:

$$X_u^t = \frac{K_E F X_0}{K} + \frac{K_E K_a F X_0}{(K_a - K)} \left(\frac{-e^{-K_a \cdot t}}{K_a} + \frac{e^{-Kt}}{K} \right) \qquad \text{(bu)}$$

Plot of X_u^t vs. Time (t): A carefully drawn **plot of X_u^t vs. shall normally provide the so-called Urinary Excretion Curve** as illustrated in *Figure 3.18*.

Thus, at a specific situation when the 'Total Drug' has ultimately been duly excreted from the body, i.e., at $t = \alpha$, Equation (bu) gets reduced to:

$$X_u^\alpha = \frac{K_e F X_0}{K} \qquad \text{(bv)}$$

where,

X_u^α = Total amount of unchanged drug duly excreted in urine at an **infinite time (i.e., t_a).**

Therefore, one may quite judiciously and skillfully develop an 'appropriate equation' which critically describe the amount of the drug to be excreted vs. time based on **Equations (bu) and (bv).**

Furthermore, the total amount of an unchanged drug excreted in time at **an infinite time (i.e., ta)** given by X_u^α **minus the amount of drug being excreted in time 't' (i.e., X_u^t)** is represented by the following equation:

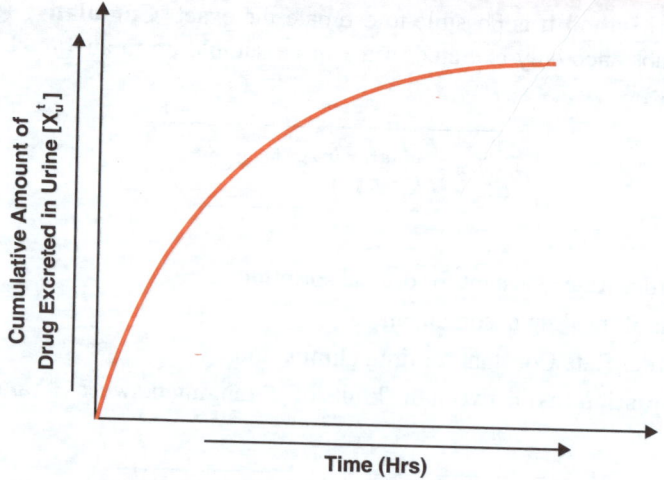

Fig. 3.18: A Plot between Cumulative Amount of Drug Substance Excreted in Urine *vs.* Time.

$$X_u^\alpha - X_u^t = \frac{X_u^\alpha}{(K_a - K)} (K_a \cdot e^{-Kt} - K \cdot e^{-K_a t})$$ **(bw)**

Pharmacokinetic Parameters of a Drug: A plot of log X_u^t *vs.* *t* is usually employed to calculate the ensuing **Pharmacokinetic Parameters** of a drug, as described in Figure 3.19.

However, the residual line may be drawn by using the method of residuals, the slope of which is found to be equivalent to $-K_a/2.303$. hence, in **Equation (bv)**, if the values of *F* and X_o are known, one may calculate 'K_e' quite easily.

Practice Problems: Let us look into the following *two* representative practice problems:

Problem I: Ceftizoxime was administered to an adult subject at a dose of 2 g *via* IV route, and was duly advised to consume *two* glassfuls of water at the time of administration and again 2 hr later so as to induce urination. Eventually, the 'subject' voided at two different intervals, *viz.* 2.5 and 7 hr. The urine sample collected at 2.5 hr contained 1.44 g of ceftizoxime, and the one collected at 7 hr contained 490 mg. the observed serum concentration (mgL) as a function of time was found to be described by the respective 'bi-exponential equation'.

$$C = 64.8\, e^{-3.5 hr^{-1}t} + 83.8 e^{-0.47 hr^{-1}t}$$

(i) **What would be the actual calculated renal clearance values for each of the two urinary excretion time intervals?**

Solution: As we know that $CL_R = At/AUC$, where both **At and AUC** designate specifically the stipulated time duration.

Hence, at 2.5 hr: AUC (0-2.5 hr) = 141.7 mgL^{-1}

$\therefore$
$$CL_R = \frac{1440}{141.7} = 10.16 \text{ L hr}^{-1}$$

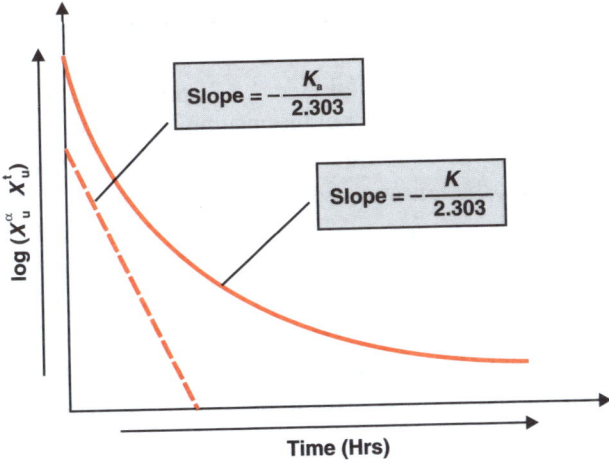

$$\text{Slope} = -\frac{K_a}{2.303}$$

$$\text{Slope} = -\frac{K}{2.303}$$

Fig. 3.19: A Plot between log $(X_u^a - X_u^t)$ *vs.* Time (hr).

$$CL_R \; \frac{10.16 \times 1,000}{60} = 169.3 \text{ mL m in}^{-1}$$

Likewise, at 7 hr: AUC (2.5-7 hr) = 48.5 mg L^{-1}

∴

$$CL_R \; \frac{490}{48.5} = 10.1 \text{ L hr}^{-1}$$

or

$$CL_R \; \frac{10.1 \times 1,000}{60} = 168.3 \text{ mL m in}^{-1}$$

(ii) What will be the corresponding 'Total Body Clearance' and 'f_u' values?

Solution It is known that the **Total Body Clearance (CL_T):**

$$CL = \frac{\text{Total amount of 'drug' unchanged}}{\text{Area under the plasma-level time curve}}$$

$$= \frac{2,000}{196.8} = 10.16 \text{ L hr}^{-1} = 169 \text{ mL m in}^{-1}$$

i.e.,

$$CL = 169 \text{ mL m in}^{-1}$$

since,

$$CL = CL_R; \text{ hence } 'f_u' \approx 1$$

Problem 2: A 'drug substance' is administered *via* IM route to a healthy subject and the following two data obtained (Table 3.11):

- **plasma concentration of the drug substance (mg mL) and**
- **time (hr)**

Calculate the absorption rate constant and order of the absorption process precisely from the above data.

Solution: The **Wagner-Nelson Method** (*see 4.3.2 under Part III in this section*) may be applied for the assessment of the exact order of the ensuing absorption phenomenon. It also helps in the calculation of the Absorption Rate Constant.

In this particular instance, the following equation is employed:

$$\frac{A_t}{V_d} = C_t + K \int_0^t C \cdot dt$$

First of all a **semi-log plot between plasma drug concentration *vs.* time must be prepared;** and, therefore, the **'slope'** of the so-called **'Terminal Linear Segment of the Plotted Graph'** is found to be equivalent to $\left[-\dfrac{K}{2.303} \right]$:

Table 3.11. Time *vs.* Plasma Drug Concentration	
Time (hr)	**Plasma Drug Concentration (mg mL^{-1})**
0.25	0.65
0.50	1.2
0.75	1.8
1.0	2.4
1.5	3.5
2.0	4.4
3.0	6.0
6.0	5.5
12.0	2.4
18.0	0.9
24.0	0.5

i.e.,

$$\text{Slope} = 0.0651$$

$$K = 0.0651 \times 2.303 = 0.15 \text{ hrs}$$

The **Biological Half-Life ($t_{1/2}$)** is calculated as follows:

$$t_{1/2} = \frac{0.693}{0.15} = 4.62 \text{ hrs}$$

On the basis of the above *two* given values, *e.g.,* **Plasma Concentration of the Drug Substance (mg mL)** and **Time (hr),** one may calculate the following determinations, such as:

$$\int_0^t C \cdot dt; \quad K \int_0^t C \cdot dt; \quad \frac{A_t}{V_d}; \quad \text{and} \quad \frac{A_\alpha}{V_d} - \frac{A_t}{V_d}$$

All these six determinants are arranged together in Table 3.12.

Explanations of 3rd to 6th Columns in Table 3.12: These specified columns may be further expatiated as below:

3rd Column $\left[\int_0^t C \cdot dt\right]$: It clearly exhibits the area under the **Curve (C)** *vs.* **Time Curve** duly calculated in a sequential manner right from $t = 0$ to each steps of the time points by the help of the recognized Trapezoidal Rule.

4th Column $K \int_0^t C \cdot dt$: It vividly shows that each of the preceding areas multiplied **by K**.

5th Column [A_t/V_d]: It refers to the sum total of the values given in the **2nd** and **4th Columns** as per the following expression:

$$\frac{A_t}{V_d} = C_t + K \int_0^t C \cdot dt$$

However, $\dfrac{A_\alpha^*}{V_d}$ is the maximum value in the **5th Column (10.00).**

Table 3.12. Values of Six Determinants Present in Plasma Drug Concentration

Time (hr)	Plasma Drug Concentration (mg mL⁻)	$\left[\int_0^{t_r} C.dt\right]$	$K \int_0^{t_r} C.dt$	$\dfrac{A_t}{V_d}$	$\left[\dfrac{A_a}{V_d} - \dfrac{A_t}{V_d}\right]$
0.25	0.65	0.1	0.02	0.67	0.38
0.50	1.2	0.3	0.05	1.25	0.75
0.75	1.8	0.7	0.11	1.91	8.09
1.0	2.4	1.2	0.18	2.58	7.52
1.5	3.5	2.6	0.39	3.89	6.21
2.0	4.4	4.5	0.68	5.08	5.02
3.0	6.0	9.7	1.45	7.45	2.54
.0	5.5	27.1	4.07	9.57	0.33
12.0	2.4	50.8	7.62	10.02	0.08
18.0	0.9	60.4	8.06	9.96	0.04
24.0	0.4	64.4	9.645	10.0044	-

6th Column $\left[\dfrac{A_\alpha *}{V_d} - \dfrac{A_t}{V_d}\right]$: It evidently shows the ensuing **residual existing between** A_a/V_d and A_t/V_d (*i.e.*, **each sequential value in the 5th Column**).

Now, plot the graphic representation between the following pairs, namely:

- **value in the 6th Column *vs*. time**, and
- **log of values in the 6th Column *vs*. time.**

Thus, *two different situations* may arise at this point in time:

Situation 1: When the absorption phenomenon obeys the **First-Order Kinetics**, one may eventually obtain the '**Semi Log Plot**' as a straight line having a **slope** of $-\dfrac{K_a}{2.303}$.

Situation 2: When the **Absorption Phenomenon** critically follows a **Zero-Order Kinetics**, the resulting '**Cartesian Plot**' shall invariably give rise to a **straight line having the slope equivalent to the respective Zero-Order Rate Constant.**

NOTE	**Importantly, in this particular instance, one may obtain a straight line having the 'Cartesian Plot'. Therefore, the ultimate absorption phenomenon rigidly follows the *Zero-Order Kinetics*.**

Remarks: These essentially comprise the following:

1. The aforesaid example depicts clearly the usefulness of the **Wagner-Nelson Calculation** for examining critically the exact mechanism of release profile of drugs from '**dosage forms**' **in *vivo*.**

2. **First-Order Phenomenon** is usually observed due to the **drug absorption from a solution;** whereas, any deviations from it evidently shows the **Release Pattern of the Dosage Form**.

3.6.3. *Hepatic Clearance*

Hepatic Clearance is also known as the **Hepatic Elimination of Drugs.**

Extraction Ratio (E): It refers to **the ratio of the rate of drug elimination and the rate at which the drug gains entry into the organ of elimination**. The extraction ratio designates a measure of the efficiency with which an organ of the human body actually eliminates a given drug.

Table 3.13 provides the **Hepatic and Renal Extraction Ratios** of certain important *drug substances and their respective metabolites.*

Thus, the **Organ Clearance of a Drug** may be defined as – '**the product of blood flow to the organ (Q), and the respective extraction ratio (E).**

---

* Where, $\dfrac{A_\alpha^*}{V_d} = 10.\,0$, which is the actual amount of drug absorbed from the dosage from up to time (a) divided by the volume of distribution (V_d)

Hence, the equation for the **Hepatic Clearance (CL$_H$)** is expressed as:

$$CL_H = Q_H \cdot E$$ (bx)

where, **Q$_H$ is the hepatic blood flow.**

Equation (bx) may suggest that a closer look at this '**Simple Model**' meant for **Hepatic Clearance (CL$_H$)** would be directly proportional to the respective **Hepatic Blood Flow (Q$_H$)**. However, this conclusion may not prove to be absolutely correct since the **Extraction Ratio (E)** varies inversely with **Q$_H$**. Based on the above cited facts and observations, it may be inferred that for both *qualitative and quantitative predictions of the* '**Hepatic Drug Clearance**', it must require a definitely *more* **Complex Model for Hepatic Clearance.** In fact, one may actually look for such a parameter which has got to be quite independent of any physiological factor(s).

The various types of '**Models**' have been duly proposed and tested to provide adequate mechanism for the **Hepatic Clearance of Drug Substances** which are as follows.

3.6.3.1. *Venous Equilibrium Model of Hepatic Clearance*

It has exhibited a *significant* **advantageous utility** in the critical and precise prediction of:

- **pathophysiological,** and
- **drug-induced profile.**

Table 3.13. Hepatic and Renal Ratio (*E*) of Certain Important Drug Substances and Their Respective Metabolites

S. No.	Mode of Extraction	Calculated Extraction Ratio (*E*)		
		Low	**Intermediate**	**High**
1.	**Hepatic Extraction**	Diazepam, Phenobarbitone, Phenytoin, Procainamide, Theophylline	Aspirin, Codeine, Nortriptyline, Quinidine	Propranolol, Lidocaine, Nitroglycerine, Morphine Isoprenaline
2.	**Renal Extraction**	Digoxin, Furosemide Atenolol, Tertracycline	Penicillin's (selected ones) Cimetidine	Penicillin's (selected ones) Hippuric Acid Sulphated Drugs (Several Procainamide, drugs) Glucuronides

alteration in the overall hepatic clearance. Importantly, in the **Venous Equilibrium Model,** the ultimate *hepatic extraction* is usually given by the following expression:

$$E = \frac{f_{ub}\ CL_{u,int}}{Q_H f_{ub}\ CL_{u,int}}$$ (by)

where,

f_{ub} = Unbound fraction in blood, and

$CL_{u,int}$ = Unbound intrinsic hepatic clearance.

In true sense, **Unbound Intrinsic Hepatic Clearance ($CL_{u,int}$)** evidently reflects the inherent ability of the liver to help in the removal of drug from blood in the absence of several other **Confounding Factors,** *viz* Q_H and fub. As it has already been demonstrated that the **Hepatic Clearance is the product of Q_H and *E*, hence, we may have the following expression:**

$$CL_H = \frac{(Q_H)\,(f_{ub} \times CL_{u\cdot int})}{Q_H f_{ub} \times CL_{u\cdot int}} \tag{bz}$$

Equation (bz) designing a '**Model for Hepatic Clearance**' essentially give rise to a reasonably powerful tool for predicting such vital alterations in:

- **drug clearance,** and
- **steady-state drug concentrations,**

in typical conditions when somne limiting parameters are dealt with. Following are *two* **specific instances,** such as:

    (a) **when $Q_H \gg f_{ub}$, $CL_{u.int}$, CL_H may be duly approximated by fub.$CL_{u.int}$,** and

    (b) **when $Q_H < f_{ub}.CL_{u.int}$, CL_H may be approximated by Q_H.**

Important points These essentially comprise the following:

1. **Drugs with a High f_{ub},$CL_{u.int}$ Values:** These are believed to show an obvious **Perfusion Rate-Limited Elimination,** *i.e.,* their respective **Elimination Rate** shall be exclusively limited by **hepatic blood flow.**

2. **Drugs with a Low f_{ub},$CL_{u.int}$ Values:** These are found to be absolutely independent of the **Perfusion Rate.**

Consequently, these limiting conditional ties imposed on drugs do permit us to put together several drug substances into such classified categories which predominantly show '**Identical Pharmacokinetic Parameters**'.

Examples

Following are *two* **typical examples,** namely:

Agents having an fub, $CL_{u.int} < 0.2$ L. min: These are usually classified as '**Low Intrinsic Clearance Drug Substances**'.

Agents having an f_{ub}, $CL_{u.int} > 5$ L. min: These are invariably defined as-'**high intrinsic clearance drug substances**'.

S. No.	Drugs with Low Intrinsic Clearance (f_{ub}, $CL_{u.int}$ <0.2 L. min)
\multicolumn{2}{c}{**Table 3.14. Typical Examples of Drug Substances Having Low and High Intrinsic Clearance which get Terminated Largely via Hepatic Metabolism***}
1	Antipyrine
2	Barbiturates
3	Diazepam
4	Digoxin

5	Phenytoin
6	Theophylline
7	Tolbutamide
8	Warfarin

S. No.	Drugs with High Intrinsic Clearance (f_{ub}, $CL_{u.int}$ > 5 L min)
1	Chlorpromazine
2	Encainide
3	Meperidine
4	Metroprolol
5	Propafenone
6	Propranolol
7	Tricyclic Anti-depressants
8	Verapamil

[* *Adapted From*: German AR. **Remington: The Science and Practice of Pharmacy**, 20th ed., Vol. II. Lippincott New York: 2010.]

The various specific examples of drug substances having both low and high intrinsic clearances which are duly **Eliminated** *via* the **Hepatic Metabolism** are given in *Table 3.14*.

Importantly, the venous equilibrium model for hepatic clearance represents prominently an extremely important and useful means to the precise assessment of the critical impact of all possible alterations in the **Protein-Binding Phenomenon** upon the so-called '**Hepatic Clearance**'. Reviewing **Equation (ca)** with particular reference to a drug substance showing a distinctly low intrinsic hepatic clearance, one may observe changes in the protein binding that would ultimately cause proportional changes in the hepatic clearance. Interestingly, this kind of a '**Drug**' is believed to show restrictive clearance, which means the unbound (or free) drug is largely available for clearance by the liver.

Likewise, the corresponding **High Intrinsic Hepatic Clearance Drug Substances** are found to show **Non-Restrictive Clearance.**

3.6.4. *Extra Hepatic/Non-Renal Elimination*

Enough experimental evidences have mostly affirmed the glaring fact that not only the drugs but also the **Xenobiotics** and their respective **Metabolites** are invariably excreted by such routes other than hepatic and renal. Therefore, the aforesaid '**other routes**' of elimination are usually termed as **Extra Hepatic/Non-Renal (or Extra Renal) routes of elimination.** These are essentially represented by the following means of elimination:

- **biliary excretion,**
- **exhalation,**
- **foecal excretion,**
- **intestinal excretion,**
- **excretion *via* saliva/skin,** and
- **excretion *via* milk,**

which will now be treated individually in the following sections.

3.6.4.1. *Biliary Excretion*

Biliary Excretion may be defined as 'elimination of intact drug molecules or this metabolites in the bile secretions into the GI tract where either reabsorption and/or excretion in the faeces may take place'.

It is, however, pertinent to state here that the biliary excretion is usually regarded to be the most important as well as a complementary route to both renal/hepatic elimination.

Mode of Action: The **bile production takes place by the hepatic cell lining and bile canalaculi**. First of all, the blood emanated from GI tract passes via **'liver'** which serves as the **Predominant Site of Metabolism'**. Besides, **'liver'** is responsible for the removal of:

- **drug substances,** and
- **respective metabolites,**

that may be eventually excreted in the bile before they gain access right into the general circulation.

Salient Features: These essentially include:

1. Transportation of drug substances and their respective metabolites from blood to bile happens to an **'Active Phenomenon'**.

2. Invariably, relatively **bigger drug molecules (mw>250-300)** are duly excreted via the biliary excretion.

3. **Biliary excretion** designates an extremely vital route of elimination for the specific **conjugated chemical entities (or compounds)**.

Classification of Substances Excreted *via* Biliary Excretion: In fact, these specialized substances are duly categorized into the following ***three*** classes that are solely based upon their ratio of concentration present in **Bile *vs.* Plasma.**

Class A: Substances that belong to this particular class have a **'ratio of 1'** (*i.e.*, **the ratio of concentration in bile *vs.* plasma stands at 1**). *Examples are:* **Na, K, Cl, glucose, Cs, Co, Hg and thalliumj (Th).**

Class B: Substances that belong to the specific class have a **'ratio >1'**, and it ranges between 10 and 1,000. Examples are: **bile acids, bilirubin, Pb, As and Mn.**

Class C: *Substances* that belong to this class have a **'ratio <1'**. *Examples are:* **Zn, Fe, Au, Cr, inulin and albumin.**

NOTE	1. **The Class B compounds invariably designates a large segment of such drug substances which are duly excreted by the *Biliary Excretion'*.** 2. **In reality, these compounds are excreted exclusively by means of the *'Active Transport Mechanisms'*. That is, mechanism by which such compounds belonging to either *Class A and/or Class C* normally get excreted remains to be understood completely.**

Important Features: There are two important features pertaining to the hepatic excretory mechanisms, and biliary excretion pattern, which shall now be treated briefly as under:

- **Hepatic Excretory Mechanisms:** It has been duly observed that in neonates:* That is, **newborn up to 4 weeks of age** the ensuing hepatic excretory mechanisms are not found to be developed completely on account of which certain drug invariably exhibit glaring 'toxicity'.

Quabain is a *cardiotonic* **Drug** which clearly exhibits 40-folds more toxicity specifically in neonates in comparison to the adult rats.

Ouabain

- **Biliary Excretion Pattern:** It distinctly shows appreciable variation in the biliary excretion pattern due to species; and consequently, the extrapolation of data derived from animals to humans is rendered extremely difficult to accomplish.

The release pattern of **Indomethacin, an Anti-inflammatory, Antipyretic**, and **Analgesic Drug,** usually gets excreted up to **3.8% in dogs**; whereas, monkeys excrete up to **33.6% to bile**. Besides, **52.1% gets excreted in dogs**; whereas, **monkeys excrete up to 33.6% in bile**. Amazingly, **52.1% gets excreted in dogs in the Phase II metabolite of Indomethacin; whereas, only 8.1% gets excreted in monkeys**.

Indomethacin

Enterohepatic Circulation of Bile Salts Generally, the drugs ad their respective metabolites gain entry into the duodenum *via* the common bile duct, and ultimately pass into the small intestine. In doing so, the drugs may get reabsorbed into the body from the intestine. Importantly, there are certain drugs that will be categorically reabsorbed right into the main blood steam and hence, return to the liver by the so-called **Enterohepatic**** as illustrated in *Figure 3.20*.

In this manner, the drug substance undergoes

- **further extensive metabolism, and**
- **ultimately secreted right into bile.**

---

*   **Enterohepatic**: It refers to the intestines and liver circulation of the bile salts,

**   **Neonate**: That is, **newborn upto 4 weeks of age**

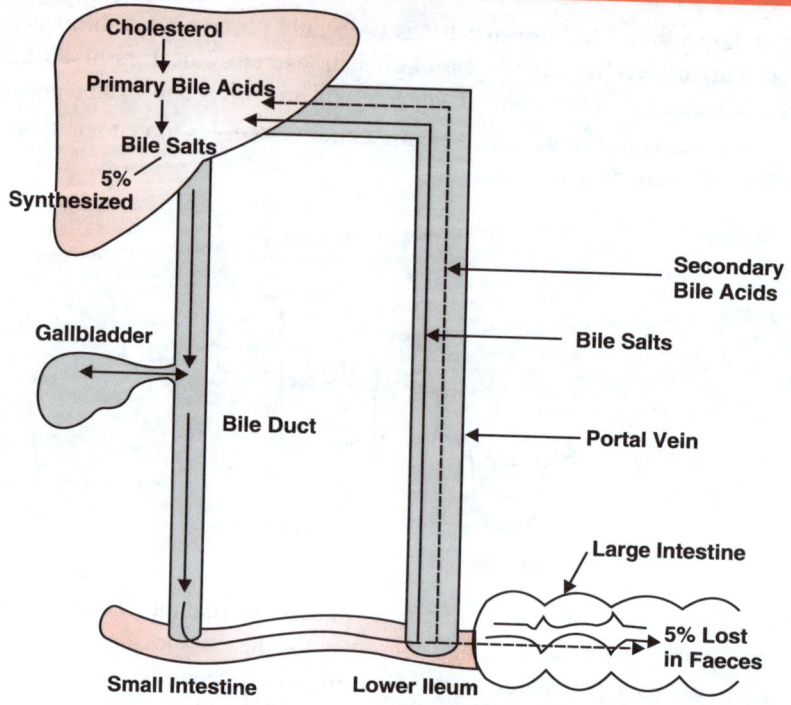

Fig. 3.20: Diagrammatic Representation of the Enterohepatic Circulation of Bile Salts. [*Adapted and Modified From*: Ward JPT *et al*. Physiology at a Glance. Blackwell Publishing, Oxford, U.K.: 2005]

And the above *two* **on-going phenomena** are usually termed 'Enterohepatic Cycling', which may eventually help in a big way in extending the duration of action of a drug substance.

Consequences of Enterohepatic Circulation: The *two* **major consequences of Entrohepatic Circulation** are as follows:

1. The '**drug**' soon after being secreted into the bile would be finally reabsorbed as an 'active' drug.

2. The '**active**' drug may be re-eliminated into the bile and get reabsorbed.

As a consequence of aforesaid sequel of events, the ensuing 'circulation' of drug substances that get actively secreted right into the bile may be eliminated primarily right from the human body via the kidneys.

Examples

Ampicillin, Penicillin, Sulpha-Drugs and the like.

Biliary function can be monitored and assessed by means of the drug **Sulphobromophthalein Sodium (a diagnostic aid for hepatic function)** is found to be eliminated more or less completely as the **parent drug in bile**.

3.6.4.2. *Exhalation**

In fact, **Exhalation** (or **Pulmonary Excretion**) is solely responsible for the critical excretion of both **gases and volatile products** *via* lungs. There are *two* **prominent roles** played mainly for the **excretion of drug substances *via* lungs**, namely:

- plasma-drug concentration, and
- blood-gas partition coefficient.

Nevertheless, the **excretion of drug substances *via* lungs** is caused exclusively due to the phenomenon of '**Simple Diffusion**'.

Examples-These essentially include:

Chloroform, Ethanol (in **Acoholic Beverages**), and **Halothane**.

Besides, it may also be observed critically that:

- gases having low solubility exhibit rapid excretion, and
- gases with high solubility in blood exhibit rather slow excretion.

Factors Influencing Exhalation: These essentially comprise the following:

1. **Pulmonary blood flow,**
2. **Rate of respiration,** and
3. **Solubility.**

3.6.4.3. *Foecal Excretion*

It has also been duly established that the **Foecal *Excretion-Designates as one of the most important routes of elimination of drug substances; and their respective metabolites.***

Following are the several recognized sources for the **Foecal Excretion**, for instance

- unabsorbed drug substances,
- biliary excretion, and
- intestinal excretion.

Interestingly, the **Actual Excretion via Faeces** is found to be absolutely of a direct nature for:

- certain specific drugs, or
- respective metabolites having little absorption or incomplete absorption.

Example

Quaternary ammonium compounds, Sucrose, Polymers (polyesters), and Cholestry-ramine:

The aforesaid **unabsorbed portion of drugs,** solely contribute to the *actual Foecal Excretion due to their inherent restricted intestinal absorption.*

In short, the **Foecal Excretion** is by virtue of the on-going **Biliary Excretion** episode.

---

* **Exhalation:** It refers to the phenomenon of breathing out (*i.e.,*) just opposite of inhalation.

3.6.4.4. *Intestinal Excretion*

In a broader perspective, the **Intestinal Excretion** is mostly important for such drug substances that predominantly possess such aspects:

- **low rates of metabolism,**
- **low renal clearance,** and
- **low biliary clearance.**

Examples

There are *two* **vital types of drugs,** namely:

- **Organic Acidic/Basic Drugs:** They do exhibit an **'Active Secretion'** specifically in the intestine, such as: **Quinine**-*an anti-malarial drug;* **Nicotine**-*an agent used for treatment of smoking –withdrawal syndrome.*
- **Drugs with Diverse Chemical Properties:** They do exhibit 'slow intestinal excretion' into the faeces, for instance: **Digitoxin**-*a Cardiotonic drug:* **Hexachlorobenzene**-*an industrial antiseptic (withdrawn since 1994 because of carcinogenicity. Dioxin (TCDD)- as defoliant in Vietnam during the 1960s, and since banned due to its carcinogenicity in 1994).*

3.6.4.5. *Excretion via Saliva/Skin*

The critical excretion of drug *via* saliva and skin (sweat) is largely due to the **'Passive Diffusion'** of the *lipid-soluble drugs.* It has been established beyond any reasonable doubt that both **Drug Substances,** and their respective **Metabolites** that are solely excreted *via* sweat are believed to cause various types of **dermatological manifestations,** such as:

- **Urticaria-** a vascular reaction of the skin duly characterized by transient eruption of slightly elevated patches which appear to be most pale or more red than the surrounding areas.
- **Dermatitis-** inflammation of the skin characterized by weeping vescicles and/or dry sealing, and,
- **Allergic Disorders-**relate to the skin rashes, severe itching (causing redness of the skin).

Example

The typical examples of **Drug Substances** that are invariably *excreted via skin (sweat)* are **Pb, Hg, Ethanol** and **Antipyrene.**

Drugs Excreted *via* **Saliva**: In true sense, the **'Basic Drugs'** are usually excreted more abundantly in saliva *vis-a-vis* the **'Acidic Drugs'**. Through most of the drug substances are duly excreted in saliva due to the **'Passive Diffusion'**, yet quite a few of them are largely secreted in the saliva actively, such as: *Penicillin, Phenytoin* and *Lithium (Li)*.

| NOTE | Drugs and their metabolites that are excreted mainly via saliva are swallowed frequently thereby enabling the entire phenomenon of absorption of the drug to start afresh. |

Sweat (Skin) Testing of Drugs is carried out for the *specific identification* of 'Drug Abuse'. **Saliva Testing of Drugs** is carried out for the **Ingestion of Narcotics**, *e.g.*, **Cocaine, Opiates, Marijuana, Amphetamines, Methamphetamines,** and **Phencyclidine.**

3.6.4.6. *Excretion via Milk*

Generally, the **Excretion of Drug Substances and their Metabolites** into the 'Milk' proves to be of great importance and concern due to the following vital reasons:

- **Every possible danger of drugs to be transferred right from 'mother' to 'infant' is through breast feeding,** and
- **Drugs excreted in cow's milk may be directly ingested by humans,** *e.g.*, **Oxytocin.**

Importantly, the critical *transfer of Drug Substances from* **Plasma to Mother's Milk** is mainly caused due to the **inherent Passive Diffusion Process; and,** therefore, solely depends on such vital factors as:

- **pK_a of the drug,**
- **pH partition existing between plasma (pH 7.4) and milk (pH 6.6),**
- **plasma concentration of the drug,**
- **lipoidal solubility profile of the drug,** and
- **molecular weight of the drug.**

Important Points: These essentially consist of the following:

1. The presence of C_a **and Fat in Milk** enable the **'Lipophilic Drugs'** to undergo *chelation* with the former and get **excreted in the milk duly.**
2. The inherent *acidic nature of Milk* in comparison to plasma, renders the weakly basic drugs to concentrate more easily in milk.
3. Excessively **High Plasma Protein** Drugs actually demonstrate relatively less secretion in **Milk,** *viz* **Diazepam.**

> **NOTE**
>
> **The actual quantum of drug substance being excreted in the breast milk is invariably in extremely small amounts but it may possibly affect a 'suckling infant' who possesses specifically:**
> - **lesser ability to metabolize the drug** and
> - **allow it to be excreted from the infants body.**

3.7. NON-LINEAR PHARMACOKINETICS

3.7.1. *Preamble*

A good number of **Therapeutically Effective Drugs** *vis-a-vis* their ensuing 'Pharmacokinetics' may be expatiated satisfactorily based upon its **First-Order Kinetics** or **Linear Kinetics.** Nevertheless, one may come across quite a few drugs that predominantly exhibit

- **Non-Linear Absorption Profile,** *e.g.*, **Ascorbic Acid,**
- **Non-Linear Distribution Pattern,** *e.g.*, **Naproxen,** and
- **Non-Linear Elimination trend,** *e.g.*, **Riboflavin.**

As we know that in the specific instance of **First-Order Kinetics** or **Linear Kinetics,** one may critically observe changes in the prevailing **Plasma-Drug Concentration** *vs.* **Time (hr)*** and are invariably found to be *directly proportional to the dose of the drug administered.* Therefore, such **Plots** (*see Figure 3.6*), *i.e.,* more appropriately 'Semi-Log Plots of Plasma Drug Concentration' *vs.* Time' shall become super imposable when necessary corrections have been duly incorporated for the '**Administered Doses of the Drug**'. Thus, the aforesaid phenomenon is invariably termed as the '**Principle of Superimposition**'.

Besides, it may be noted categorically that in such typical instances, the following **Pharmacokinetic Parameters,** for instance:

- **Volume of Distribution (V_d),**
- **Elimination Rate Constants (K_E),**
- **Plasma Half-Life ($t_{1/2}$),** and
- **Hepatic Claerance (CL_H),**

are generally found to be absolutely independent of the *actual dose of drug being administered.*

3.7.2. Michaelis-Menten Equation

The **Michaelis-Menten Equation** is also termed as the **Dose-Dependent Kinetics.** It has been duly observed the several **biological phenomena** are precisely mediated by the following *two* **vital aspects,** *viz.,*

- **enzyme systems,** and
- **transport carrier system.**

Obviously, the aforesaid *two* **systems** have restricted capacities; and, therefore, are rendered to be quite '**Saturable in Nature**'. Thus, the **Kinetic Profiles** of these undergoing phenomena are amply elaborated and described by the **Michaelis-Menten Equation,** which may be expressed as follows:

$$-\frac{dC}{dt} = \frac{V_{max} \times C}{K_m + C}$$

(cc)

where,

$-dC/dt$ = Rate of decline of drug concentration with regard to time,

V_{max} = Theoretical maximum rate of the on-going process and

K_m = Michaleis-Menten constant.

3.7.2.1. *Accounting for Deviation of Michaelis-Menten Equation*

A survey of literature would reveal that first and foremost the **Michaelis-Menten Equation** was duly employed in the investigative studies of 'Enzyme Kinetics'.

Enzyme + Substrate $\underset{K_2}{\overset{K_1}{\rightleftharpoons}}$ **Enzyme substrate complex** $\overset{K_3}{\longrightarrow}$ **Enzyme + Product**

---

*   It is due to **absorption, distribution, metabolism and elimination (ADME)** of the drug administered

Symbolically, the above may be represented as:

$$E + S \underset{K_2}{\overset{K_1}{\rightleftharpoons}} [ES] \xrightarrow{K_3} E + P \qquad \text{(cd)}$$

At this particular point in time, we may have to ascertain *three* **important assumptions,** namely:

- **ES represents a Steady-State Complex.**
- **At 'Saturation of an Enzyme',** *i.e.,* **when the substance concentration remains higher** *vis-a-vis* **enzyme concentration, all enzymes generally found as ES-complex,** and
- **Prevailing 'saturated parameters' the ultimate rate of formation of the product shall always be maximum** *i.e.,* $V_{max} = K_3 [ES]$.

At equilibrium, *i.e.,* at a steady state, we may have the following expression:

where

$$V_{\text{Formation of ES complex}} = V_{\text{Cessation of ES complex}}$$

$$V_{\text{Formation of ES complex}} = K_1 \cdot [E] \cdot [S]$$

$$V_{\text{Cessation of ES complex}} = K_2 \cdot [ES] + K_3 [ES]$$
$$= [ES](K_2 + K_3)$$

Hence, we may have:

$$K_1 \times [E][S] = [ES](K_2 + K_3) \qquad \text{(ce)}$$

On dividing **Equation (ce)** K_1, we have:

$$[E] \cdot [S] = [ES]\left[\frac{K_2 + K_3}{K_1}\right] \qquad \text{(cf)}$$

As we know that:

or

$$K_m = \frac{K_2 + K_3}{K_1}$$

where, K_m = **Michaelis-Menten Constant**

Equation (cf) may now be written as:

$$[E] \times [S] = [ES] \times K_m$$

or

$$[E] = K_m \times \frac{[ES]}{[S]} \qquad \text{(cg)}$$

It is known that [E] is the **concentration of free enzymes** *i.e.,* the quantum of enzyme actually available for the ensuing reaction, and hence, it may be expressed as:

$$[E] = [E_t] - [E_c]$$

where,

$[E_t]$ = **Concentration of total enzyme** and

$[E_c]$ = **Concentration of enzyme present in [ES]-complex.**

In this manner, **Equation (cg)** may be written as

$$[E_t] - [E_C] = K_m \times \frac{[ES]}{[S]} \qquad \text{(ch)}$$

Equation (ch) may be divided by **[ES]** to obtain:

$$\frac{[E_t] - [E_C]}{[ES]} = \frac{K_m}{[S]}$$

or

$$\frac{[E_t]}{[E_C]} - 1 = \frac{K_m}{[S]}$$

or

$$\frac{[E_t]}{[E_C]} = 1 + \frac{K_m}{[S]}$$

or

$$\frac{[E_t]}{[E_C]} = \frac{[S] + K_m}{[S]} \qquad \text{(ci)}$$

Interestingly, at this critical stage, two situations may arise namely:

Situation 1: When 'Enzyme' is saturated': It means that when the substrate concentration is higher than the corresponding enzyme concentration. Thus, we may have:

$$[E_t] = [ES]$$

Besides, the rate of the reaction is **maximum (V_{max}).).** We have already seen earlier that:

$$V_{max} = K_3 \cdot [ES]$$

Therefore,

$$V_{max} = K_3 \cdot [E_t]$$

or

$$[E_t] = \frac{V_{max}}{K_3} \qquad \text{(cj)}$$

Situation 2: When 'Enzyme' remains unsaturated: It indicates that the substrate concentration is lower in comparison to the respective enzyme concentration. Thus, we may have:

$$[E_t] \neq [E_C]$$

But,

$$V = K_3 \cdot [ES]$$

or

$$[ES] = \frac{V}{K_3}$$ (ck)

Therefore, we may have the following expression:

$$\frac{[E_t]}{[E_C]} = \frac{V_{max}/K_3}{[ES]}$$

or

$$\frac{[E_t]}{[E_C]} = \frac{V_{max}/K_3}{V/K_3}$$

or

$$\frac{[E_t]}{[E_C]} = \frac{V_{max}}{V}$$

Now, on the basis of the above derivations, **Equation (cK)** may be written as:

$$\frac{V_{max}}{V} = \frac{K_m + [S]}{[S]}$$

or

$$\frac{V_{max}}{V} = \frac{[S]}{K_m + [S]}$$ (cl)

or

$$V = \frac{V_{max} \times [S]}{K_m + [S]}$$ (cm)

Thus, **Equation (cm)** designates the **Michaleis-Menten Equation**

3.7.2.2. *Graphical Representation of Michaelis-Menten Equation*

The 'Non-Linear Pharmacokinetics' essentially involves as a necessary consequence '*V*' as the **Rate of Change of Drug Concentration (-d*C*/d*t*), and 'S' as drug concentration (C).**

Figure 3.21 illustrates the graphical representation of **Michaelis-Menten Equation.**

Figure 3.21 clearly reveals that types of **'Reaction Kinetics'** as follows:

- **First-Order Kinetics [Marked 'X']:** It may be observed that at the initial stages, where low dose levels prevail, the **change in drug concentration (-d*C*/d*t*)** is found to be linear with respect to **change in total concentration.**
- **Mixed-Order Kinetics [Marked 'Y']:** In this instance one may observe **an increase in concentration, (-d*C*/d*t*)** that is seen to be neither 'linear' nor 'independent' *vis-a-vis* the ensuing alteration in the total concentration.
- **Zero-Order Kinetics [Marked 'Y']:** ultimately, when the **total concentration** remains to be very high (*i.e.*, **high-dose levels**), **(-d*C*/d*t*)** is found to be absolutely independent of the prevailing **total concentration of the drug substance.**

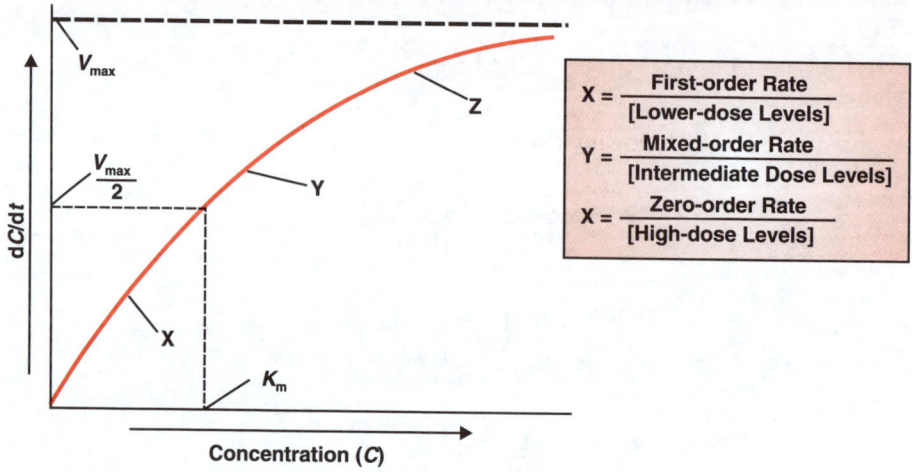

Fig. 3.21: A Graphical Plot Showing the Michaleis-Menten Equation.

Let us take into consideration the following *three* **typical situations:**

Situation 1: When $K_m = C$:

Here, **Equation (cc)** becomes

$$-\frac{dC}{dt} = \frac{V_{max} \times C}{2 \times C}$$

or

$$-\frac{dC}{dt} = \frac{V_{max}}{2} \qquad \text{(cn)}$$

In other words, the **Michaelis-Menten constant, K_m,** is equivalent to the drug concentration at which:

- **rate of process,** or
- **rate of reaction**

is almost equal to one-half of the '**Theoretical Maximum Rate**' of the reaction.

Situation 2: When $K_m > C$:

It shows evidently that K_m is reasonably greater than C, therefore, for the sole purpose from a practical angle, we may have the following expression:

$$K_m + C \simeq K_m$$

If that is so, **Equation (cc)** will be rendered to

$$-\frac{dC}{dt} = \frac{V_{max} \times C}{K_m} \qquad \text{(co)}$$

However **Equation (co)** is very much akin to the first-order elimination of the drug substance, wherein, the **First-Order Rate Constant $K_E = V_{max}/K_m$.**

Observations: There are *three* **important observations** from the above statement of facts:

- **Elimination:** The critical elimination of an array of drugs invariably follow the **First-Order Reaction Kinetics,** which suggests explicitly that '**the plasma-drug concentration prevailing at the site of reaction remains lower than K_m**'.
- **Exceptions:** The aforesaid phenomenon do have certain glaring exceptions, *e.g.*, **Ethanol, Salicylates,** and **Phenytoin**.
- **Deviations:** There are certain prominent deviations duly observed in certain typical case of drug toxicities, which could eventually result from the '**abnormally high concentration of drug**' in the body.

Situation 3: When $K_m < C$:

In other words, the drug concentration is found to be sufficiently greater than K_m. therefore, for practical purposes, we may have:

$$\boxed{K_m + C \simeq K_m}$$

Thus, **Equation (cc)** becomes

$$\boxed{-\frac{dC}{dt} = V_{max}} \qquad \text{(cp)}$$

Based on **Equation (cp),** one may conclude that the '**rate of reaction**' usually comes into play at a **constant rate** V_{max}, and the former is found to be absolutely independent of the drug concentration. Hence, it is more or less identical to the **Zero-Order Kinetics'**.

Example

Ethanol and its respective metabolism process.

3.7.3. *Drug Elimination by Capacity-Limited Process*

Let us look into the typical instance when an **IV administered drug** in a subject gets adequately eliminated by means of the **capacity-limited process.**

Equation (cc) is as:

$$\boxed{-\frac{dC}{dt} = \frac{V_{max} \times C}{K_m \times C}}$$

Rearranging **Equation (ca),** we have:

$$\boxed{V_{max} \times dt = -\frac{dC}{C}(C + K_m)} \qquad \text{(cq)}$$

Integrating **Equation (cq),** we get

$$\boxed{V_{max} \cdot t + I = -C - K_m \cdot \ln C} \qquad \text{(cr)}$$

where, **I = Integration constant.**

Now, at **Time** $(t) = 0$, $C = C_0$; and hence, we have:

$$\boxed{I = C_0 - K_m \cdot \ln C} \qquad \text{(cs)}$$

Substituting **Equation (cs)** in **Equation (cr)**, we get:

$$t = \frac{(C_0 - C)}{V_{max}} + \frac{K_m}{V_{max}} \left(\ln \frac{C_0}{C} \right) \qquad \text{(ct)}$$

Changing to the '**Common Logarithm**' we may obtain:

$$\log C = \log C_0 + \frac{(C_0 - C)}{2.303 \, K_m} - \frac{V_{max}}{2.303 \, K_m} \qquad \text{(cu)}$$

However, from Equation (cu) one may get a plot between **Log Plasma Drug Concentration** *vs.* **Time (*t*)**, which would give rise to a curve having its *terminal linear segment* with a slope equivalent to $V_{max}/2.303 \, K_m$ as illustrated in *Figure 3.22*.

NOTE	In the drug elimination phenomenon by the capacity-limits process, one may conveniently calculate the two kinetic parameters, V_{max} and K_m, by various laid down techniques.

3.7.4. *Important Recognized Plot Variants in Non-Linear Pharmacokinetics*

· There are, in fact, *four* **Important Plot Variants** with regard to the **Non-Linear Pharmacokinetics**, namely:

- **Lineweaver-Burk Plot (or doubled-reciprocal plot),**
- **Hanes-Woolf Plot,**
- **Woolf-Augustinsson-Hofstee Plot,** and
- **Direct Linear Plot,**

which will be treated individually in the following sections.

3.7.4.1. *Lineweaver-Burk Plot (or Doubled-Reciprocal Plot)*

The **Lineweaver-Burk Plot** refers to-'**the straight-line plot obtained when the reciprocal of the velocity of an enzyme reaction is plotted against the reciprocal of the substance concentration**'. In other words, it designates the straight line duly obtained from the reciprocal of the **Michaelis-Menten Equation** and is also known as the '**Doubled-Reciprocal Plot**'.

In the course of an intensive prolonged research, it becomes almost necessary and important to estimate precisely the **Rate of Change of Plasma-Drug Concentration with Time**. Therefore, in order to accomplish the critical objective, the '**Blood Samples**' are normally withdrawn at different pre-determined time intervals and ultimately, the data is plotted graphically. Thus, one of this most abundantly utilized plot is termed as the **Lineweaver-Burk Plot**. It is a plot of *two* entities:

$$\frac{1}{dC/dt} \quad vs. \quad \frac{1}{C_m}$$

(where C_m represents the plasma-drug concentration at the midpoint of the ensuing 'Sampling Profile')

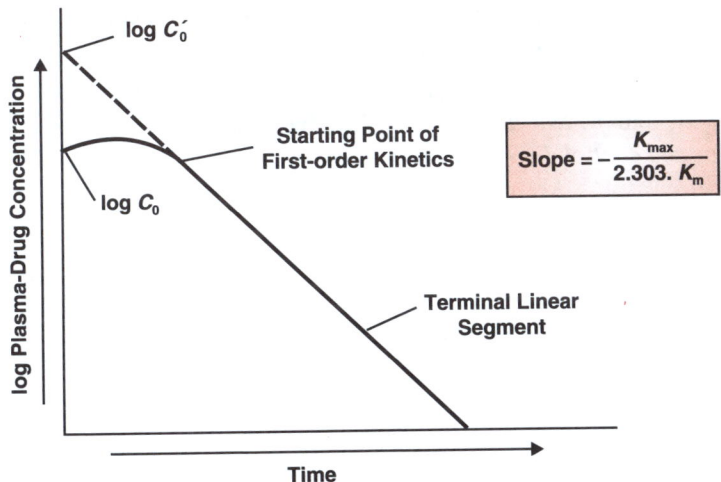

Fig. 3.22: A Plot between Plasma-Drug Concentration *vs.* Time (hr) Drug being Administered *via* IV Route with Capacity-Limited Process.

Figure 3.23 depicts the graphical representation of the **Lineweaver-Burk Plot.** Let us take the reciprocal of **Equation (cc):**

$$\frac{1}{dC/dt} = \frac{K_m}{V_{max} \cdot C_m} + \frac{1}{V_{max}} \qquad \textbf{(cv)}$$

(where C_m **is the plasma-drug concentration at the midpoint of the sampling interval).**

Now, a plot of the **Reciprocal of dC/dt vs. Reciprocal of C_m** gives rise to a *straight line* (*Figure 3.23*) having the following *two* **components:**

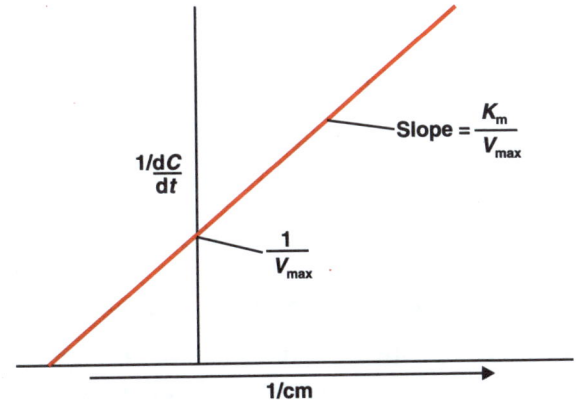

Fig. 3.23: Graphical Representation of Lineweaver-Burk Plot (or Doubled-Reciprocal Plot).

$$\boxed{\begin{array}{c} \textbf{Y-Intercept} = 1/V_{max} \quad \textbf{and} \\ \textbf{Slope} = K_m/V_{max} \end{array}}$$

Variants in Lineweaver-Burk Plot: There are *three* **prominent variants** in the **Lineweaver-Burk Plot** which shall be treated separately in the following sections:

1. **Identification of Competitive Enzyme Inhibition:** *Figure 3.24(a)* shows a plot between **1/V and 1/(D),** wherein the *two* **extrapolated lines from the point of intersection,** *i.e., each for the inhibitor and control diverge from each other.*

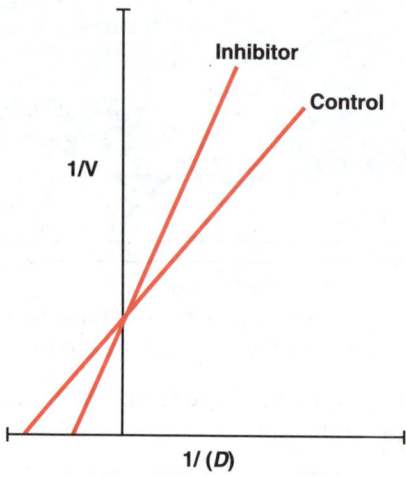

Fig. 3.24(a): Lineweaver-Burk Plot to Identify Competitive Enzyme Inhibition.

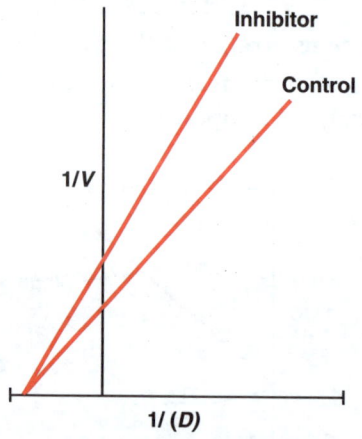

Fig. 3.24(b): Lineweaver-Burk Plot to Non-Identify Competitive Enzyme Inhibition

2. **Identification of Non-competitive Enzyme Inhibition:** *Figure 3.24 (b)* depicts a plot between **1/V and 1/(D)** wherein the *two* **extrapolated lines** from the points of interception on the **Y-axis (*i.e.,* 1/V, inhibitor and control, diverge from each other.**

3. **Identification of Uncompetitive Enzyme Inhibition:** *Figure 3.24 (c)* illustrates a plot between **1/V and 1/(D),** wherein the *two* **extrapolated lines** from two different point on the **X-axis (*i.e.,* 1/CD) have *two* points of intersection on the Y-axis (*i.e.,* 1/V) that are almost parallel to each other.**

3.7.4.2. *Hanes-Woolf Plot*

It has been observed that many a times in the **Doubled-Reciprocal Plot, the 'Plotted Points'** appear to be too closed to one another. Hence, to circumvent this sort of problem, the **Hanes-Woolf Plot** is employed.

It is solely based on the following equation:

$$\left[\frac{C_m}{dC/dt}\right] = \frac{K_m}{V_{max}} + \frac{C_m}{V_{max}} \tag{cw}$$

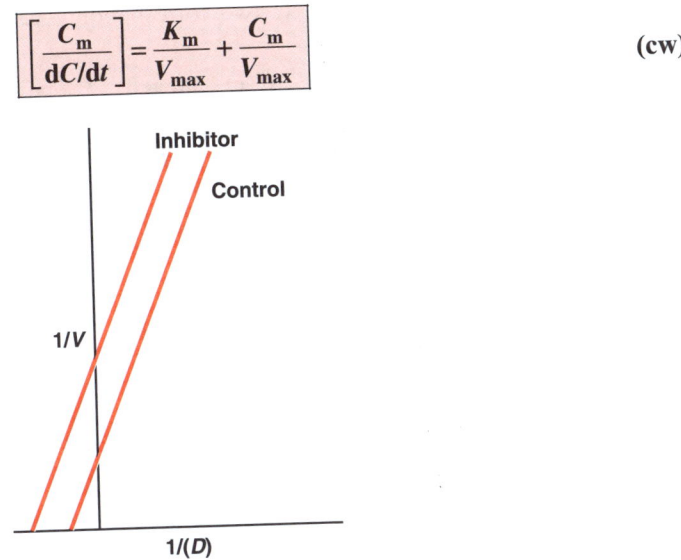

Fig. 3.24 (c) Lineweaver-Burk Plot to Identify Uncompetitive Enzyme Inhibition.

Equation (cw) is duly formed by the rearrangement of **Equation (cv)**. Hence, based on **Equation (cw)**, the observed plot of $\frac{Cm}{dC/dt}$ *vs.* C_m shall turn out to be a **straight line having the following** *two* **components.**

$$\text{Slope} = 1/V_{max} \quad \text{and}$$
$$\text{Y-Intercept} = K_m/V_{max}$$

3.7.4.3. *Woolf-Augustinsson – Hofstee Plot*

In a further attempt to overcome the appearance of **Doubled-Reciprocal Plot** and the **Closeness of 'Points'**, the **Woolf-Augustinsson-Hofstee Plot** came into being. It is exclusively based on the following equation:

$$\frac{dC}{dt} = V_{max} - \frac{(dC/dt) \cdot K_m}{C_m} \tag{cx}$$

Now, based on **Equation (cx)** the *graphical plot* of $\frac{dC}{dt}$ *vs.* $\frac{dC/dt}{Cm}$ will appear to be *straight line* having the following *two components*:

$$\text{Slope} = -K_{\text{m}} \quad \text{and}$$
$$\text{Intercept} = V_{\text{max}}$$

3.7.4.4. *Direct Linear Plot*

The **Direct Linear Plot** comes into being when *two* **altogether different dosing rates**, *viz.* DR_1 and DR_2, invariably give rise to two corresponding steady states designated as C_{ss1} and Css_2

Figure 3.25 clearly illustrates a '**Direct Linear Plot**' designating steady-state concentrations when the drug substance is duly administered at *two* **different rates.**

In Figure 3.25, the points between C_{ss1} and Dr_1 and C_{ss2} and DR_2 are carefully joined to obtain **straight lines.** Now, the point of intersection of these *two* **straight lines** is duly extrapolated along the **Y-axis** (*i.e.*, the DR-axis) to obtain V_{max}; and likewise along the **X-axis** (*i.e.*, the $C_{ss\text{-axis}}$) to get K_{m}.

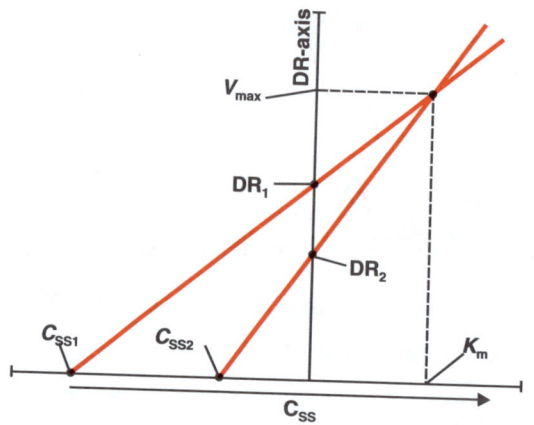

Fig. 3.25: A Direct Linear Plot Showing Steady-State Concentrations (C_{ss}) when Drug is Administered 1`at Distinctly *two* Different Rates.

3.8. Pharmacokinetic Profiles of Some Specific Examples from Various Classes of Drugs

Perhaps it would be worthwhile to examine the *reported* **Pharmacokinetic Profiles** of at least representative typical example belonging to the following **Class of Drugs** with particular reference to these cardinal aspects:

- **chemical structure, name, uses,**
- **pharmacokinetic profiles in animal models,**
- **experimental procedure,**
- **analytical protocol,**
- **results and discussion,** and
- **summary.**

Following are the selected **'Classes of Drugs'** that have been discussed briefly by citing the example of a specific example:

- **Antihypertensive,** *e.g.*, *Captopril,*
- **Antiarrhythmics,** *e.g.*, *Procainamide Hydrochloride,*
- **Antianginal drugs,** *e.g.*, *Nitroglycerine,*
- **Antineoplastic agents,** *e.g.*, *Fluorouracil,* and
- **Antibiotics,** *e.g.*, *Piperacillin Sodium*

The aforesaid **'Drugs'** have been treated individually in the following sections.

3.8.1. *Antihypertensives*

Captopril (Singhvi *et al.*, 1981)*

Captoril

-[(2S)-3-Mercapto-2-methyl-1-oxopropyl]-L-proline [= sites labeled with ^{14}C]

Brand Name: Capoten [Squibb].

Captopril is a potent, orally active, specific inhibitor of the enzyme that catalyzes the **Conversion of Angiotensin I to Angiotensin II.** It has been shown clinically to be an **effective antihypertensive agent.**

Pharmacokinetics of Captopril in Dogs and Monkeys: Captropil is a chemically unstable thiol compound in **Biological Samples** and undergoes *rapid auto-oxidation to form the disulfide dinner of the parent compound; and some other products.* To minimize such processes, **Captopril** was converted to its **N-Ethylmaleimide derivative in Blood, Urine and Bile during or immediately after sample collection.**

Experimental Procedure: Clinical Protocol-[^{14}**C] Captopril was universally labeled with carbon 14 in the Proline Moiety. A non-ionic surfactant (Triton X-14), a tissue solubilizer (Soluene-350), and N- Ethylmaleimide were used.** Other chemicals were reagent grade. Three male adult purebred **Beagles** (dogs) and three male adult **Rhesus Monkeys** were fasted overnight prior to the study, hydrated orally with water, anaesthesized with intravenous **Pentobarbital Sodium**, intubated with an endotracheal catheter and maintained under-anaesthesia by *constant intravenous infusion of Pentobarbital Sodium.*

Steady-state concentrations of unchanged **Captopril** in the blood were determined. Constant intravenous infusion doses were maintained for 4 hr in *three anaesthetized dogs and three anaesthetized monkeys.* [^{14}C] **Captopril** was infused, using a constant infusion pump after which **5% Manitol** was given, and the animal was kept under anaesthesia for an additional 6 hr.

---

* Singhvi SM *et al.: J. Pharm. Sci.,* **70** (10): 1108-1111, 1981

Urine and Blood samples were collected every **30 minute during [^{14}C] Captopril Infusion, for 3 hr after the end of infusion; and then every 1 hr for the next 5 hr.** A blood sample was withdrawn at the mid-point of each collection. All samples were tested with **N- ethylmaleimide; and analyzed for total radioactivity and unchanged Captopril.**

Analytical Protocol Blood and **Urine Samples** were analyzed using a **Thin-Layer Radiochromatographic Assay (TLRA)** for **Captopril.** This method is quite specific for unchanged **Captopril** and has a **limit of detection of 10 ng mL^{-1}**.

Results and Disscussion: The **Pharmacokinetic Profile** was evaluated exclusively on data obtained for unchanged **Captopril** in *blood, urine* and *bile* during the **Steady-State and the Post-Infusion Phase**. A **Semi-Logarithmic Curve** was obtained from the plot of concentrations of *unchanged* **Captopril** in blood versus time. **The bi-exponential decline of blood Captopril concentrations indicates that the drug exhibit characteristics of a *two*-compartment open model, with elimination occurring from the central compartment.**

The results of the various pharmacokinetic parameters were averaged for all three animals. The **Volume of Distribution [V_d] of Captopril was higher in the monkey (3.61 kg^{-1}) than in the dog (2.51 Kg^{-1}); the Volume of the Central Compartment (V_1) was about the same (0.51 kg^{-1}) for both species. The Values for Distribution Rate Constants (K_{12} and K_{21})** were comparable for both species. However, the overall **Elimination Rate Constant (K_{CL}) in the Monkey (2.6 hr^{-1})** was about twice that found in the **Dog (1.3 hr^{-1}) due to higher renal clearance in the monkey.**

The body and renal **Clearance Values (in mL kg hr^{-1}) of Captropil in the Monkey 1135 (CL$_T$), 944 (CL$_R$) were much greater than the corresponding values for the Dog 605 (CL$_T$), 341 (CL$_R$)**, primarily because **the net tubular secretion of Captropil was three times higher in the monkey than in the dog.**

The **Terminal Half-Life ($t_{1/2}\beta$) Value** was slightly higher in the **Dog than in the Monkey, 2.8 and 2.2** hr, respectively.

Summary: The disposition of **Captopril** in **Dog and Monkeys** following intravenous infusion of the drug was studied to gain a good understanding of **Captopril Pharmacokinetics**; and to provide information for **Properly Designing Pharmacokinetic Studies in Humans. Captopril** appeared to exhibit characteristics of **a *two*-Compartment Open Model** in both the **Dog and Monkey.** The difference between the total **Body Clearance and Renal Clearance of Captopril** in both species was primarily due to the **Metabolic Clearance of Captopril.** The large values of **Volume of Distribution (V_d)** obtained indicated extensive distribution of **Captopril** throughout the body.

3.8.2. *Antiarrythmics*

Procainamide Hydrchloride: [BP, BPC] (Kamath et al., 1981)*

Procainamide Hydrochloride

4-Amino-N-(2-diethylaminoethyl) benzamide hydrochloride.

* Kamath BL *et al.: J. Pharm. Sci.*, **70**: 667-669, 1981

Brand Names: Procan® (Parke-Davis); Pronestyl Hydrochloride® (Squibb).

Procainamide Hydrochloride is an effective **Antiarrythmic Drug.**

Pharmacokinetics of Procainamide and N-Acetylproclainamide in Rats: ^{14}C-Labelled Procainamide and ^{14}C-Labelled N-Acetylproclainamide (*the major metabolite of proclainamide in humans*) as hydrochloride salts were diluted with **Unlabelled Drugs.**

Clinical Protocol: Eight male rats were used as subjects. Each animal received **Procainamide** (75 mg kg^{-1}) and **N-Acetylprocainamide** (86 mg kg^{-1}) intravenously according to a *two*-way cross-over design. Four of the eight rats received **Procainamide** first, while the other four received N-Acetylproclainmide. The day before the drug was administered, a cannula was inverted into the jugular vein of each rat under light ether anaesthesia.

The **Drug Solutions** were administered intravenously through the jugular cannula after an overnight fast. Water was freely available at all times. **Serial blood samples (0.4 mL each)** were withdrawn at different time intervals after drug administration. After each withdrawl, 0.4-0.5 mL of normal saline containing 1% Heparin Solution was infused to replace the lost volume. **Plasma** was separated and frozen immediately. **Urine and Faeces** were collected for 48 hr and Frozen until they were assayed. The *second* phase of the study was performed after a **lapse of 3-7 days.**

Analytical Methods: The **Total Radioactivity** in Urine was determined directly via a **Liquid Scintillation Counter (Model 2425)**. The **Total Radioactivity** in the Faeces was measured after homogenization (**Polytron Homogenizer**), and combustion in an **Oxidizer (Model B306)**. The **Procainamide** and **N-Acetylprocainamide** concentrations in plasma and urine were determined by a specific **High Performance Lipid Chromatographic (HPLC) method.**

The **plasma concentration time plate** of Procainamide and N-Acetylprocainamide for each rat was fitted to **mono-and bi- Exponential Equations**, respectively, using **Non-Linear Least Squares Regression Analysis**. The **Elimination of N-Acetylprocainamide** is described by a *two*-**Compartment Open Model.**

Results and Discussion: After dosing with **Procainamide, 84% and 5%** of the *Total Administered Radioactivity* were eliminated in *Urine* and *Faeces*, respectively. **Forty-nine percent** of the amount recovered in urine was **Unchanged Procainamide,** and **20%** was **N-Acetylprocainamide**. As much a **31%** was excreted in an *unidentified form*. After dosing with **N-Acetylprocainamide 90.5%** and **3.2%** of the *Total Administered Radioactivity* were eliminated in *Urine and Faeces*, respectively. Of the amount recorded in urine, 80% of the dose was unchanged N-Acetylprocainamide and the remainder was unidentified. Only traces of **Procainamide** were found in the Urine of three rats after **N-Acetylprocainamide administration.**

The mean **Elimination Half-Life of the N-Acetylated Metabolite of Procainamides** was **2.22 hr**. The *mean values* for the **Biological Half-Life of Procainamide and N-Acetylprocainamide were 0.658 and 2.13 hr;** showing that **the latter was about three times the former value**. There was little difference in the values of the **Volume of Distribution of either drug-4.60 and 3.28 L kg^{-1}** for **Procainamide and N-Acetylprocainamide** respectively. The **Renal Clearance of Procainamide** was **1.92 L hr^{-1} kg^{-1}**, *twice as large as that of* N-Acetylprocainamide, **0.880 L hr^{-1} kg^{-1}.**

Summary: Procainamide (I) is metabolized partially to **N-Acetylprocainamide (II)** in rats but is **excreted mainly unchanged (~50% of the dose)** in the **Urine**. A small portion (3%-5%) of the intravenous dose of both drugs was eliminated in the **Faeces indicating Biliary Secretion** status perceptively.

The investigation of **Comparative Pharmacokinetics in rats** showed that the **Biological Half-Life of II is ~ *three* times longer than that of I in rats**. The **Volume of Distribution of** these drugs is quite similar. The **Renal Clearance of I** (1.92 L hr^{-1} Kg^{-1}) is twice as large as that for **II** (0.929 L hr^{-1} Kg^{-1}).

In summary, the **Elimination of I and II** when given individually to rats can be described by **one-and-two-Compartment Open Models,** respectively.

3.8.3. *Antianginal Drugs*

Nitroglycerine (McNiff *et al.*, 1981)*

$$CH_2ONO_2$$
$$|$$
$$H{-}C{-}ONO_2$$
$$|$$
$$CH_2ONO_2$$

Nitroglycerine

1,2,3-Propanetriol trinitrate

Brand Name: Nitroglyn® (Key Pharmaceuticals).

Other Names: Glyceryl Trinitrate, Glonoin, Trinitrin, Sublingual Nitroglycerine has been used extensively for the relief of acute attacks of **Angina Pectoris**. Recently, it was shown to be effective in patients with **Congestive Heart Failure (CHF)** following **Myocardinal Infraction.**

3.8.4. *Pharmacokinetics of Nitroglycerin after Intravenous Infusion in Normal Subjects*

3.8.4.1. *Experimental Procedure*

Clinical Protocol: Eight healthy, non-smoking male adult volunteers were used as subjects. Prior to this study and at least one week before receiving the **Nitroglycerine Infusion,** each subject was *pre-Screened for* Nitroglycerine Hypersensitivity by Sublingual Administration of 0.15 mg doses of Nitroglycerin (USP Tablets) at different times for a total dose of 0.6 mg. Subjects who did not show any **adverse reactions or nitrate hypersensitivity** were included. **Nitroglycerin Solution** was supplied in **10 mL ampules containing 5 mg of Nitroglycerin in a Buffered Solution of 10% ethanol. To 100 mL of Normal Saline (0.9%), 5 mL of this solution was added in a glass intravenous container just before use.**

Nitroglycerin Solution was infused into a *peripheral forearm vein through a* **Polyter Catheter (Angiocath) at a flow rate of 0.764 mL min^{-1} for 32 min.** Disposable plastic syringes, previously determined not to cause drug loss, were used to draw blood samples through a peripheral vein cannula in the arm not used for infusion. The cannula was then flushed with **Heparin (100 U mL^{-1}) in 0.9% Sodium Chloride.** Samples (5 mL) were drawn at 0 (*just prior to Infusion*) and at various times. The plasma was transferred **to silanized glass culture tubes,** immediately *centrifuged, separated* and *then placed on ice for storage at −20°C.*

---

* McNiff EF *et al.*: *J. Pharm. Sci.,* **70**: 1054-1058, 1981

Analytical Protocol Plasma Samples were assayed in duplicate according to GLC procedure.

Results and Discussion: Plasma Nitroglycerine Kinetics is characterized by rapid disappearance and an apparently large plasma clearance. The **Plasma Half-Life of Nitroglycerine** determined from this study was **2.8 ± 0.9 min**. This value indicates a result of both **Blood Degradation** and **Organ Metabolism of Nitroglycerin,** the latter most probably by the liver (**Maier** *et al.*, **1981**)*

The **Apparent Plasma Clearance** determined in this study ranged from **0.31 to 1.03 L min^{-1} kg^{-1} corresponding to values of total body clearance of 29.8-78.3 L min^{-1}.**

Substantial *inter-subject variability in* Nitroglycerin Kinetics was observed in this study. In certain subjects (but not all), the **Plasma Nitroglycerine Concentrations** approached apparent steady-state values.

By using the **Apparent Clearance Values** obtained, an apparent **Volume of Distribution of 3.3 ± 1.2 L kg^{-1}** can be estimated. Minor fluctuations in **Nitroglycerin** content in the **Non-plasma (tissue) Compartment**, which may result from a host of **Internal and External Stimuli,** could cause dramatic fluctuations in **Plasma Nitroglycerine Concentrations**.

The **Mean Half-Life Value of ~2.8 min reflects in vivo spontaneous blood degradation of Nitroglycerin in humans**. This *rapid degradation* is due to spontaneous hydrolysis or enzymatic breakdown of **Nitroglycerin**.

Summary: Eight normal subjects received a **dose of ~0.6 mg IV of Nitroglycerin at a rate of 18 mcg min^{-1}. Plasma Concentrations** of intact drug during and after the infusion were determined using a **GLC Method. Intra- and Inter-subject Variability in Nitroglycerin Plasma Kinetics was substantial.** Generally, **Plasma Nitroglycerin Disposition** was characterized by:

1. **A large Apparent Plasma Clearance**

$$(0.3 - 1\,\text{L min}^{-1}\,\text{kg}^{-1})$$

2. **A large Volume of Distribution**

$$(\sim 3\,\text{L kg}^{-1})$$

3. **A rapid Plasma Half-Life (~3 min).**

In conclusion, **Nitroglycerin Kinetics** is characterized by **Apparent Extensive Tissue Distribution and Rapid Plasma Clearance** perceptively.

3.8.5. *Antineoplastic Agents*

Fluorocuracil (Philips *et al.*, **1980)****

Fluorouracil
5-Fluoro-2,4 (1H, 3H)-pyrimidinedione

---

* Maier GA *et al.*: *J. Pharm. Sci.*, **70:** 1057, 1981.

** Philips TA *et al.*: *J. Pharm. Sci*, **69:** 1428-1431, 1980.

Brand Names: Efudex® (Hoffmann-La Roche); **Adrucil®** (Adria)

Fluorouracil is of *palliative value* in certain types of **Carcinoma**, particularly of the **Breast** and the **Gastrointestinal Tract (GIT)**.

3.8.6. PHARMACOKINETICS OF ORAL AND INTRAVENOUS FLUOROURACIL IN HUMANS

3.8.6.1. *Experimental Procedure*

Clinical Protocol: The subjects were 11 female patients undergoing therapy for **Breast Carcinoma** and **Postmastectomy**. The subjects were ambulatory and were being treated under the conditions of a multicentre trial to examine the *benefits of* **Cyclic Adjuvant Chemotherapy in both Node-Positive and Node-Negative Operable Breast Cancer. Node-Positive patients** received **Fluorouracil by intravenous injection**, while **Node-Negative patients** were **dosed orally**. Since each subject received either **Oral or Intravenous Fluorouracil**, it was not possible to examine **Fluorouracil Kinetics** after oral and intravenous doses in the same person.

Intravenous doses of 250 mg of Fluorouracil were administered in 5 mL of water for injection into a forearm vein over 30 s. **Oral Doses of Fluorouracil** were administered in 10 mL of water for injection followed immediately by 90 mL of orange juice. No dietary restrictions were applied. **Blood samples (10 mL)** were taken from a forearm vein in the arm, not used for drug administration in the intravenous study, and were placed in **Heparinized Tubes**. Plasma was promptly separated and stored at **-20°C** until it was assayed.

Analytical Protocol: Fluorouracil was extracted from plasma using a **High-Performance Liquid Chromatographic (HPLC) system**. The solvent was 10^{-2} **M Phosphate Buffer (pH 5.5). Uridine** was used as the **Internal Standard**. The lower limit of detection was **0.1 mcg mL^{-1}**, and neither commonly occurring **undersides nor drugs** other than **Fluorouracil** being taken by the subjects interfered with the *chromatographic peaks of* **Fluorouracil or Uridine**.

Results: Individual plasma levels of **Fluorouracil** were obtained from the **Intravenous and Oral Doses**. Following *intravenous dosing*, **Plasma Fluorouracil Levels** at the 5-min sampling varied from 6.4 to 29.5 mcg mL^{-1} with a mean value of 13.4 mcg mL^{-1}. **Drugs levels, declined monoexponentially. The Mean Half-Life of Fluorouracil in plasma was 6.3 min, the Mean Distribution Volume was 0.2 L Kg^{-1}, and the Plasma Clearance was 1410 mL min^{-1}.**

Following oral dosing, peak plasma levels of **Fluorouracil** ranged from **4.4 to 14.3 mcg mL^{-1}** with a *mean value of* **8.3 mcg mL^{-1}**. The **Mean Half-Life** of *Drug Elimination* was **7.2 min**, while the **Absorption Half-Life Time** was **3.4 min**. This value indicates fast absorption of **Fluorouracil** under the conditions employed in this study.

Discussion: The Mean Distribution Volume for Fluorouracil of 0.2 L Kg^{-1} and the Plasma Clearance of 1410 mL min^{-1} are consistent with previously reported values of 0.35 L Kg^{-1} and 1441 mL min^{-1} obtained in three patients (Garrett *et al.*, 1977)* and of 0.25 L Kg^{-1} and 1265 mL min^{-1} obtained in eight patients (McMillan *et al.*, 1978)**

---

*   Garrett ER *et al.*: *J. Pharm. Sci.*, **66**: 1422, 1977.

** McMillan WE *et al.*: *J. Pharm. Sci.*, **38**: 3479, 1978.

Cohen *et al.* (1974)* suggested that the nature of **Fluorouracil Absorpotion** may not only *depend on* the **vehicle with which the drug is administered but also be influenced by the degree of Hepatic involvement. Garrett *et al.* (1977**)** obtained prolonged plasma levels of **Fluorouracil** from plasma after oral and intravenous doses to patients with relatively normal liver function.

The results obtained in the present study are consistent with the **Hypotheses (Cohen *et al.*, 1974*Garrett *et al.*, 1977**)** Absorption of **Fluorouracil** from the oral doses to subjects who had no **discernible hepatic involvement** was efficient and rapid. Although the clinical protocol prevented intravenous and oral doses being given to the same subjects, thus, preventing direct comparisons within an individual, the plasma data nevertheless indicate that the **oral dose was approximately 28% available as unchanged drug.**

Furthermore, the data obtained in this study indicate that circulating levels of oral fluorouracil may be as reproducible between individuals as those obtained from intravenous doses.

Summary: The **Pharmacokinetics of Fluorouracil** was examined after *single* **250 mg intravenous doses** and **500 mg Oral Doses** to female patients with **Breast Cancer**. In five patients who received intravenous **Fluorouracil**, the mean plasma level of **Unchanged Drug was 13.4 mcg mL^{-1}**, the **Elimination Half-Life was 6.3 min**, and the **Plasma Clearance was 1410 mL min^{-1}**. In six patients who received oral fluorouracil, the mean peak value of unchanged drug in plasma was 8.3 mcg mL^{-1} and the elimination half-life was 7.2 min. The *Overall Bioavailability of* **Oral Fluorouracil** as unchanged drug was **28%**; and the variation in **Plasma Drug Levels** between individuals was similar following **oral and intravenous doses.**

3.8.7. *Antibiotics*

Piperacillin Sodium (Batra *et al.*, 1983)***

Piperacillin Sodium

Sodium (2S, 5R, 6R)-6-[(R)-2-(4-ethyl-2,3-dioxo-1-1piperazinecarbamido)-2-phenylacte-amidol]-3, 3-dimethyl-7-oxo-4-thia-1-azabicyclo [3.2.0] heptane-2-carboxylate.

Brand Name: **Pipracil**® **(American Cyanamid Co.)**

Piperacillin is a novel *semi-synthetic Pencillin* that possess broad spectrum anti-bacterial activity against *Gram*-**negative** and *Gram*-**positive pathogenic bacteria**, including **anaerobes**. In certain cases, a **Piperacillin** and **Gentamicin** *combination* would be preferred to obtain a **Synergistic Effect.** To evaluate the toxicity of these *two* **drugs when administered alone or in**

---

* Cohen JL *et al*: Cancer Chemother.Rep., **58**: 724, 1974.

** Garrett ER *et al.*: *J. Pharm, Sci.*, **66**: 1422, 1977.

*** Batra VK *et al.*: *J. Pharm, Sci.*, **72**: 894-898, 1983.

combination, a one-month study was undertaken in dogs. Since **Aminoglycosides** can interact with α-**LactamAntibiotics**, the study was designed to allow the serum concentrations to be *analyzed* **Pharmacokinetically**.

3.8.8. PHARMACOKINETICS OF PIPERACILLIN AND GENTAMICIN FOLLOWING INTRAVENOUS ADMINISTRATION TO DOGS

3..8.8.1. *Experimental Procedure*

Clinical Protocol: Six groups of 18-20 month-old **Beagle Dogs** (two males and two females in each group) were utilized for the study. The weight range was **9.4-12.3 kg for the males** and **7.9-9.6 kg for the females**.

Drug solutions, made prior to each dose, were administered twice daily (~5 hr apart) over a 5 min period with an **Infusion Pump (Respond, 2000)** calibrated using the **Specific Syringes, solutions** and **tubing employed**. Doses administered were adjusted to the body weight twice a week. The **concentration of Piperacillin Solution** in sterile water for injection, expressed as free acid, was **250 mg mL^{-1}**. The **Gentamicin Solution was made in concentrations of 1 and 2 mg mL^{-1} using sterile isotonic saline**. For drugs that received both drugs, the solutions of **Piperacillin** and **Gentamicin** were prepared independently and mixed in the infusion flow during administration.

Serum Samples were obtained from one dog per sex-group prior to infusion and at various times following the commencement of the infusion during the *First* (**Phase 1**) and *Last* (**Phase 2**) weeks of dosing. **Urine samples** were collected for two consecutive days from all dogs during the first and last weeks of the study.

Analytical Protocol: Antibiotic concentrations were determined by the **Disk Diffusion Method**. The *assays* **for Pipecerallin** were performed with **Sarcina lutea (ATCC 9341)** (*indicator organism*) *grown* on antibiotic **Medium No. 1^5** to which **0.6% sodium polyanethole sulphonate was added to inhibit Gentamicin activity. The limit of detection was 0.16 mcg mL^{-1}**. The *assays for* Gentamicin were performed with *Bacillus subtilis* (ATCC 6633) grown on **Mycin Agar to which 1,000 kinetics units of penicillinase were added per milliliter of medium to inactivate the Piperacillin. The limit of detection was 0.16 mcg mL^{-1}**.

Results and Discussion: Following administration of **500 mg kg^{-1} of Piperacillin alone**, the mean serum concentration at the *end of the infusion in* **Phase I** was **2,475 mcg mL^{-1}; after 5 min, it declined rapidly and biexponentially. In Phase 2**, no *detectable levels of Piperacillin were present before the start of the infusion*. At the end of the **Infusion, the serum concentration was 4,200 mcg mL^{-1}, a level higher than that seen in Phase I.** After 5 min, serum concentrations were about the same magnitude as observed in Phase I. Simultaneous administration of **Gentamicin** did not change the **serum Piperacillin** levels to any significant extent.

The *time course of both* **Piperacillin** and **Gentamicin** in the dog serum could be described by a two-**Compartment Open Model**. The **Pharmacokinetic Parameters**, except the **Volume of Distribution of the Central Compartment (V_c)**, of both the drugs in Phase 2 were not different from those in Phase 1. Even though V_c dropped significantly in Phase 2, no statistically significant change was observed either in the **Volume of Distribution at steady (V_{dss}) or the Overall Volume of Distribution (V_d). *The reason for the lower V_C in the second phase is not* yet fully known.**

Since the *two* **drugs** were given in combination, it was considered of interest to compare the pharmacokinetics of the **Piperacillin** with that of **Gentamicin**. Based on the data from both phases, the half-life of piperacillin was 24 min, the body and renal clearance were 49 and 22 mL min^{-1}, respectively, and the **Volume of Distribution** at steady state was **228 mL kg^{-1}**. The corresponding values for **Gentamicin** were 70 min, 33 and 19 mL min^{-1}, and 314 mL kg^{-1}, respectively. Compared with **Gentamicin, Piperacillin showed a shorter Half-Life and a larger Body Clearance.** There were **no statistically significant differences** either in the **Volume of Distribution or in the Renal Clearance of the two Drugs.**

Summary: Piperacillin Sodium was administered intravenously to dogs, alone or in combination with **Gentamicin, twice a day (~5 hr apart) for 36-37 days. Neither there was any significant affect of Gentamicin on the Pharmacokinetics of Piperacillin, nor the Pharmacokinetics of Gentamicin changed significantly when Pipercaillin was administered simultaneously. However, the urinary recovery of Gentamicin decreased significantly when it was co-administered alone or in combination with piperacillin clearly indicates that the inter-action between Piperacillin and Gentamicin occurred after excretion,** *i.e.*, **either in the urinary bladder or in the collection container.**

SUGGESTED READINGS

Benet LZ et al. (Eds) : **Pharmacokinetic Basis for Drug Treatment.** Raven, New York:1984.

Davies SS, Prichard BNC (Eds) : **Biological Effects of Drugs in Relation to Their Plasma Concentration** MD : University Park Press, Baltimore 1973.

D'Argenio DZ (Ed.) : **Advanced Methods of Pharmacokinetics and Pharmacodynamic Systems Analysis** Plenum Press, New York: 1991.

Gibaldi M, Perrier D : **Pharmacokinetics**, 2nd ed. **Marcel Dekker** New York: 1982.

Pecile A, Rescigno A : **Pharmacokinetics, Mathematical and Statistical Approaches to Metabolism and Distribution of Chemicals and Drugs,** Plenum Press, New York: 1988.

Reidenberg MM, Erill S (Eds) : **Drug-Protein Binding, Esteve Foundation Symposium** I. Praeger Publ. New York: 1986.

Shargel L, Yu ABC : **Applied Biopharmaceutics and Pharmacokinetics.** Appleton and Lange, Norwalk, CT 1993.

Welling P, Tse F : **Pharmacokinetics**, Marcel Dekker, New York 1993.

Chapter 4

CLINICAL PHARMACOKINETICS

4.1. INTRODUCTION

Clinical Pharmacokinetics relates to-'**the application of critical phenomenon of** *Pharmacokinetics* **to the safe and effective therapeutic management of the individual patient'.**

Another school of thought entails vehemently that the '*normal dosage regimen*' and its expected results are invariably a so-called *Statistical Best Guess*-which we generally recognize as:

- **Usual Dosage Regimen;** and
- **Actions and Adverse Reactions.**

In usual practice, however, the **Clinicians** (*Physicians*) do believe *per se* that: "**each individual patient is different; and hence, the ensuing *Practice of Medicine* makes a critical attempt to altogether anticipate and avoid either:**

- the '*Non-average Complications*'; or
- **ensure to adjust the therapy solely based upon observations made a *posteriori*".**

As-to-date, a dedicated and meticulous attempt has been made to accomplish by all means the so-called:

"**Safe and effective management of *Drug Therapy* episode in the individual patients do designate the most preferred and dramatic means whereby the science (discipline) '*Pharmacokinetics*' has made a logistic and enormous contribution to improve upon the '*Medical Practice*' across the globe".**

In a broader perspective, the so-called '**Dosage Regimens**' for an array of '**Drug Substances**' may be easily and conveniently adjusted quite **safely and effectively** by making use of the typical-'**Symptomatic End Points**'; however, there are certain recognized **Important Agents** for which it is indeed **not ideal at all.**

Points to Ponder: These essentially include:

1. There are a host of '**Agents**'-that do require the following *two* extremely important requirements perceptively:

- **individual blood-level determinations;** and
- **critical adjustment of the *Dosage Schedule* so as to "*titrate*'-the patient with the intended '*Drug*'.**

2. There are *four*-'typical Drug characteristic features'-which are intimately associated with the above logical approach (*in '1' above*), such as:

   ❑ '**Drug**' is needed critically;

   ❑ Response is related in a far-better way to the respective **plasma-concentration** *vis-à-vis* to the **Drug Dosage Regimen**;

   ❑ Narrow-range does prevail between:

   • minimum required blood level, and

   • the one which is likely to produce **Adverse Effects**, and

   ❑ Broad-spectrum of variability does occur in the so-called **Inter-patient Blood levels** being obtained from the **Identical Dosage Regimens**.

> **NOTE**
>
> **(1) Obviously, today's '*state-of-the art*' with respect to a specific '*Drug Therapy*' is nothing but a highly specialized dynamic area.**
>
> **(2) Explicitly, the intricate '*problems*' associated with each of these examples virtually differ perceptively; and hence, their respective *chemical solutions* do differ as well.**
>
> **(3) Nevertheless, ideally it would be to define the ensuing '*Problems*' first; and then to '*Review*' the suitable '*Kinetic Approaches*' to address to its solutions intelligently and judiciously.**

In a broader perspective, the **Clinical Pharmacokinetics** is solely concerned with the phenomenon of applying the **Pharmacokinetic Principles** and **Pharmacodynamic Aspects** to aid in the correct and proper '**dosage-regimens' for the individual patients**.

However, at this point in time, it would be quite necessary to have a clear concept of the following *two* **terminologies frequently encountered in the present context**, namely:

• **How does the body react to the drug (*i.e.*, Pharmacokinetics)?** It usually relates to the study and understanding of such critical factors that actually determine the time course of drug that appears eventually within the human body, *viz.* **absorption, distribution, metabolism** and **excretion (ADME).**

Estimation-In most cases, the actual concentration of a drug substance in plasma shall provide a crucial reflection of those present in the tissues of the body. It also encompasses such typical sites where the desired/undesired effects are duly elicited.

• **How would the drug react to the body (*i.e.*, Pharmacodynamics)?** It is normally concerned with the ensuing time course of a drug substance inside a human body. Besides, it relates to the specific study of establishing the relationship among the following *three* **cardinal aspects,** namely.

➢ **Drug Concentration,**

➢ **Pharmacological Activity Profile,** and

➢ **Toxicological Response.**

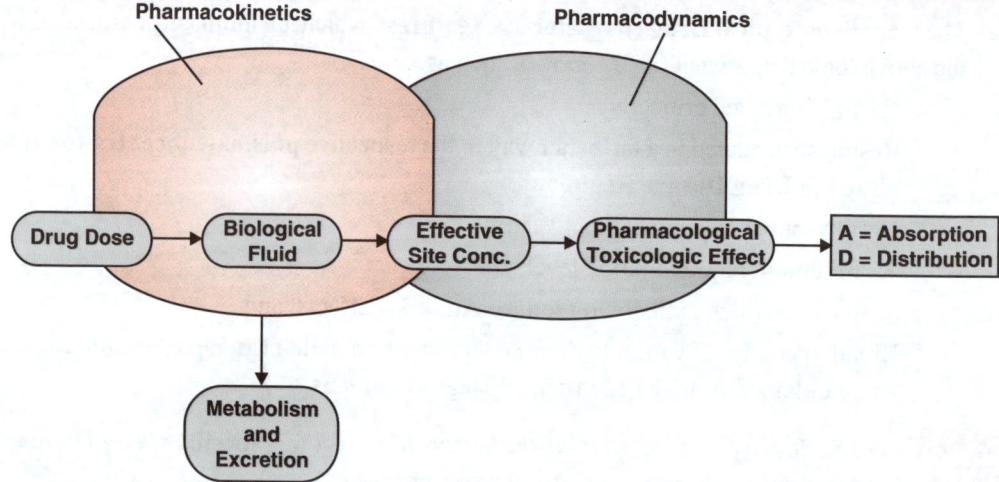

Fig. 4.1. Diagrammatic Representation of Clinical Pharmacokinetics in Relation to Phenomenon of using Pharmacokinetic Principles and Pharmacodynamic Aspects to Aid in the Selection of a Suitable Drug Dosage Regimens for Individual Patients.

Figure 4.1 shows the integrated relationship of the **Clinical Pharmacokinetics** closely concerned with the phenomenon of utilizing important aspects as given under:

- **Pharmacokinetic Principles,** and
- **Pharmacodynamic Criteria,**

in order to help in the most judicious selection of the appropriate **Drug Dosage-Regimens** meant for the **individual patients.**

It has been established beyond any doubt that for several **drug substances** there exists a unique relationship between:

- **Drug Response,** and
- **Plasma-drug Concentration.**

Importantly, the emergence of **Intra-and Inter-individual Variability in Pharmacokinetics appears to be of immense value,** when such drug substances in which the ensuing **Plasma Concentrations** *overlap with those needed for desired clinical effect. In addition, the observed 'Variability in Pharmacokinetics' may invariably come into play due to the following *five* important aspects,** such as:

- **Genetic influence,**
- **Disease conditions,**
- **Ageing phenomenon,**
- **Drug-drug interactions,** and.
- **Environmental factors (*viz.* industrial pollutants, cigarette smoking etc.)**

4.1.1. *Scope of Pharmacokinetics*

The **Scope of Pharmacokinetics** relates to the time course of drug concentration in a human body after its administration due to an array of its parameters. In true sense, the information

---

* Usually in conjunction with '**toxic effects**'

obtained from the **Pharmacokinetics of a Drug (D_1) helps in anticipating (predict) the Pharmacokinetics of another drug (D_2).** A survey of literature pertaining to the **Pharmacokinetic Behavioural Pattern** of a particular drug substance amalgamated with certain critical and vital **Pharmacodynamic Parameters,** *e.g.,* the '**Therapeutic Index:** *of the same may be effectively put to several meaningful applications.

Following are the *ten* **important applications of the Pharmacokinetics Principles**; namely:

1. Development and design of '**Newer Drug Molecules'** showing excellent inherent features, such as:
   - **extensively modified therapeutic efficacy.**
   - **lesser side effects,** and
   - **fewer toxic effects.**

2. Design and development of an '**Optimized Formulation'** for better and usefulness of the **Drug Product** (or **Dosage Form**).

3. Effective **development and design of such unique formulations** as:
   - **controlled-release formulation,**
   - **targeted-release formulation,**
   - **ocular-release formulation,**
   - **transdermal-release formulation,**
   - **iontophoretic-release formulation,**
   - **mucoadhesive-release formulation,**
   - **supramolecular-release formulation,** and
   - **oral-transmucosal-release formulation.**

4. Proper selection of the **most appropriate and preferred route for drug administration** *e.g.,* **IM, IV, oral, transdermal, subcutaneous.**

5. **Choice of most suitable drug** for an individual by a physician.

6. Predict and clearly explain the following *two* **undesired aspects:**
   - **drug-drug interactions **and
   - **drug-food interactions***.

7. Perceptive design of the most suitable '**Multiple-dosage Regimen'** *i.e.,* **sustained-release formulations** (usually a **Tablet or Capsules**)-wherein, the release pattern of the drug is duly extended over a stipulated span of time.

8. Most precise and classical '**Therapeutic Drug Monitoring'** in specific individual patients, *e.g.,* **Time-controlled Secondary Pharmaceutical Products** (*dosage forms*) *vs.* **Chronopharmacology.**

Examples

Time-released formulation of theophylline [Theo-24®]:

---

* **Therapeutic Index:** It refers to the quantitative comparison of a therapeutic effect and an untoward effect of a drug in the human body. Alternatively, the ratio of the maximum tolerated dose of a drug to its minimum curative dose is termed as the therapeutic index.

** Such as **Ca^{2+} and Tetracyclines** cause chelation of the bivalent cation.

*** Grape fruit juice (containing Xenobiotics) inhibit drug-metabolism, thereby leading to prolonged drug action plus serious adverse effects [Murray M: *Clin Pharmacokinetics*, 23: 132, 1992]

The **drug product** duly attained the *requisite* **therapeutic drug concentration** during the night and remarkably avoided toxic effects during the day (when the drug was administered at 1500 hrs).[*]

1. Effective and preventive dosage adjustments in the event of an observed:
   - **changed physiology,** and
   - **drug interactions.**
2. Mainly aimed at accomplishing the utmost **desirable Therapeutic Objective(s).**

4.1.2. *Therapeutic Objective(s)*

The **Therapeutic Objective** is invariably referred to such cardinal factors that predominantly:
- **control and manage,** or
- **cure the disease condition,**

in the *least possible time-frame with bare minimum side-effects by the careful and judicious usage of the* **Least Quantum of Drug'.** As-to-date, tremendous thrust and effective research-oriented efforts are geared towards:
- **new drug development,** and/or
- **structural modifications,**

so as to afford an improved **Pharmacokinetics Characteristic Feature and Enhanced Glaring Efficacy.**

Besides, there are quite a few well-recognized and widely accepted **'Drug Product design'** endeavours across the globe that are solely aimed at:
- **an optimized bioavailability of 'Active Drug',** and
- **improved control/cure of human ailments** *via* **targeted or controlled-release formulations.**

Following are certain aspects that critically meet the **'Therapeutic Objectives'** in an efficient and effective manner:

1. Correct choice of route of administration of **'Drug'** to allow the **'Active Drug'** to have an access to the **'site of action'** in both sufficient quantum and faster mode.
2. Choice of an appropriate **'drug substance'** is solely dependent upon attaining an **'optimum therapy level'** by striking a proper balance between the desired and undesired effects.
3. Co-administration of many drugs simultaneously to a patient may ultimately cause perceptive change in the observed **'Pharmacokinetic Profile of a Drug',** that could be due to the **drug-drug interactions taking place.**

 NOTE   **Therefore, a proper judicious understanding of the interaction makes easier the appropriate and rational usage of drugs that are intended to be co-administered to a patient (under the close supervision of a physician).**

Some Typical Problems in Clinical Pharmacokinetics

In order to understand explicitly the so-called intricacies involved with **some typical problems in Clinical Pharmacokinetics,** let us consider the particular instance of **Phenytoin (diphenylhydantoin)**-as one of the most commonly used-**'Anticonvulsant Drugs'.**

[*] Smolensky *et al.*: *Chronobiol.Intl.*, 4 (3): 435-437, 1987.

Nevertheless, the precise and effective control and management of the **'epileptic seizures'** is observed to be:

"**more reliably correlated with the** *'Anticonvulsant Plasma Levels'* **in comparison to the respective 'dose' used**".

Besides, the *average dosage regimens* being adminstered certainly do not take into account the observed **patient-variability separately** at all. In fact, the actual-'**Plasma-level Monitoring' of Phenytoin (and other 'anticonvulsant drugs')** is invariably recognized and practiced as: "**the recommended approach in the so-called establishment of the** *optimum-dosage-regimen profile* **for each patient separately**".

Table:4.1 records the range of **Optimal Plasma Concentrations** duly established for a good number of selected 'Anticonvulsant Drugs':

\multicolumn{3}{c}{**Table: 4.1. The Observed Optimal Therapeutic Plasma Levels for some Selected Anticonvulsant Drugs:**}
S. No.	**Name of Anticonvulsant Drug**	**Range [Amount (mcg or $mg.mL^{-1}$)]**
1.	Carbamazepine	4-10; 6-12 mcg
2.	Clonazepam	~30-60; 15-50 ng
3.	Ethosuximide	40-80; 40-110 mcg
4.	Diazepam	>400-500; > 600 ng
5.	N-Desmethylmethsuximide[*]	10-40 mcg
6.	Phenobarbital	10-30; 10-25 mcg
7.	Phenytoin	10-20 mcg
8.	Primidone	5-10 mcg
9.	Valproic Acid	~60-80; > 50 mcg.

1. As reviewed in: Eadie MJ: *Clin Pharmacokinet.,* 1:52, 1976.
2. An **'Active Metabolite'** of Methswaimide.

Individual Patients: It has been duly observed that:

- problems that are associated intimately with *individual patient* variation in the so-called *Phenytoin Plasma Levels*-has necessitated an intensive research; and
- individual patient variability in *Phenytoin Plasma Concentration* may be duly attributed to one or more specific reasons.

Following are the *four* **cardinal recognized reasons**-which could be typical and critical for the individual patient variability in the *'Phenytoin'*-Plasma concentration:

- ➤ **Nonlinear Kinetics,**
- ➤ **Bioavailability**
- ➤ **Drug-Interactions,** and
- ➤ **Compliance,**

which would be discussed separately in the sections that follows:

4.1.2.1. *Nonlinear Kinetics*

In the particular instance of **Phenytoin** one may observe critically that **< 2% of the administered dose** gets duly excreted in the urine as *'Intact Phenytoin'* perceptively. Martin *et al.* (1977)* reported that the so-called *'Primarily Metabolite' para*-Hydroxyphenylphenyl **hydration (HPPH)** usually accounts *for 70-80% of the entire given dose of Phenytoin*. Importantly, in the majority of patients the phenomenon of **Phenytoin Elimination** is observed to be:

"**Nonlinear following the** *therapeutic dosage regimen* **perhaps due to the partial saturation of the so-called** *para*-**Hydroxylation Metabolic Pathway**".

NOTE	A dose of 300 mg Phenytoin administered once daily is quite often being recommended for: • adequate Seizure control, and • minimum 'Side-Effects'.

4.1.2.2. *Bioavailability*

Importantly, **Phenytoin** (a *cyclic imide*) having **dissociation constant pka≈g*** *i.e.,* almost insoluble in water.

Example: **Phenytoin Sodium** gets dissolved up to **1 g in 66 mL of water**; however, the *resulting solution* appears to be '**turbid**' unless and until the **pH is duly adjusted to >11.7.**

NOTE	Hence, the *'drug'* (Phenytoin Sodium) gives rise to a crucial *solubility problem* at the physiological pH (in a human body).

Remarks: Nevertheless, the '**drug**' is absorbed largely right from the *proximal segment* of the small intestine-wherein, the rate is found to be rather *slow and variable*-having:

't_{max} **values ranging between 4-24 hours**'.*

Amazingly, in a classical '**Single-dose Investigative Study**' of 100 mg Capsules of Phenytoin Sodium-the *'Elimination Phase'* was apparently found to be of the **First Order**; and thus, following a fair comparison of **AUC-Values** perceptively-that eventually varied from between **92-131% of the Innovator's Product.****

4.1.2.3. *Drug Interactions*

A plethora of *Pharmacokinetic Drug Interactions* involving **Phenytoin** may be found in various scientific literatures; however, only a few proved to be of relevant and significant clinically.

Importantly, based on the scientific revelations and literature survey one may always bear in mind that:

"**drugs may eventually either** *depress* **or** *elevate* **the ensuing** *'Phenytoin Levels'*; **and thus, to some extent the reported** *variability profile* **in the subjects could be apparently attributed to the differences in their actual** *Drug Therapy Episode*".

---

* Melikian AP *et al.*: **Bioavailability of Eleven Phenytoin Products,** *J Pharmacokinetic Biopharm.,* 5: 133, 1977.

** Davies SS and Prichard BNC [Ed]: **Biological Effects of Drugs in Relation to their Plasma Concentrations,** University Park. Press, Baltimore (USA), 227, 1973.

4.1.2.4. *Compliance*

Importantly, when a '**patient**' fails to understand comprehensively the so-called:

"prophylactic nature of the on-going treatment",

– it would definitely pose a *serious problem* perceptively.

Comments: Interestingly, the absolute-'**absence of seizures**' quite often provides the ultimate basis for '**non-compliance**' in the mind of the concerned subjects. Thus, it is widely recognized as the **well-documented problem with Phenytoin particularly***.

Lund (1973) vehemently pronounced that the ultimate results are indeed found to be absolutely typical thereby showing that:

"nearly 32% of 276 subjects showed levels <10 mcg.mL^{-1} very much at the prescribed (recommended) dose levels of *5.6 ± 1.8 (SD)* mg.Kg^{-1}daily".

Besides, only **36.6%** showed values in the range between **10-20 mcg.mL^{-1}**; whereas, **11.6% (35 subjects)** were more than **20 mcg mL^{-1}** and *six* of these subjects specifically showed such **side-effects** as:

- **Ataxia**
- **Nystagmus** and
- **Somnolence.**

> **NOTE** However, the '*Compliance*' was duly tested in particularly the so-called: *Low-Plasma-Level Patients.*

4.2. DOSAGE REGIMENS: DESIGN-MODALITIES-AND IMPLEMENTATION

Preamble

Dosage Regimen strictly regulated the amount of '**Drug**' and '**Schedule for Administration**' to a patient.

Dosage Form (or **Drug Product**) refers to-'**the pharmaceutical preparation intended for use by or administration to a patient with a minimum of further processing, *e.g.*, Tablet, Capsule, Elixir, Suspension, Injectables etc'.**

Dosage Range represents the *maximum and minimum Dose* to achieve a therapeutic benefit without any toxic effects.

Dosage Rules essentially consist of the following *four* **important aspects, such as:**

- **Rules for calculating dosage-especially for children,**
- **Clark's Rule-weight in pounds times adult dosage divided by their age plus 12 times the adult dosage equals the respective child dose,**
- **Young's Rule-age in years divided by the age plus 12 times the adult dosage equals the child dose, and**
- **Body Surface Area (BSA) Rule- BSA in m^2 (of child) divided by the average adult BSA (1.73 m^2) multiplied by the adult dosage equals the child dose.**

The *design modalities*, and *implementation* of **Dosage Regimens** shall now be discussed appropriately in the following sections:

4.2.1. Design of Dosage Regimens

In actual practice, the dosage regimens could be categorized into the following *two* **types:**

- **optimal single dosage regimen,** and
- **optimal multiple dosage regimen,**

which will be discussed briefly in the following.

4.2.1.1. Optimal Single Dosage Regimen

An optimal single dosage regimen may invariably provide an '**effective treatment**'. Nevertheless, the actual prevalent illness in most cases are found to be longer enough *vis-a-vis* the ensuing therapeutic effect caused by an optimal single dose.

Examples

1. **Albendazole** (an '**anthelmintic**') is given once only to children for deworming.
2. **Antiemetics, Hypnotics**, and **Analgesics** are given in a single dose to produce an effective treatment.

4.2.1.2. Optimal Multiple Dosage Regimen

In certain specific instances, *viz.* **Prolonged Illness (tuberculosis, pernicious anaemia, chronic diabetes, essential hypertension etc.)**, it becomes almost mandatory to have drugs on a repetitive basis stretched duly over a certain stipulated length of time which depends solely on the critical '**nature of ailment**'.

Therefore, to accomplish a successful therapy, the design of an '**Optimal Multiple Dosage Regimen**' is an absolute necessity. Hence, an **Optimal Multiple Dosage Regimen** may be defined as – '**a predetermined protocol wherein the drug is required to be administered in appropriate doses having** enough frequency level, which precisely ensures adequate maintenance of the plasma concentration very much well within the proposed **Therapeutic Window**[*] during the entire period of therapy'.

Examples

The following are a few classical examples:

1. **Antibiotics, Antihypertensive, Antibacterials, Antituberculosis**: These drugs do essentially require a minimum level of effective concentration to be maintained at all times, so as to accomplish the **Best Therapeutic Efficacy** (*i.e.*, **drugs with Broad-Therapeutic Indices**).
2. **Phenytoin, Cephalosporin, Xylocaine**: These drugs with **Narrow Therapeutic Indices** must be administered in such a manner that their **toxic concentration (level) is not exceeded.**

---

[*] **Therapeutic Window**: It refers to a definite protocol devoid of any excessive fluctuation and drug accumulation in the body.

Designing a Dosage Regimen: In designing a **Dosage Regimen**, the following *two* **important aspects** should be taken into consideration; namely:

- **Pharmacokinetic Parameters of the 'Drug'**: It is largely found to remain constant in the course of therapy, *i.e.,* when the **dosage regimen** gets duly established. However, if one observes any type of change during therapy, the **dosage regimen** is rendered '**Invalid**'.
- **Basic of Calculations for Dosage Regimen**: These typical calculations are solely based upon:
  - ➢ **Open one-compartment model,** and
  - ➢ **Two-comaprtment model,**

in case, one makes use of ô (*i.e., dosage interval*) instead of K_E (**elimination constant**), and $V_{d.ss}$, *i.e.,* apparent volume of distribution at steady state instead of V_d (apparent volume of **distribution**).

Doses Size: Dose Size usually refers to the **quantity or volume of a medicinal agent** intended to be taken at one time (*unit dose*) or *in a given time interval, e.g.,* **Daily Dose.** In a broader perspective, it may be ascertained that the **actual apparent magnitude** of:

- **therapeutic response,** and
- **toxic response,**

depends exclusively on the '**Dose Size**'.

Important Points

1. **Dose Size** calculations mostly need a comprehensive knowledge for the critical '**quantum of drug**' being absorbed effectively soon after the administration of each dose.
2. Greater variations between $C_{SS.max}$ and $C_{SS.min}$ may be observed with greater dose size in the course of:
   - **each and every dosing period,** and
   - **ultimately causing probability in 'toxicity'.**

Figure 4.2 shows the diagrammatic representation of the direct influence of dose size upon the ensuing **Plasma-Concentration-Time Profile** soon after the following *two* **events**, namely:

- **oral administration of 'Drug',** and
- **administration at 'Fixed Schedules of Time'.**

Explanation

The various steps involved are as follows:

1. The plot between the observed **Plasma-Drug Concentration (mcg mL^{-1})** *vs.* **Time (hrs)** at different **Dosing Intervals (T)** clearly shows *three* zones marked by **X, Y and Z** (*see Figure 4.2*).
2. The **X-zone** relates to the **Longer-Dose Profile** with matching longer variations that critically exhibits the ensuing **therapeutic and toxic responses**.
3. The **Y-zone** represents the **optimum dose profile with therapeutically successful and effective responses.**

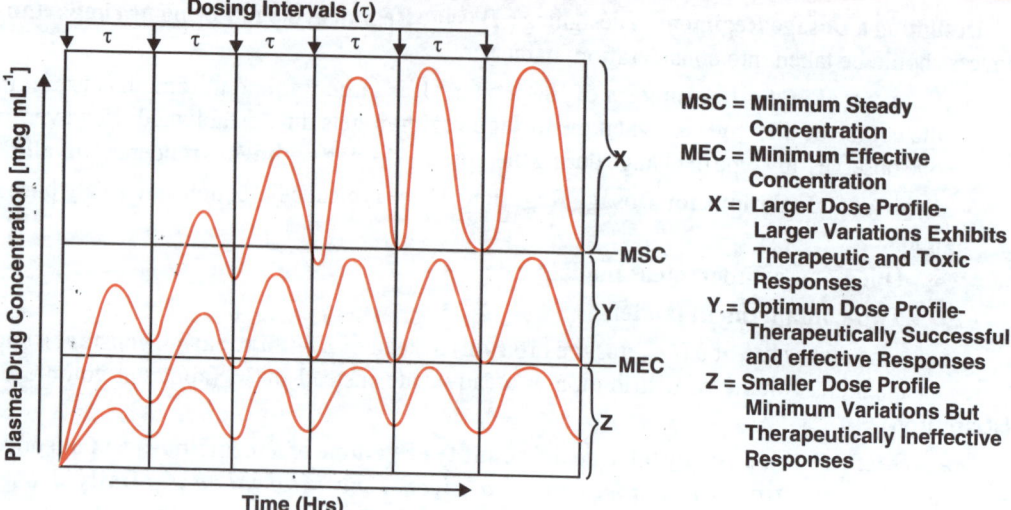

Fig. 4.2: Diagrammatic Representation of Dose Size Influence upon Plasma-Drug Concentration vs. time Profile soon after Administration of a Drug at Fixed Dosing Intervals (T) of Time (hrs).

4. The **Z-zone** designates the particular **smaller dose profile with minimum variations, while showing almost ineffective therapeutic responses.**

Dosing Frequency: It is known that the '**Dosing Interval**' refers to –'**the time elapsed between the administration of consecutive doses of a drug**'. Importantly, the **Dosing Interval** (*which is the inverse of the Dosing Frequency*) is usually calculated based on the **plasma half-life** ($t_{1/2}$) **of the drug.** In a situation, where the specific '**Dose Interval**' is enhanced while the dose remains unchanged, one may critically observe the following values, namely:

C_{max}-**decreases**

C_{min}-**decreases**

C_{av}-**decrease, and**

C_{max}/C_{min} **ratio-increases.**

> **NOTE**   When the specific 'dose interval' is reduced (*i.e.,* dsoing frequency increased), the above values of C_{max}, C_{min}, C_{av} and C_{max}/C_{min} ratio become just the 'opposite'.

In addition, the reduced dose interval profile may result in a significant accumulation of drug in the human body leading to toxicity status.

Figure 4.3 illustrates the diagrammatic profile pertaining to the influence of the '**Dosing Frequency**' upon the **Plasma-Drug Concentration-Time profile** duly obtained soon after the oral administration of the '**Fixed Doses of a Drug**'.

Explanation

The following are the different sequential steps involved:

1. The graphic plot between **Plasma-Drug Concentration (mcg mL^{-1}) vs. Time (hrs)** at varying **Dosing Frequency** explicitly shows *three* distinct zones marked by X, Y and Z (*see Figure 4.3*).

2. The **X-zone** designates the **High-Dosing Frequency ($\tau <_{1/2}$)** with lesser variations that exhibits both *therapeutic and toxic responses*.

3. The **Y-zone** relates the **Optimum-Dosing Frequency ($\tau = _{1/2}$)**, and proves to be successful therapeutically.

4. The **Z-zone** represents the **Low-Dosing Frequency ($\tau >_{1/2}$)** with large variations and turns out to be **unsuccessful therapeutically**.

Salient Features: It is quite necessary to sustain a proper balance between the *two* **components**, namely:

- **Dose Size,** and
- **Dosing Frequencies.**

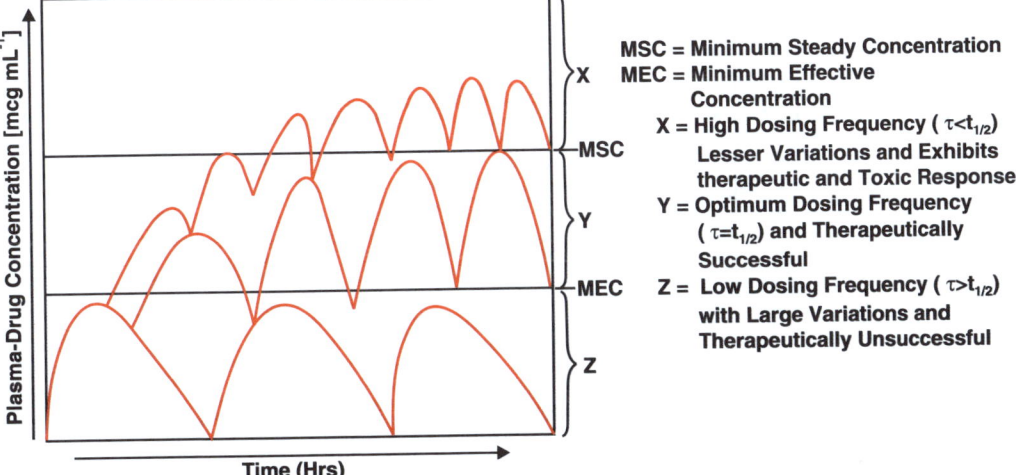

MSC = Minimum Steady Concentration
MEC = Minimum Effective Concentration
X = High Dosing Frequency ($\tau < t_{1/2}$) Lesser Variations and Exhibits therapeutic and Toxic Responses
Y = Optimum Dosing Frequency ($\tau = t_{1/2}$) and Therapeutically Successful
Z = Low Dosing Frequency ($\tau > t_{1/2}$) with Large Variations and Therapeutically Unsuccessful

Fig. 4.3: Diagrammatic Representation of Dosing Frequency Influence upon Plasma-Drug Concentration-Time Profile Obtained Soonafter the Oral Administration of Fixed Doses of a Drug.

In order to accomplish the *two* **most sought after requirements,** *viz., Safely and Efficacy.* However, one may not obtain such a status simply by administering relatively **'Higher Doses at a Less Frequency'. Importantly, the administrations of rather doses at frequent intervals do produce definitely lesser variations.**

Explanation

Digoxin, a cardiac glycoside, has a **Narrow Therapeutic Index;** and, therefore, is administered most preferably in small doses only at **frequent intervals (normally $< t_{1/2}$ of the drug),** so as to accomplish:

- **a therapeutic profile having the least variations,** and
- **very much similar to the profile obtained with either,**
  - ➤ **controlled-drug release system, or**
  - ➤ **constant rate infusion.**

Accumulation of Drug in Multiple Dosing In order to understand the intricacies associated with the **accumulation of drug in Multiple Dosing System,** accomplished after **IV Multiple**

Dosing *with the dosing interval equivalent to one plasma half-life ($t_{1/2}$) of the drug, one may consider the amount of drug duly present in the body-time as depicted in* Figure 4.4.

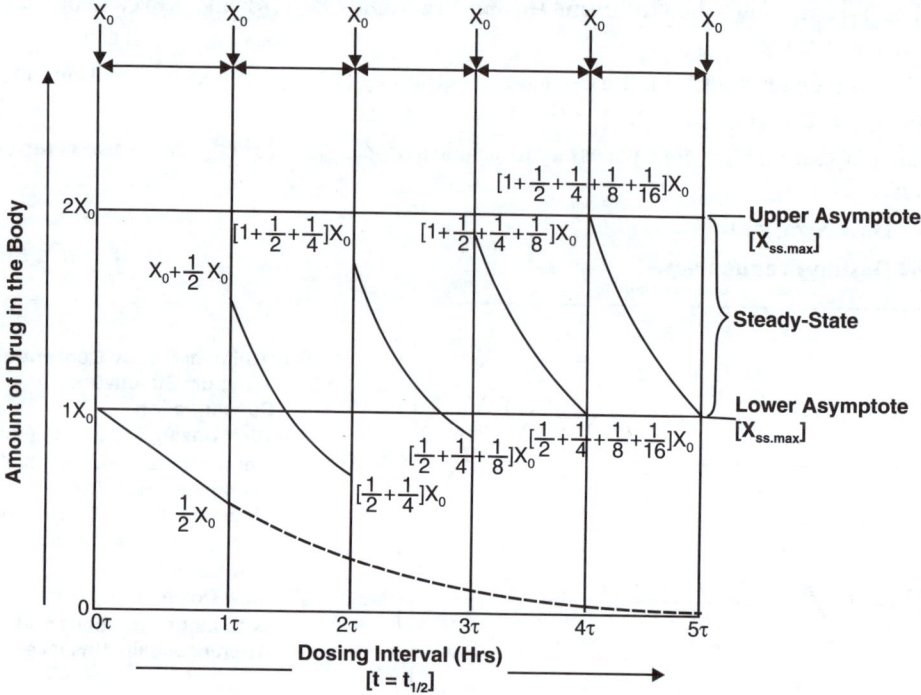

Fig.4.4: Diagrammatic Representation Showing Accumulation of Drug in the Body with Multiple Dosing Regimen of IV Bolus having Dosing Interval Equivalent to One Plasma Half-life of the Drug.

NOTE   **Approximately *five* plasma half-lives are essentially required for accomplishing the 'steady state'.**

Explanation

The various cardinal steps involved in Figure 4.4, showing the **accumulation of drug in a Multiple-Dosing System,** are as follows:

1. Immediately after the administration of the very **first dose, X_o, at $\tau = 0$,** the quantum of drug available in the body shall be $X = 1X_0$.

2. Now, at the **next dosing-interval,** will be the quantum of drug remaining in the body, *i.e.,* $X = \frac{1}{2}X_0$.

3. Likewise, the administration of the **subsequent IV dose helps to raise the body content to a level equivalent to $X = X_0 + \frac{1}{2}X_0$,** *i.e.,* accumulation of drug takes place in the body. Thus, it suggests explicitly that the phenomenon of '**accumulation**' comes into play due to the fact that drug from the corresponding previous doses has not yet been removed completely.

4. Since the quantum of drug in the body slowly gets enhanced because of accumulation, the respective elimination rate also increases in a proportionate manner until it accomplishes:

➤ **a steady state**, or

➤ **reaches a plateau state**

in a critical situation when the **Rate of Drug gaining adequate entry into the body almost equals to the Rate of Exit of Drug.**

5. Consequently, at the steady state, the **observed maximum values ($X_{SS.max}$), and minimum values ($X_{SS.min}$) do show a tendency to approach the respective asymptotes strategically located at the plateau**, *viz.* '**Upper Asymptote**' and '**Lower Asymptote**'.

6. Importantly, at the **plateau, $X_{SS.min} = 1X_0$**, and **$X_{SS.max} = 2X_0$**, which means that $X_{SS.min}$ equals the quantum of drug present in the body soon after the administration of the **First-Dose**; whereas, $X_{SS.max}$ **clearly equals twice the first dose**. Besides, we may have the following *two* expressions:

$$X_{SS.max} - X_{SS.min} = X_0$$

and

$$X_{SS.max}/X_{SS.min} = 2$$

7. The above observations hold good only in a situation **when $\tau = t_{1/2}$, and the drug is administered *via* the IV route.**

8. **When $\tau < t_{1/2}$, the extent of accumulation is greater and *vice versa*.**

Remarks: The concluding remarks include:

1. The degree up to which a drug gets accumulated duly in the body in the course of **Multiple Dosing Designates** a function of:

   - **dosing interval,**
   - **elimination half-life**, and
   - **independent of dose-size**

2. The degree up to which a drug shall get accumulated irrespective of any dosing interval in a subject may be duly derived based upon the **relevant informations obtained with a single dose.**

It is invariably represented by the so-called '**Accumulation Index (Rac)**' as given by the following expression:

$$Rac = \frac{1}{1 - e^{-K_E t}} \qquad \text{(a)}$$

Reachable Time for Achieving Steady State in Multiple Dosing: It has been established beyond any doubt that the reachable time needed for a steady state solely depends on the plasma half-life ($t_{1/2}$) of the drug substance. In fact, the desired plateau is accomplished in nearly *five* **plasma half-lives in a specific situation when $K_a > K_E$** (*i.e.*, the **First Order Rate Constant** is greater than the **Elimination Rate Constant**). In other words, the rate at which the '**multiple-dose steady-state**' is attained satisfactorily may be estimated by K_E (*i.e.*, the **Elimination Rate Constant**).

Interestingly, the time taken to reach the above cited **multiple-dose steady state** is found to be absolutely independent of the following *three* **critical aspects; namely:**

   - **dose size,**
   - **dosing interval**, and
   - **number of doses.**

Multiple Dosing Profile: The most fundamental objective of the therapeutic treatment by a drug is to attain rapidly and maintain reasonably the ensuing **Plasma-Drug Concentration** within the limits of the **'Therapeutic Range'** with least possible observed fluctuations.

Example

Oral Multiple Dosing Regimens: In this typical instance, after the administration of the first dose one may notice an enhancement in the **Plasma-Drug Concentration Level** which is immediately followed by a *distinct peak level*, and ultimataly a *decline in the Plasma-Drug Concentration.*

The administration of the **Second Dose** further increases the level of **Plasma-Drug Concentration** and attains a level higher than in the **First-Dose**. Nevertheless, there shall be a continuous increase unless and until a **steady-state Plasma-Drug Concentration** is duly accomplished, as depicted in Figure 4.5.

Evidently, one may prominently observe a **'Steady State'** as and when the input and output of the drug substance stands to be **'equal'**.

Calculation of Drug Accumulated in Human Body after the First Dose: It may be calculated easily by using the following expression:

$$R = \frac{1}{1 - e^{(-0.693\tau)/t_{1/2}}}$$ (b)

where,

R = Accumulation factor,[*] and

τ = Dosing interval.

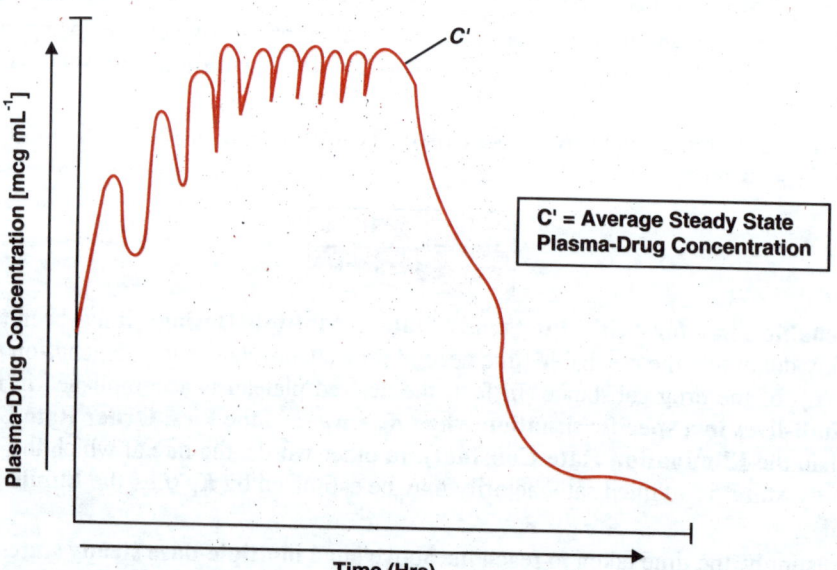

C' = Average Steady State Plasma-Drug Concentration

Fig. 4.5: Schematic Representation of the Plasma-Drug Concentration-Time Profile soonafter Multiple Dosing Regimen.

---

[*] **Accumulation Factor:** It solely depends on *two* **vital parameters**, viz. **Dosing interval** and **Plasma half-life** $(t_{1/2})$.

First-Order Kinetics: On the basis of the **First-Order Kinetics,** *nearly 90% of the average steady-state* **Plasma-Drug Concentration** shall be attained very much within the *four* **Plasma Half-Lives.** Importantly, the realistic time span needed to actually approach the 'steady state' shall depend solely upon the **Plasma Half-Life of the Drug.** However, it has been observed from various experimental investigative studies that the **average steady-state plasma-drug concentration ($\cancel{E}$)** would depend exclusively on the following *four* important factors; namely:

- X_0, *i.e.,* the 'maintenance dose',
- F, *i.e.,* the fraction of the 'absorbed dose',
- $\hat{O}$, *i.e.,* the 'dosing interval', and
- C_L, *i.e.,* the 'clearance'.

Thus, we may have the following expression for **(C)**:

$$C' = \frac{F\, X_0}{C_L \tau} \tag{c}$$

we also know that

$$X_0 = \frac{C'V_d \tau}{1.44 F\, t_{1/2}}$$

Putting the value of X_0 in equation (c) we have

$$C' = \frac{1.44 \cdot F \cdot X_0 \cdot t_{1/2}}{V_d \cdot \tau} \tag{e}$$

where

V_d = **Volume of Distribution.**

But AUC = Area Under the Plasma-Drug Concentration *vs.* the Time Curve after a single maintenance dose. Therefore, **Equation (d)** may be written as

$$C' = \frac{AUC}{\tau} \tag{e}$$

i.e., the **average steady-state plasma-drug concentration (C) is equal to area under the plasma-drug concentration *vs.* time curve (AUC) divided by the 'dosing interval (τ)'.**

4.2.2. Average Drug Concentration vs. Body Content from Multiple Dosing to Steady State

4.2.2.1. Preamble

It may be observed that the overall **Average Drug Concentration** prevailing at a **Steady State ($C_{ss.av}$)** serves as a function of the **Maintenance Dose (X_0), fraction of dose absorbed (F), dosing interval ($\hat{o}$), and clearance (CL-R) of the drug,** that may be expressed as:

$$C_{ss.av} = \frac{F \cdot X_0}{CL_R \cdot \tau} \tag{f}$$

or

$$C_{ss.av} = \frac{1.44 F \cdot X_0 \cdot t_{1/2}}{V_d \cdot \tau} = \frac{AUC \, (single \, dose)}{\tau} \tag{g}$$

where,

Factor 1.44 = Coefficient for the reciprocal of 0.693 in **Equation (g)**, and

AUC = Area Under the Curve following a **'single maintenance dose'**.

Hence, **Equation (g)** may be employed to Calculate the **Maintenance Dose of a Drug Substance** to accomplish its predetermined concentration. We already know that:

$$X = V_d \cdot C$$

hence, the body content at a steady state is given by the following expression:

$$X_{ss.av} = \frac{1.44 \cdot F \cdot X_0 \cdot t_{1/2}}{\tau} \tag{h}$$

Interestingly, **Equation (h) suggests clearly that the aforesaid Average Values do not represent the arithmetic mean of** $C_{ss.max}$ **and** $C_{ss.min}$ **by virtue of the known fact that the ensuing plasma-drug concentration declines exponentially.**

In a broader perspective, there are *three* **important aspects** with particular reference to the *average drug concentration vs.* **body content from the multiple-dosing system to the steady-state,** namely:

- **Loading and maintenance doses,**
- **Maintenance of drug level within the therapeutic range,** and
- **Perfect design of dosage regimen based upon the plasma-drug concentration.**

which will discussed individually in the following sections.

4.2.2.2. *Loading and Maintenance Doses*

Loading Dose refers to-**'the administration of a drug in a larger initial dose than the usual one to speed entrance into the circulating blood'.** It is also known as the **'Bolus Dose'** or 'priming dose'.

Maintenance Dose entails the *Periodic Dose* following the **'Loading Dose'** given earlier to keep the **Drug-Plasma Concentration very much within a Therapeutic Range** perceptively.

Example

Chloroquine Phosphate [250 mg tablets: Lariago®]: The *anti-malarial drug* is first administered orally as four tablets (≡ to 1000 mg of drug) on the day 1 as the Loading dose which is followed by two tablets each on the day 2, day 3 and day 4, respectively, as the Maintenance Doses.

It actually takes almost *five* **plasma half-lives ($t_{1/2}$) to attain the Therapeutic Activity Level**; and, therefore, the time taken would be very long for such drugs having a **Long Plasma Half-Life** (see **Accumulation of Drug Multiple Dosing** *in this section and Figure 4.4*). Thus, it is quite feasible to obtain a plateau immediately by giving a dose which provides the ultimate desired steady state almost instantaneously well before starting the respective **Maintenance Doses (X_0)**, *i.e.,* the '**Loading Dose ($X_{0.L}$)**. It is duly expressed by the following simple equation:

$$X_{0.L} = \frac{C_{ss.av} \cdot V_d}{F} \qquad \text{(i)}$$

where,

- $C_{ss.av}$ = Average drug concentration at a steady state (C_{ss}),
- V_d = Volume of distribution, and
- F = Fraction of dose absorbed.

Dose Ratio: The '**Dose Ratio**' may be defined as '**the ratio of Loading Dose to Maintenance**, *i.e.,* $X_{0.L}/X_0$**. As a guiding rule, the dose ratio has three variants;** namely:

- $X_{0.L}/X_0$ = [2.0 when $\tau = t_{1/2}$,
- $X_{0.L}/X_0$ = Lesser than 2.0 when $\tau > t_{1/2}$ and
- $X_{0.L}/X_0$ = Greater than 2.0 when $\tau < t_{1/2}$.

It may be observed critically that in a situation when the **Loading Dose** is not optimum, *i.e.,* it either remains too low or too high, the **Steady State (C_{SS})** may be accomplished within nearly *five* **Plasma Half-Lives** in a similar manner to when absolutely '**no loading dose**' is being administered, as illustrated in Figure 4.6.

NOTE	1. The above-mentioned Equations (f), (g) and (h) and the explanatory discussions so far are applicable only to such drugs which predominantly follow up the 'one-compartment open model kinetics' having the first-order disposition. 2. However, the 'multi-compartment models' shall deal with more complex equations.

Exaplanation

Various important aspects of Figure 4.6 are as follows:

1. The **Plasma-Drug Concentration**-Time profiles of drugs having **Dose Ratio either equal to 2** (*shown by bold-line curves*) **or less than 2** (*exhibited by dotted-line curves*) **are lying generously between Minimum Steady-Concentration (MSC), and Minimum Effective Concentration (MEC).**

2. The **Plasma-Drug Concentration**-Time profiles of drugs having **Dose Ratio more than 2** (*shown by normal-line curves*) **usually are located between the Maximum Steady Concentration and Minimum Steady Concentration.**

3. The '**Loading Dose**' ($X_{0.t}$) is given duly at 'zero' hrs; whereas, the subsequent '**maintenance doses (X_0)**' at the definite **Dosing Intervals ($t_{1/2}$).**

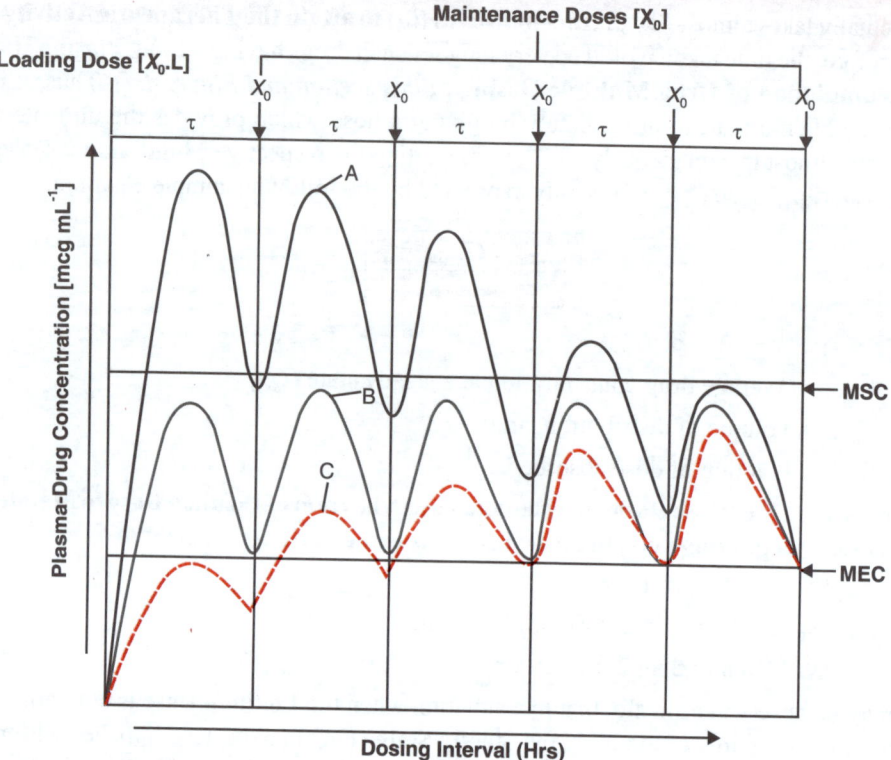

Fig. 4.6. Diagrammatic Representation of Plasma-Drug Concentration-Time Profiles obtained when Dose Ratio Remains>2(A), 2 (B) and <2(C).

4.2.2.3. *Maintenance of Drug Level Within the Therapeutic Range*

In the overall case, convenience or difficulty in the proper and adequate maintenance of drug level concentration within the **Therapeutic Window** (*or Range*) depends exclusively on the following *three* **critical aspects,** namely:

- **therapeutic index of the drug,**
- **plasma half-life of the drug,** and
- **convenience of dosing.**

In usual practice, it is primarily a difficult task to maintain and sustain such a crucial 'Drug Level' particularly for a drug possessing:

- **short plasma half-life (< 3 hrs),** and
- **narrow therapeutic index (*e.g.,* Heparin),**

On the basis of the fact that the 'Dosing Frequency' should necessarily be $< t_{1/2}$.

Selected Examples: These consist of:

1. **Drugs with High Therapeutic Index**: For drugs having a **Large Therapeutic Index** ($>>TD_{50}/ED_{50}$), *e.g.,* **Penicillin** ($t_{1/2}= 0.g$ hrs), it will be rather safe as well as common to administer doses in excess (often nearly 10 time excess) of that which is needed minimally to obtain the desired **therapeutic response.**

NOTE   In this specific instance, bioavailability fails to change the Therapeutic Index.

1. Importantly, **Penicillin** can be administered '**Less Frequently**' *i.e.,* every 4-6 hrs; however, the **Maintenance Dose** should always be larger so that the **Plasma-Drug Concentration** *remains above the minimum inhibitory level.*

2. **Drugs with Low Therapeutic Index: Drugs with a Low Therapeutic Index,** *e.g.,* **Warfarin,** may be administered at dose intervals ranging between **1 and 3 Plasma Half-Lives ($t_{1/2}$).** As the dose of **Warfarin** is increased, one may observe that a relatively **larger segment of the patients respond**[*] until almost all patients respond as shown in Figure 4.7.

NOTE   When the '*Therapeutic Index*' is low, it is quite possible to have a range of concentrations at which point both the effective as well as toxic responses invariably overlap, *e.g.,* certain patients show a haemorrhage condition; whereas, others show the desired two fold prolongation of the prothrombin time.

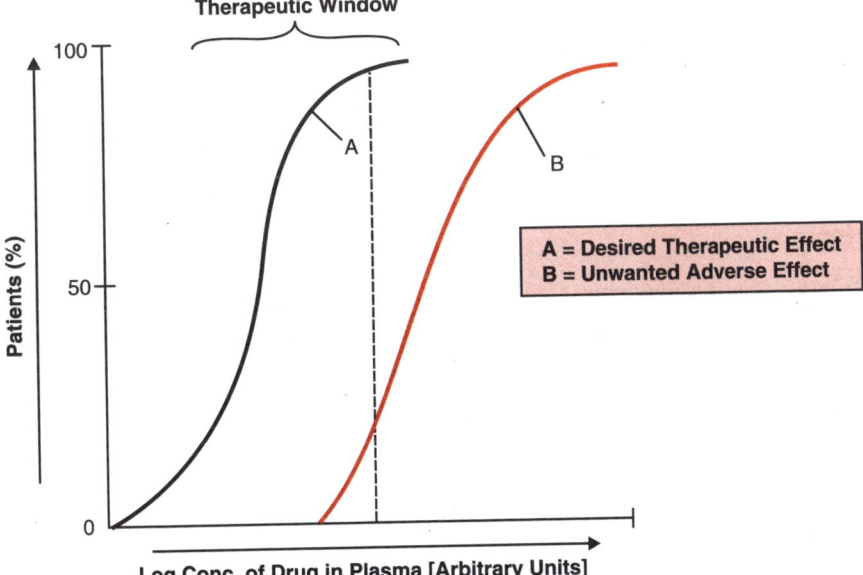

Fig. 4.7: Diagrammatic Representation of the Cumulative % of Patients Responding Plasma Levels of Warfarin.

Other Examples: Commonly used **Low Therapeutic Index Drugs** include: **Hypoglycaemic agents, Digoxin, Anti-arrhythmics, Aminoglycosides, Xanthenes, Cytotoxic and Immunosuppressive Drugs.**

4.2.2.4. *Perfect Design of Dosage Regimen Based Upon the Plasma-Drug Concentrations*

Preamble Till late 1960-s practically all patients were treated with the '**same dosage of a specific drug**'. Obviously, there was absolutely no coveted status for the **Pharmacokinetic** and **Pharmacodynamic** Variability in the introduction of **drug therapy.**

* For '**Warfarin**', the desired response appears as a *two fold increase in the* **Prothrombin Time.**

Koch-Weser (1975)[*] carried out an intensive and extensive survey, for a period of 3 years extending from 1970 to 1972, with particular reference to the **'Phenytoin Dosages'** recommended for the critical prevention of seizure in nearly 200 ambulatory patients; and duly observed that almost 92% of the patients actually received the **usual dose of 300 mg day^{-1}**.

Remarkable Observation: Koch-wester's observation was really remarkable in the sense, since phenytoin designates a quintessential example of a specific drug substance having significant inter-patient variability quotient in the so-called **Clinical Response**.

Till date, **Clinician**[**] while initiating a particular dosage regimen critically takes the following aspects into consideration:

- **patients age,**
- **size (body weight),**
- **disease condition,** and
- **concomitant (connected) drug therapy.**

Exceptional Examples: These essentially consist of:

1. **Theophylline** (a *diuretic*) is normally prescribed at higher than **'usual mg kg^{-1}doses'** for children and smokers; whereas, lower than **'usual doses'** is recommended for patients with a history of **Congestive Heart Failure (CHF),**

2. There are certain specific drug substances that are mostly prescribed at a much reduced doses for patients having a history of **Impaired Renal Function.**

Examples

    Antibiotics (Cephalosporins, Ofloxacin, Norfloxacin); Digoxin, Lithium etc.

3. **Elderly Patients: They are usually recommended with more conservation dosages of Hypnotics (Barbiturates), Anti-anxiety Drugs (Reserpine, Chlorpromazine)** etc.

Design of Dosage Regimen may be carried out effectively provided the following parameters are known:

- **therapeutic range of the drug substance,**
- **apparent volume of distribution (V_{d}-),**
- **clearance (C_L),** and
- **plasma half-life ($t_{1/2}$) of drug substance.**

In fact, these parameters actually render a great help in maintaining the drug concentration within the therapeutic range, that could be further expressed explicitly as:

- **Upper limit designated as C_{upper},** and
- **Lower limit designated as C_{lower}.**

Thus, one may accomplish readily the **Maximum Dosing Interval (T_{max})** *that solely depends upon the following* **two critical conditions**; such as:

- **therapeutic index (C_{upper}/C_{lower} ratio),** and
- **elimination half-life of drug,**

---

[*]   Koch-Weser *J: Eur .Clin.Pharmacol.,* **9**: 1,1975.

[**]   **Clinicians**: A staff member providing technical medical services, especially a physician, also a pharmacist or nurse associated with patient care system.

which may be expressed by the following equation:

$$\tau_{max} = \frac{2.303 \log (C_{upper}/C_{lower})}{K_E} \qquad \text{(j)}$$

As we know, $K_E = 0.693/t_{1/2}$, therefore, equation (j) may be re-written as

$$\tau_{max} = \frac{2.303 \log (C_{upper}/C_{lower})}{0.693/t_{1/2}} \qquad \text{(k)}$$

or

$$\tau_{max} = 3.32 \cdot t_{1/2} \cdot \log (C_{upper}/C_{lower})$$

It may be argued logically from **Equation (k)** that the ensuing **'Dosing Interval (τ)'** thus selected is invariably of a smaller value in comparison to τ_{max}. hence, it follows that the anticipated **Maximum Maintenance Dose $[X_{0max}]^*$** may be duly expressed as:

$$X_{0max} = \frac{V_d (C_{upper} - C_{lower})}{F} \qquad \text{(l)}$$

Where,

V_d = Apparent volume of distribution and

F = Fraction of drug absorbed.

On the basis of the above facts and observations, it is now possible to arrive at the **Maintenance Dose (X_0)**, and the **Average Steady-state Condition $(C_{ss.av})$** as follows:

$$X_0 = \left(\frac{X_{0max}}{\tau_{max}}\right) \tau \qquad \text{(m)}$$

$$C_{ss.av} = \frac{(C_{upper} - C_{lower})}{2303 \log (C_{upper} - C_{lower})} \qquad \text{(n)}$$

4.2.3. *Individualization*

In a broader perspective, the **Drug Dosing Profile** and/or **Dosing Adjustments** *are invariably based upon the logistic calculations related to the population data.*

Inter-Subject Variability: It refers to-'**the production of appreciably large differences in the pharmacologic response by using the 'same dose of a drug' in altogether different individuals.** Alternatively, it explicitly pronounces that the definite dose needed to cause a specific **Pharmacologic Responses Dose** varies from one individual to another.

Individualization of a dosage regimen demands the **Rational Drug Therapy** to fulfill the patients requirements specifically. Importantly, the **Clinical Pharmacokinetics** makes use of the

---

* That is, X_{0max} may be obtained from each and every τ_{max} (maximum dosing interval).

underlying **Pharmacokinetic Principles** in the *skillful design of dosage regimens for the individual patients*.

The inter-subject variability is essentially of *two* **sources** in the drug responses, namely:

1. **Pharmacokinetic Variability**: It is generally caused due to the ensuing differences in the concentration of drug at the site of action. Besides, certain differences prevailing in the **absorption, distribution, biotransformation (metabolism), and excretion (ADME)** are also equally responsible for the **Pharmacokinetic Variability** profile.

2. **Pharmacodynamic Variability**: It is exclusively attributed to the **Actual Pharmacological Responses** that predominantly varies from one individual to another at a given specified dose.

4.2.3.1. *Objectives of Individualization*

First and foremost, an insufficient therapeutic response certainly demands a higher dosage regimen; whereas, the inherent **Drug-Related Toxicity** critically calls for a definite **Lower Dosage Regimen.** Therefore, in order to help the phenomenon of individualization, it is absolutely necessary to make the availability of drug in the respective **Drug Products (or *Dosage Forms*)** with **varying dose strengths**, *e.g.,* **Losartan Potassium [Tozaar®]** an *antihypertensive agent available as 25 and 50 mg* **Tablets. Azithromycin [Azibest®]-*an antibiotic available in 100, 250 and 500 mg Tablets.***

Interestingly, the number of dose-strength availability of a drug depends exclusively on the following *two* **major criteria,** namely:

- **therapeutic index of the drug,** and
- **extent of inter-subject variability.**

NOTE   **In reality, smaller therapeutic index and larger inter-subject variability shall lead to a greater number of dose-strength dosage forms for a 'drug'.**

4.2.3.2. *Important Steps for Individualization*

Having assumed that practically **'all subjects'** do essentially require the same plasma-drug concentration range for the **therapeutic effectiveness**, the following are the *three* **steps intimately involved in the desired individualization of the Dosage Regimen,** namely:

- **Determination of Pharmacokinetic Parameters:** It is required to determine in an individual subject

  ➢ **pharmacokinetics parameters,** and
  ➢ **respective population values,**

in order to find out the degree of variability observed. **Evidently, greater the accountability of variations, better would be the probabilities of achieving the desired therapeutic objective.**

- **Variability *vis-a-vis* Measurable Characteristic Features:** Such attributing characteristic features comprise: age factor, weight, and above all the critical renal/hepatic ailment.

- **New Dosage Regimen Designing:** It is accomplished on a continuous basis from the available **'Collected Data'.**

Conclusively, the 'Design of Newer Dosage Regimens' necessary implicates such adjustments as: **Dosage Profile, Dosage Interval,** and a **Combination of Both,** *i.e.,* **dosage-dosage in val.**

Drug Dosing Profile in Obese Patients It is quite evident that the *apparent* **Volume of distribution** (V_d) of the drug is solely dependent on the *body weight,* **since the latter is directly related to the volume of the body fluids.** Thus, the **'Ideal Body Weight (IBW)'** of either sex may be calculated from the following expressions:

$$IBW_{Men} = 50 \text{ kg} \pm 1 \text{ kg/2.5 cm}$$
[Both above or below 150 cm in height]

(o)

$$IBW_{Women} = 45 \text{ kg} \pm 1 \text{ kg/2.5 cm}$$
[Both above or below 150 cm in height]

(p)

> **NOTE** **A person is regarded as obese if the body weight is found to be more than the 'ideal body weight' (IBW).**

Importantly, in obese people, the corresponding ratio between the lean to adipose tissue is significantly small, since a major proportion of the body fat changes the *apparent* **Volume of Distribution** (V_d) of the drugs critically. Besides, the **Extracellular Fluid (ECF)** present in the *adipose tissue* is found to be appreciably small *vis-a-vis* the lean tissue of the **obese subjects.**

Important Generalizations: Following are some of the important generalizations pertaining to both drug distribution and dose adjustments particularly in obese people:

1. **Digoxin (a Cardiac Glycoside):** It fails to cause an even distribution of the drug in the 'excess body space' substantially. As there is no alteration in the V_d; hence, the **Drug-Dose** to be given must be calculated on the **IBW basis.**

2. **Gentamycin (a Polar Antibiotic):** The drug invariably gets distributed **in the excess body space of the obese patients** to a limit that stands to be much less *vis-à-vis* the **lean tissues.** Therefore, the **Drug Dose** must be relatively lesser based on **per kg body weight,** but more than that of the **IBW basis.**

3. **Caffeine and Theophylline (Diuretics), Lidocaine (Local Anaesthetic), Lorazepam (Anxiolytic):** These drugs exhibiting similar, degree of distribution for both **adipose and lean tissues** certainly require that the dose to be administered must be calculated on the **total body weight.** In this way, the apparent dose of the drug may appear to be higher. However, due to the *inherent higher V_d,* the administered dose will be the same based on **per kg total body weight.**

4. **Diazepam (anti-skeletal muscle spasms), Phenytoin (antiepileptic agent):** Importantly, the **lipid-soluble drugs** like **Diazepam** and **Phenytoin** do exhibit *appreciable distribution particularly in the adipose tissue* (**fat deposits**) thereby registering **higher V_d for obese patients.** The above explanation suggests that relatively larger drug dose shall be needed on the basis of **total body weight.**

Drug Doses Calculations for Neonates, Infants and Children: On a broader perspective, it should be understood quite explicitly that the **neonates, infants, and children** *essentially require* *an altogether different* **Dosage Regimen duly calculated, on population basis, for the adults.** In reality, the glaring differences in the **Dosage Regimen** are on account of the following facts, namely:

- **total body surface area (TBSA),**
- **total body weight (TBW),** and
- **extracellular fluid (ECF),**

duly *calculated on per kg body weight basis.*

It has been adequately established that in **neonates, infants,** and **children,** *the actual body surface area shows a reasonably good correlation with the realistic dosage requirement with such physiological aspects,* namely:

- **cardiac output,**
- **glomerular filtration rate (GFR),** and
- **renal blood flow.**

Variants in Calculated Doses for Neonates, Infants and Children: Following are the *four different means* generally adopted to **Calculate the Respective Doses for: neonates, infants** and **children;** namely:

- **Young's Rule,**
- **Clark's Rule,**
- **Fried's Rule,** and
- **Mosteller's Equation (or Square Metre Surface Area)**

which will be treated individually in the following sections:

1. **Young's Rule**: It is applicable for children 2 years and above.

$$\left[\frac{\text{Age (yr)}}{\text{Age (yr)} + 12}\right] \text{adult dose} = \text{child's dose (approx.)} \tag{q}$$

2. **Clark's Rule**: It is also suitable for children 2 years and above.

$$\left[\frac{\text{Weight (lb)}}{150}\right] \text{adult dose} = \text{child's dose (approx.)} \tag{r}$$

3. **Fried's Rule**: It is meant for infants up to 2 years age.

$$\left[\frac{\text{Age (months)}}{150}\right] \text{adult dose} = \text{infant's dose (approx.)} \tag{s}$$

4. **Mosteller's Equation (or Square Metre Surface Area)**: The **Surface Area (SA)** *in square metres* may be calculated by the help of **Mosteller's Equation**:

$$\text{SA (in m}^2) = \frac{(\text{height . weight})^{1/2}}{60} \tag{t}$$

$$\left(\frac{\text{SA of child}}{\text{SA of child}}\right) \text{adult dose} = \text{child's dose (approx.)} \qquad \text{(u)}$$

The '**Average Body SA**' of an adult is **1.73 cm^2**, therefore, **Equation (u)** may be written as

$$\left(\frac{\text{SA of child}}{1.73}\right) \text{adult dose} = \text{child's dose (approx.)} \qquad \text{(v)}$$

In case the dose of the drug is prescribed clearly as the **quantum of drug per body SA (m^2)**, one may calculate the individual dose as:

$$\text{Dose} = (\text{amount of drug m}^{-2}) \times \text{body SA (m}^2) \qquad \text{(w)}$$

In addition, a relationship also prevails between **body SA and body weight**, which may be expressed as

$$\text{SA (m}^2) = \text{body weight (kg)}^{0.7}$$

Therefore, it is possible to **Calculate the Child's Dose** (approximately) as given by the following expression:

$$\text{Child's dose (approx.)} = \left[\frac{\text{body wt. of child (kg)}}{70}\right]^{0.7} \cdot \text{adult dose} \qquad \text{(x)}$$

Based on **Equation (x)** one may conclude that since the '**Total Body Weight (TBW)**' as observed in the *neonates* is only **30% greater than the adults,** one may derive that:

- **apparent volume of distribution (V_d) specifically for the water-soluble drug substances is relatively much more *vis-a-vis* in infants,** and
- **apparent volume of distribution V_d particularly for the most fat-soluble drug substances remains significantly smaller in infants,**

which actually determines the **Dose-Adjustment** most logically and methodically.

Haemodialysis: Haemodialysis refers to-'**the process of separating macromolecules from ions and low molecular weight compounds in solution by the difference in their rates of diffusion *via* a semi-permeable membrane through which crystalloids pass readily but colloids pass slowly or not at all**'.

The **Haemodialysis** is invariably carried out in severe cases of '**Renal Failure**', *i.e.,* in '**uremic patients**', in order to remove such substances as:

- **urea,**
- **creatinine,**
- **uric acid,**
- **phosphate,** and
- **other endogenous waste products.**

Importantly, **Haemodialysis** may also bring forth:

- **drug loss from the body,** and
- **essentially need 'additional dose adjustments'.**

Factors Influencing Haemodiazability of a Drug: There are *five* important factors influencing **Haemodiazability of a drug,** namely:

1. **Aqueous Solubility of Drug:** The lesser the aqueous solubility of a drug, the lesser would be its **Dialyzability Profile.**

2. **Blood Flow:** Likewise, lesser is the **blood flow in the body,** lesser shall be the observed dialyzability of the drug substance administered.

3. **Dialyzate Flow:** The lesser is the **Dialyzate Flow Rate,** lesser will be the dializability of a drug administered in the body.

4. **Molecular Dimension:** The greater the **Molecular Dimension,** lesser would be the haemodiazability of a drug administered.

5. **Volume of Distribution (V_d) or Protein Binding:** The greater the **Volume of Distribution (V_d)** or more the drug undergoes protein-binding, lesser shall be the observed dializability profile of a drug substance.

Calculation for Fractionally Removed Drug by Haemodialysis: The fraction (*f*) of the drug being removed by **Dialysis (or Haemodialysis)** may be calculated as follows:

$$f = \left[\frac{t_{1/2} - (t_{1/2})d}{t_{1/2}}\right](1 - e^{-0.693T}/(t_{1/2})d)$$

where,

f = Fraction of **'drug'** being removed by dialysis,

$t_{1/2}$ = Plasma half-life of **'drug'** without dialysis,

$(t_{1/2})d$ = Plasma half-life of **'drug'** while dialysis is on and

T = Duration of dialysis.

Obviously, to maintain (and also sustain) the **Therapeutic Concentration** with regard to the quantum of drug removed from the body by **dialysis,** it must be replaced by the same amount at the **'end of the dialysis'**; and this can be calculated as follows:

$$X_d = f \cdot C\,K.V_d$$

where,

X_d = Amount of drug being removed from the body by haemodialysis,

f = Fraction of 'drug' removed by dialysis,

C = Pre-dialysis of plasma-drug concentration and

V_d = Apparent volume of distribution.

NOTE

1. **Peritoneal Dialysis:** It refers to-*'the dialysis pertaining to the peritoneum (i.e., the serous membrane lining the walls of the abdominal and pelvic cavities), and resembles closely to 'haemdialysis'.* **In this instance, the peritoneal membrane is being employed; whereas in haemodialysis, the synthetic membrane is used. Irrespective of the underlying fact that the peritoneal membrane happens to be much more permeable, the 'Peritoneal Dialysis' appears to be critically less effective in comparison to 'haemodialysis'. Perhaps the most plausible explanation for this anomaly being that 'Lipophilicity' is essentially required to a certain extent for enabling the process of** *dialysis by the peritoneal membrane.*

2. **Haemoperfusion Method:** An almost identical methodology, the *'haemoperfusion method'* **is invariably carried out in the critical removalof a drug substance in a specific instance of** *'drug overdose'.*

The phenomenon of **Haemoperfusion** refers to-'the passing of large volumes of blood over an extracorporeal absorbent substance (*i.e.,* a substance occurring outside the human body) so as to remove the toxic products'.

Drug Dosing in Elderly Patients: In usual practice, the **Drug Dosing Level** must be reduced appreciably in the elderly patients due to the significant overall decline in:

- **body metabolism,** and
- **general functionality.**

It has been duly established that the following *two* **aspects**, such as:

- **decrease in 'Lean Body Mass',** and
- **increase in 'Body Fat',**

invariably come into play even up to **100% in elderly patients** *vis-a-vis* **young adults**. Following Table no. 4.2 is a comparison between **the Drug Dosing Profile in elderly and Young Adults.**

S. No.	Elderly Patients	Young Patients
	Table 4.1. Drug Dosing Profile in Elderly and Young Adults	
1.	Higher-peak alcohol levels are observed due to smaller volume of total body water.	Normal peak alcohol levels are observed
2.	Apparent volume of distribution (V_d) for a water- soluble drug (viz.paracetamol) may get reduced, and that of a lipid-soluble drug (*viz*.diazepam) may get increased.	V_d has practically no effect either for water-soluble or lipid-soluble drug.
3.	Age-related alterations in both hepatic and renal functionalities significantly change the overall clearance of drugs [CL_R and CL_H].	No such changes are usually observed.
4.	Since there is a progressive decline in the renal function, the actual dosage regimen of drug substance which are excreted unchanged in urine largely must be minimized significantly.	Not applicable at all.

Patient's Maintenance Dose with Same $C_{ss.av}$: The evolution of a **generalized equation** which *allows proper calculation of the maintenance dose for a patient of any age* (**with neonates and infants as exceptions**) with a view to obtain same '$C_{ss.av}$' is given by the following expression:

$$\text{Patient's maintenance dose} = \frac{\text{(wt. in kg) } 0.7 \text{ (140 - age in years)}}{1660} \times \text{adult dose}$$

Drug Dosing in Hepatic Disease: In a broader perspective, disease states do give rise to major variations in the observed '**drug response**'. Amazingly, the *two* **well-known Bioactive Processes,**

- **Pharmacokinetics,** and
- **Pharmacodynamics,**

pertaining to several drug substances are critically changed due to various disease conditions, except than the one that is under treatment.

It has been amply substantiated that the observed influence of the prevailing **Hepatic Disorder** upon:

- **drug availability,** and
- **drug disposition.**

appears to be absolutely unpredictable perhaps by virtue of an array of such '**effects**' which is produced by an **impaired liver** (or *liver ailments*) as follows:

- **reduced drug-metabolizing enzymes,**
- **drug-protein binding,** and
- **ultimate hepatic blood flow.**

Therefore, it becomes quite necessary to establish a correlation between the following *two* **critical aspects,** such as:

- **changed drug pharmacokinetics,** and
- **observed hepatic function.**

and this turns out to become a rather difficult task.

Example

In reality, there are a good number of different pathways which a '**drug**' may follow for its ultimate ensuing metabolism, and, obviously each of them gets affected to an altogether different level in the particular instance of a hepatic disease. In usual practice, the physician normally should minimize the **drug-dosage level** in such patients having an observed '**Hepatic Dysfunction**' record, based upon the following *two* **criteria,** namely:

- **reduced hepatic clearance,** and
- **increased drug availability.**

Drug Dosing in Renal Disease: The following *two* **important aspects** may be observed in patients having a history of '**Renal Failure**', namely:

- **increased plasma half-life ($>>1t_{1/2}$) of a drug,** and
- **decreased renal clearance [CL_R],**

i.e., the '*drug*' gets excreted mostly via excretion. Evidently, in such a situation, the **drug-dosing adjustment must take care of the following** *two* **critical requirements of a patient with 'Renal Failure' or 'Renal Impairment' profiles,** namely:

- **renal functional ability,** and
- **fraction of unchanged drug excreted *via* urine.**

However, one such method termed as '**Active Tubular Secretion (ATS)**' has been discussed under *A.4 in part IV.*

Based on both intensive and extensive '**Clinical Pharmacokinetics**' studies have actually put forward *two* **additional techniques**, such as:

- **Dose adjustment upon total body clearance (TBC),** and
- **Dose adjustment upon elimination rate constant and/or plasma half-life.**

which are discussed separately in the following sections.

1. Dose Adjustment upon Total Body Clearance (TBC):

Let us write *Equation (f)* as follows:

$$C_{ss.av} = \frac{F \cdot X_0}{CL_R \cdot \tau}$$

Now, the *above equation may be re-written* as follows:

$C_{ss.av}$	F	$1/CL_R$	X_0/τ
↑	↑	↑	↑
Maintained as =	Presumed •	Reduced due to •	'Adjustment'
as 'Normal'	to be 'Constant'	'Disease State'	Required Urgently

Hence, in a particular **Renal-Failure Patient**, if one considers the above values as: CL_{R1}, X_{01} and τ_1, **respectively,**[*] one may write the above equation for the **Dose-Adjustment** upon **Total Body Clearance (TBC)** designated as follows

$$C_{ss.av} = \frac{X_{01}}{CL_{R1} \cdot \tau_1}$$

Rearranging **Equation (ab)** with respect to **Drug-Dose** and **Drug-Dose Interval after due adjustment,** we may have the following equation:

$$\frac{X_{01}}{\tau_1} = CL_{R1} \cdot C_{ss.av}$$

It is, however, appropriate to state that **Equation (ac)** helps a lot in the **Critical Adjustment of the Dosage Regimen** by affecting these *three* aspects:

- **reduction in drug-dosage amount,**
- **enhancement in drug-dosing ,** and
- **a thoughtful combination of both.**

---

[*] F is presumed to be constant.

2. Dose Adjustment upon Elimination Rate Constant and/or Plasma Half-Life:

Let us write **Equation (g)** as follows:

$$C_{ss.av} = \frac{1.44\, F \cdot X_0 \cdot t_{1/2}}{V_d \tau}$$

The *above equation may be rewritten* as follows:

$C_{ss.av}$	$1.44F/V_d$	$t_{1/2}$	X_o/τ
↑	↑	↑	↑
Maintained as as'Normal'	**Presumed to be 'Constant'**	**Reduced due to 'Disease State'**	**'Adjustment' Required Urgently**

In case, one may assign the values $t_{1/2}'$, X'_0 and τ representing the specific instance for a **typical renal-failure patient,** we may have the following *modified version of the above equation* as:

$$C_{ss.av} = \frac{t_{1/2}' \cdot X_0'}{\tau'}$$

Rearranging **Equation (ad)** with regard to **Drug-Dose and Drug-Dose Interval** after due adjustment, one may arrive at the following equation:

$$\frac{X_0'}{\tau'} = \frac{C_{ss.av}}{t_{1/2}'}$$

Conclusive Remarks: These essentially include:

(a) The causation of a **prolonged plasma half-life ($t_{1/2}$)** of a drug substance is mainly due to the significant lowering of the renal-function activity; and the actual time taken to obtain the desired plateau:

- **usually takes longer time**, and
- **relates to extent of renal dysfunction.**

(b) Interestingly, these patients are invariably recommended with an appropriate **'Loading Dose'**.

4.2.3.3. *Individualization Clinical Experience and Optimization Based upon Plasma-Drug Concentration (C)*

Preamble: A critical survey of literature has revealed that there are quite few glaring examples of well-controlled prospective studies in order to illustrate that the individualization of:

- **initial drug-dosing regimens**, and
- **monitoring of plasma-drug concentrations (C),**

so as to optimize the **Drug-Dosage Levels** do result in a much *better and improved drug therapy.* Nevertheless, if this type of evidences were a mandatory requirements, the following surgical procedures might not be even available as to date:

- **cardiac bypass surgery (CBS),**
- **liver transplants (LTs),** and
- **several other clinical procedures.**

Obviously, in the specific absence of the so-called **Controlled Prospective Studies**, the most values of:

- **individualization,** and
- **optimization,**

concerned with certain **Drug Therapies** should be based absolutely on 'Clinical Experience' perceptively.

Anti-Arrhythmic Drugs: A majority of **anti-arrhythmic drugs exhibit** a *narrow therapeutic window thereby making room for an extremely careful titration of dosage regimen.* **Woosley (1988)**[*] critically observed that the plasma concentration monitoring with respect to the anti-arrhythmic agents is quite valuable. However, it is either overemphasized or misused in the process of decision making. He also pointed out categorically that there should be a sound, accurate and dependable relationship occurring between:

- **plasma-drug concentration,** and
- **drug action.**

i.e., a relationship regarded to be much more closer than the one existing between **Drug Dosage and Drug Action.**

1. **Quinidine:** It is found to be useful for **prophylaxis** and **critical treatment of atrial as well as ventricular arrhythmias.**

Important Points These essentially comprise:

- Nearly 80% of an IV dose of quinidine gets metabolized in the liver; and it shows a plasma half-life ($t_{1/2}$) ranging between 6 and 7 hrs.
- Maintenance doses of quinidine may essentially be minimized by one-third to one-half in patients having a history of **Cardiac Heart Failure (CHF)**[**] **(Ueda and Dzindzio, 1981).**
- Usual/normal dosages of quinidine when administered to patients on such enzyme-inducing drugs as Phenobarbital, phenytoin and rifampin, one may observe low-and sub-therapeutic blood levels. It necessitates, therefore, a higher than the usual dosages of quinidine in a patient.

> **NOTE**
> Quinidine being basic in nature and mostly bound to α-1-acid glycoprotein (AAG), its concentration could vary largely. In this manner, the 'free-drug concentration' rather than the 'total-drug concentration' may be found to be more intimately related to the ultimate pharmacologic effect.

[*] Woosley RL: *Am. J. Cardiol.,* **62**: 9H, 1988.
[**] Ueda CT and Dzindzio *BS: J. Clin. Pharmacol.,* **11**: 571,1981.

2. **Lidocaine**: It is considered to be the drug of choice as an **anti-arrhythmic agent** for:
   - **short-term management of ventricular arrhythmias-when administered *via* IV route,**
   - **acute myocardinal infraction (MI)-given IV,** and
   - **used prophylactically soon after myocardial infarction either to minimize or prevent the chances of primary fibrillation or tachycardia.**

Individualized Lidocaine Infusion Rates: The lidocaine infusion rates may also be individualized which is solely based upon the population data duly obtained from the patients with different extent of heart failure. **Lopez *et al*. (1982)** [*] successfully compared the **Plasma-Lidocaine Levels** in:
   - **a 'control group'** and
   - **an 'experimental group'.**

who eventually received an '**Adjusted Lidocaine Regimen**' entirely based upon whether the patient had a heart failure or no heart failure.

Control Group Patients: They were administered with a dose profile having a usual conventional approach, *i.e.*, being administered with an infusion at the rate of **1-4 mg min⁻¹** *entirely based on a clinical judgement.*

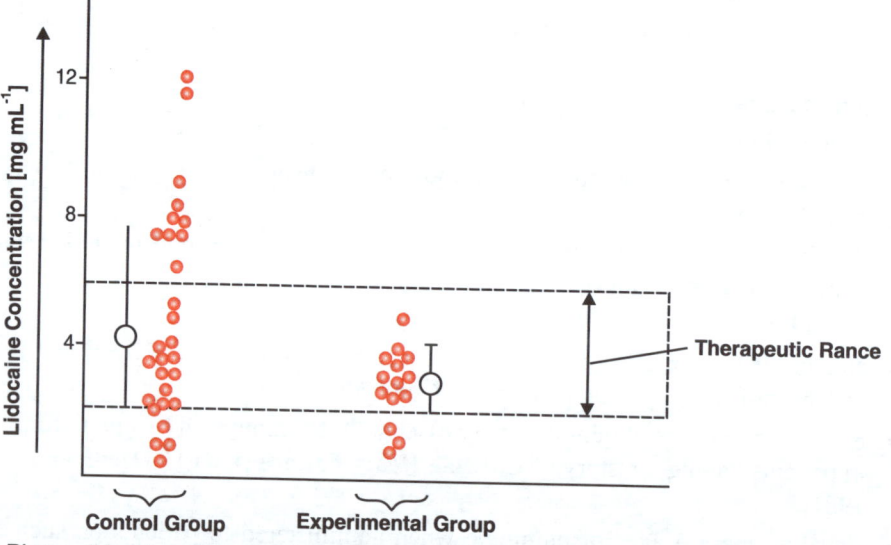

Fig. 4.8. Plasma lidocaine Concentrations: in Control Group-Dosing based on Clinical Judgement; and Experimental group-received an Adjusted Lidocaine Dosage Regimen: based on the Presence/Absence of Heart Failure. [*Adapted from*: **Lopez LM *et al. Themp.Drug Monit*.,4 ,27, 1982**]

Experimental Group Patients: These patients having '**No Heart Failure**' [*i.e.*, **Class** I] duly received **Lidocaine 12-35 mcg min⁻¹ kg⁻¹ body weight.**

The results obtained from **Control Group** and **Experimental Group** patients are depicted in Figure 4.8.

Vertical Bars: Represents mean ±1 'Standard Deviation' for Control & Experimental Grooups. Interestingly, the above cited **Individualized Lidocaine Infusion Rates Approach** has certain **meritorious advantages** for the following *two* vital aspects:

---

[*]   Lopez LM *et al*.: *Ther. Drug Monit*., **4**: 271, 1982.

- **certain particular patients remarkable,** and
- **even extendable to some patients having Class III or IV heart failures.**

4.2.4. Drug Monitoring and Drug Therapy

4.2.4.1. Preamble

Ideally, the rationale concept in '**drug therapy**' essentially needs the individualization of the **drug-dosage regimen based on an individual patient.** Therefore, '**Monitoring of Drug Therapy**' **predominantly involves the critical evaluation of drug response in a specific individual at the drug-dosage regimen recommended.**

4.2.4.2. Therapeutic Endpoint

In reality, the most articulated management of the **drug-dosage regimen** essentially involves an explicit clinical response invariably termed as the therapeutic endpoint. Nevertheless, the close and effective monitoring of the ensuing **Therapeutic Endpoint** appears to be very simple and easy for several drug substances, such as:

- **Anti-hypertensives,** *viz.*Atenolol, Propranolol,
- **Oral Hypoglycaemics,** *viz.* **Tolbutamide, Glyburide, Glipizide,**
- **Anti-anginal Drugs,** *viz.* **Nifedipine, Verapamil, Dilitazepam,**
- **Analgesics,** *viz.* **Aspirin, Sulindac, Ketoprofen, Piroxicam.**
- **Anti-coagulants,** *viz.* **Heparin, Lepirudin, Danaparoid,** and
- **Anti-hyperlipedemics,** *viz.* **Lovastatin, Gemfibroal, Colestipol, Ezetimibe.**

4.2.4.3. Toxic Endpoint

There are a host of drugs for which the observed '**Therapeutic Endpoint**' never remains explicitly clear; and, therefore, the respective toxic concentrations are usually found to be just a little more than the corresponding '**Therapeutic Concentrations**'. Thus, for such specific drugs, the '**toxic endpoint**' is duly considered for the intended therapeutic regimens, for instance, the dryness of mouth in response to treatment with '**Atropine**' (used as an anti-spasmodic agent).

4.2.4.4. Importance of Monitoring Drug therapy

These essentially include:

1. It can be accomplished by closely monitoring the **Plasma-Drug Concentrations** (*i.e.,* **Pharmacokinetic Monitoring**). However, this particular approach is extremely beneficial when
   - '**therapeutic point' is either absent or possesses no definite value,** and
   - **probabilities pertaining to 'clinical failures' are significantly high due to either pharmacokinetic variabilities or unpredictable absorption.**
2. It is absolutely useful in deciding the '**Drug-Dosage Regimen**' in the critical presence of either **renal or hepatic insufficiency.**

3. It may be understood clearly that the **phenomenon of monitoring drug therapy** must be regarded just as an '**aid**', and not as an '**alternative substitute**' for the **careful clinical observations in the management of drug therapy.**

4.2.4.5. Variants in Drug Monitoring and Drug Therapy

There are *three* **well-known variants in drug-monitoring and drug-therapy**, namely:

- **therapeutic monitoring,**
- **pharmacodynamic monitoring,** and
- **pharmacokinetic monitoring,**

which will be discussed briefly in the following sections.

Therapeutic Monitoring: Therapeutic Monitoring approach refers to the management plan that involves rigorous monitoring of the intensity as well as incidence of the *two* **most important effects:**

- **therapeutic effects,** and
- **undesired adverse effects.**

Examples

Sublingual Glyceryl Trinitrate Patches relates to the critical prevention of a pre-empted attacks of angina or shortening of duration of pain when attack occurs actually.

Pharmacodynamic Monitoring: There are some typical instances wherein the ensuing pharmacologic activity profiles of a particular drug substance may be measured with a reasonable precision, and subsequently, employed as a good guide to the prevailing therapeutic phenomenon. Nevertheless, the ultimate observed response could possibly correlate or may not do so with respect to the therapeutic effect.

Example

- **Insulin**-its ability to lower the blood-glucose level;
- **Propranolol, Atenolol**-their ability to reduce blood-pressure;
- **Ferrous Sulphate, Ferrous Glucoate (Hematinicxs)**-their ability to cause enhancement of haemoglobin levels in the circulating blood.

Pharmacokinetic Monitoring: The typical approach that essentially engages in **monitoring the plasma-drug concentration** very much within a **Targeted Drug Concentration** range is invariably termed as the targeted concentration strategy. A further extension based upon the underlying principle that the '**free drug**' is strategically located at the site of action remains in perfect equilibrium with the quantum of drug substance duly present in plasma. However, the above strategy is specifically useful in the following three instances:

- First, when the '**Therapeutic Endpoints**' are rather difficult to expatiate or afford to lack significantly:

NOTE   **Phenytoin-its ability to control and management of epileptic seizures.**

- Second, when the major aim and objective remains to maintain the overall therapeutic effect so as to accomplish the '**optimized usage of the drug**' and
- Third, when the chances of the therapeutic failure appears to be pretty *high vis-a-vis* with drugs with markedly predominant characteristics, such as:
  - ➢ **low therapeutic indices,**
  - ➢ **erratic absorption pattern,** and
  - ➢ **appreciable pharmacokinetic variance**[*].

In short, it may be summed up that the successful applicability of the **Pharmacokinetic Monitoring** requires prominently a complete knowledge related to the **Pharmacokinetic Conditions** of the drug entity, namely:

- Circumstances under which these conditionalities are prone to be changed, and to the extent these may be altered,
- Usage of a sensitive, accurate and specific analytical procedure to be adopted for the estimation of the drug concentration.

Example

Typical examples of drugs substances being **Monitored Pharmacokinetically** are

- **Digoxin,**
- **Gentamycin,**
- **Phenytoin,** and
- **Theophylline**

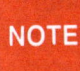 **NOTE** | Importantly, the above strategy appears to be very useful in proceeding with an individualized therapy in such patients having either a *hepatic or renal impairment* which critically necessitates the *initiations of the dose adjustments.*

4.3. Single Dose Bioequivalence Study: Design and Relevant Statistics

4.3.1. Preamble

Bioequivalence refers to-'**the specific property of having the same biological effects of that to which a drug product was compared**'.

Bioavailability is defined as-'**the rate and degree of absorption of a drug from a drug product (dosage form) into the inner compartments of the body**'.

In true sense, an elaborate study of **Biopharmaceutics** provides substantial evidential proof that the following *two* **vital aspects**, namely:

- **method of manufacture,** and
- **ultimate formulation of a drug product,**

are solely responsible for the **Marked Bioavailability of the Drug.**

---

[*] **That is, when the drug is employed in Multiple-Drug Therapy Mode.**

1. **Variants in Bioavailability Studies**: The **Bioavailability Studies** are of *two types*, namely:

Type-1-It essentially involves a logical and precise assessment related to the **Bioavailability of a New Drug Product (Dosage Form).** In other words, the respective **Pharmacokinetic Parameters** following various routes of administration of the 'New Drug Entity' are duly achieved, and employed subsequently in the meticulous development of **an Optimized Dosage Regimen.** It ultimately enables the *appropriate formulation of a* 'New Drug' meant for a pre-determined intended route of administration, and assessment of its 'Bioavailability.

Type-2- This particular type of **Bioavailability Study** critically causes to participate the eventual comparison of:

- a 'Test Formulation', and
- a 'Reference Standard Drug Product',

which enjoys the reputation of a *proven safety and efficacy*. Interestingly, this highly specific investigative studies are usually termed as the **Bioequivalence Studies'.**

2. **Switchability:** When *two* **Drug Products** are regarded to be absolutely **Bioequivalent** to each other, it obviously suggests that the delicate relationship occurring between **Drug-Concentration'** and **'Time-Profiles'** happen to be so close and similar that they fail to exhibit any sort of differences in their:

- **therapeutic effects,** and
- **adverse effects.**

Therefore, '**Switchability**' prevailing among the various *marketed Dosage Forms* is indeed a matter of great concern, *i.e.,* a patient must enjoy the liberty and freedom to exchange the drug product with another only if they are **Bioequivalent** to one another.

NOTE	The above concept and ideology holds good only if various strict and mandatory laws stipulate that all new drug products must be both safe and efficacious in nature.

3. **Elicitation of Therapeutic Effect:** In order to accomplish a reasonably good elicitation of the desired **Therapeutic Effect,** the **Drug Substance** (*i.e.,* an **active entity**) must be:

- **specifically delivered at the very site of action,**
- **critically delivered in an effective concentration,** and
- **effectively delivered during the desired period.**

Importantly, it becomes quite necessary that the overall performance of the **Drug Product** including the 'drug' remains totally reproducible in the body so as to anticipate in the **Uniform Therapeutic Effect.** Therefore, it is absolutely essential that the actual **Bioavailability of the 'Drug' in a Dosage Form** is well established and also remains perfectly reproducible. In the recent past, both **Bioavailability** and **Bioequivalence** have mustered an *ever-growing attention, indulgence,* and *involvement* because there exists an avalanche of 'Generic Drugs'[*] in the **pharmaceutical trade across the globe.**

4. **Abbreviated New Drug Application (ANDA):** In true sense, the 'Bioequivalence Study' represents an extremely important segment of **ANDA** that needs to be submitted to the **Food**

---

[*] **Generic Drugs:** they broadly refers to a 'chemically equivalent copy' of a branded-drug product whose patent has expired.

and **Drug Administration (FDA)** by a perspective **'Pharmaceutical Manufacture'** who intends to launch a **'Generic Drug'** in the market.

5. **Intricacies of Bioequivalence**: Following are some of the vital intricacies of **Bioequivalence**:

   (a) **Bioequivalence may not prove to be a simple and straightforward phenomenon for a majority of drug substance.**

   (b) **A plethora of drugs are usually recognized to be quite notorious for showing the Bioequivalence features explicitly.**

   (c) **Satisfactory Bioequivalence properties could be seen with a host of dosage forms comprising: Aspirin, Tolbutamnide, Tetracycline, and Vitamins produced by different manufacturers.**

   (d) **Bioequivalence-related problematic issues of 'Digoxin' are indeed of great importance due to its inherent narrow therapeutic index. Likewise, a host of other drugs essentially having narrow therapeutic index also pose similar type of intricate bioequivalence problems.**

NOTE	**The AdHoc Committee on Drug Product Selection of the American Pharmaceutical Association published a List of Drugs which exhibit bioequivalence exclusively.**

Therefore, based upon the above statement of facts, the **'Drugs'** have been judiciously categorized into *three* **following sections,** namely:

- **high-risk potential**
- **moderate-risk potential,** and
- **low-risk potential.**

Table 4.3 records a few selected **'Drugs'** belonging to each of the aforesaid categories:

Table 4.3. Selected Drug Substances with Three Different Types of Bioequivalence Potentials					
S. No.	**Low Risk Potential**	**S. No.**	**Intermediate Risk Potential**	**S. No.**	**High Risk Potential**
1.	Acetaminophen (Paracetamol)	1.	Amphetamine	1.	Aminophylline
2.	Codeine	2.	Ampicillin	2.	Aspirin (in high doses)
3.	Hydrochlorothiazide	3.	Chloramphenicol	3.	Bishydroxycoumarin
4.	Ephedrine	4.	Chlorpromazine	4.	Digoxin
5.	Isoniazid	5.	Digitoxin	5.	Phenytoin
6.	Meprobamate	6.	Erythromycin	6.	Para-Amino salicylic acid
7.	Penicillin V	7.	Griseofulvin	7.	Prednisolone
8.	Sulfisoxazole	8.	Prednisone	8.	Prednisone
		9.	Penicillin G	9.	Quinidine
		10.	Pentobarbital	10.	Warfarin

6. **Important Definitions:** It would be worthwhile to understand fully a few important terminologies and definitions before proceeding deep into the various glaring aspects of the 'Bioequivalence Study':

- **Drug Product (or Dosage Form): A Drug Product** refers to-'a dosage form suitable for marketing and dispensing to patients, *e.g.*, Tablets, Capsules, Oral Solutions, Injectables etc., comprising the active substance (or drug) either with or without the inactive ingredients (*viz.*excipients).

- **Pharmaceutical Equivalents [Syn: Genetric Equivalent]:** When a **Drug Product** that contains the same active ingredients (S) and is found to be absolutely identical in

  ➤ **Dosage Form,** and

  ➤ **Potency,**

to '**Another Drug Product**' but may not be equal either in **Pharmacological or Therapeutic Response** by virtue of the **Dosage-Form Effects.**

In reality, the '**Pharmaceutical Equivalent**' may essentially consist of altogether different range of the '**Inactive Ingredients**', for instance: **Colour, Flavour, Excipients and Shape.** Obviously, the observed differences in *three* different **Drug Product Variants** (*see Table 4.1*) made of a number of manufacturers may also give rise to *distinct* variance in the **Absorption Pattern** *in vivo*.

- **Pharmaceutical Alternative: The Pharmaceutical Alternative** refers to-'a drug product that contains the same therapeutic moiety/potency, and is administered by the same route, but differs in the kind of salt, ester or dosage form'.

Obviously, *two* **dosage** forms are regarded to be **Pharmaceutical Alternatives** if they comprise the *same drug molecule but in different chemical form, i.e.,* present in either:

➤ different salt (*viz.* **Ferrous Fumarate-Ferrous Gluconate; Chloramphenicol, Succinate, and Chloramphenicol Palmitate),** or

➤ different dosage form or strength (**Tablets of 25, 50 and 100 mg).**

- **Bioequivalents:** *Two* **Drug Products** are usually regarded to be **Bioequivalent**, only if:

  ➤ they happen to be pharmaceutical equivalents or alternatives, and

  ➤ they exhibit the Same Bioavailability after being administered with the same molar dose.

Evidently, their overall effects in terms of their inherent safety and efficacy shall remain the same.

- **Therapeutic Equivalent: The Therapeutic Equivalent** refers to-'a **Chemical Equivalent** which when administered at the *same dosage level* will definitely provide the *same therapeutic effect*-as measured by the control of a specific symptom, sign or ailment.

- **Essentially Similar Products:** A **Drug Product** is regarded to be '**essentially same**' to the **Original Product** (*i.e.,* the **Innovator Product'**) provided it possesses the similar 'qualitative' and 'quantitative' composition in terms of the following aspects; namely:
  - ➢ **drug substance,**
  - ➢ **formulation type,** and
  - ➢ **bioequivalence**
4. **Aims and Objectives of Bioavailability Studies**: Following are **the *four* cardinal aims and objectives of Bioavailability Studies:**
- Preliminary stages of development of an **appropriate dosage form (drug product)** for a new drug entity.
- Estimation of related influence of such aspects as:
  - ➢ excipients,
  - ➢ patient-associated factors and
  - ➢ probable interaction with other drug substances upon the efficiency of absorption ultimately.
- Critical development of '**Newer Formulations**' of the existing substances.
- Strict control of quality of a '**Dosage Form**' specifically in the early stages of marketing so as to establish exactly the influence of such factors as
  - ➢ processing modalities and
  - ➢ storage and stability on drug absorption process.

4.3.2. Bioequivalence Study Parameters

It has been duly proved that two products to be '**Bioequivalent**' only when they explicitly demonstrate:

- **similar rate (speed),** and
- **degree of drug release pattern.**

Furthermore, the quantum of drug molecules released and also the **Rate** (speed) at which the same are released must be similar by all means. However, in the *vivo* studies of two different drug products with respect to their characteristic features the following parameters need to be taken into consideration:

- **Area Under the Curve (AUC): AUC** refers to- **the area under the plasma-drug concentration time curve, and provides adequate information concerning the quantum of drug present in plasma, *i.e.,* the degree of release'.**
- C_{max}" It represents the maximum **Plasma-Drug Concentration**. However, C_{max} partially depends upon the **Rate of Drug Release** from the **Drug Product** (*i.e.,* the **Formulation**).
- T_{max}: It critically involves the *actual time required to reach maximum* **Plasma-Drug Concentration**. T_{max} necessarily dependent upon the **Rate of Drug Release from the Dosage From** (*i.e.,* from the Formulation).
- $T_{1/2}$**:** It designates the **Plasma-Half-Life of a Drug**. $T_{1/2}$ also provides the required information pertaining to the drug substance from, the body.

Additional Parameters: There are, in fact, *ten* **Additional Parameters** that are invariably studied in a **Bioequivalence Study Profile,** namely:

- **Normalized C_{max},**
- **Mean residence time (MRT),**
- **Plasma peak trough fluctuation (%),**
- **Area under blood/plasma time-concentration curve (AUC),**
- **Mean absorption time (MAT),**
- **Plateau time (PT),**
- **Half-value duration (HVD),**
- **Time above the average concentration ($T_{above}\ C_{avg}$),**
- **Percentage swing (%S), and**
- **Area under curve fluctuation (AUCF),**

which will be discussed briefly as follows.

1. **Normalized C_{max} :** C_{max}, *i.e.,* the **Maximum Plasma-Drug Concentration (mcg mL^{-1})** and t_{max}, *i.e.,* the **Maximum Time Interval (hrs)** are known to exhibit **highly significant intra-subject incidence of variability;** and, therefore, it critically necessities the usage of the '**Normalized C_{max}**' in certain typical instances. However, the '**Normalized C_{max}**' may be calculated by means of the following expression:

$$\text{Normalized } C_{max} = \frac{C_{max}}{\text{AUC}} \qquad \text{(af)}$$

where,

AUC = Area under the curve and

C_{max} = Maximum plasma-drug concentration.

Several investigative studies have logically established that the '**Normalized C_{max}**' invariably exhibits relatively lesser '**Intra-subject Incidence of Variability**' *vis-a-vis* 'C_{max}'.

2. **Mean Residence Time (MRT):** The **MRT** gives a reasonably good idea with regard to the time a drug molecule remains in the body before its elimination from the body. To calculate MRT precisely, first the critical **Area Under the Moment Curve (AUM C$_{0-\infty}$")' is divided by 'area under the curve (AUC$_{0-\eta}$)',** as given under:

$$\text{MRT} = \frac{\text{AUM } C_{0-\infty}}{\text{AUC}_{0-\infty}} \qquad \text{(ag)}$$

AUM C$_{0-t}$: It is usually calculated from the product of time and the concentration of drug against the time, and product by the **Elimination Rate Constant (K_E).**

Therefore, we may have

$$\text{AUM } C_{0-\infty} = \text{AUC}_{0-\tau} + \text{AUM } C_{t-\infty} \qquad \text{(ah)}$$

Table 4.4 records the **data of the product of time-concentration at different time intervals (hrs).**

Calculate **AUC** from the values of the product of time concentration against the time (hrs). it will yields the **AUM C_{0-24}**. Now, dividing the last product of time concentration, *i.e.*, 78 at 24th hr by K_E shall be given by **AUM $C_{24-\infty}$**. Thus, we may have

$$\boxed{\text{AUM } C_{0-\infty} = \text{AUM } C_{0-24} + \text{AUM } C_{24-\infty}}$$

3. **Plasma Peak Trough Fluctuation (%):** In usual practice, the plasma trough fluctuation (%) parameter is largely employed in the **Study of Bioequivalence** for the **sustained-release drug products exclusively.** Importantly, the **Sustained-Release Formulations** are designed in a manner so as to maintain a **Steady-State Plasma-Drug Concentration** *specifically meant for* **Extended Time Periods.** Evidently, the Critical Bioequivalence Study of the 'Sustained-Release Drug Products' generally involves an elaborative comparison with regard to the **Steady-State Plasma-Drug Concentrations** duly accomplished from two altogether different dosage forms. Hence, in this particular instance, one may have to take two additional parameters into consideration, namely:

- C_{min}, *i.e.*, **the lowest plasma-drug concentration just prior to the next dose to be administered,** and
- **PTF%,** *i.e.*, **the plasma-drug concentration percentage change observed between the two dose administered is duly calculated by the following equation:**

$$\text{PTF\%} = \frac{C_{max} - C_{max}}{C_{max}} \qquad \text{(ai)}$$

where, C_{avg} is the average plasma-drug concentration during the closing duration.

S. No.	Time (hrs)	Product of Time Concentration (mcg mL^{-1})
\multicolumn{3}{c}{Table 4.4. Product of Time-Concentration and Time (hrs)}
1	0	0
2	1	2
3	2	11
4	3	20
5	4	31
6	6	64
7	9	69
8	12	45
9	24	78

4. **Area Under Blood/Plasma Time Concentration Curve (AUC):** AUC refers to-'the Pharmacokinetic Integral Expression directly proportional to a specific amount of material undergoing a change.

Example

AUC of blood level *vs.* Time is directly proportional to the **actual quantum of drug absorbed** from a 'Single-Dose Over Infinite Time'.

Explicitly, **AUC** provides a measure of quantity of the drug present in the body at a particular duration. **Determination of AUC:** The *two* most prevalent methods invariably employed to *determine the AUC* are:

- **Trapezoidal Rule,** and
- **Estimation of AUC from Blood/Plasma Level Equations,**

which would be discussed briefly in the following sections.

1. **Trapezoidal Rule:** The **Blood Level Time Curve** may be described by the help of a series of **Trapezoids**[*] - which are eventually determined by each and every concentration time point. In fact, it is possible to find out the **Area of a Trapezoid,** which is equal to **one-half the product of the sum of the concentrations, and the time difference.**

Let us assume that the concentrations of a 'Drug X' duly present in plasma at different time intervals in a volunteer are as stated under:

S. No.	Time (hrs)	Product of Time Concentration (mcg mL^{-1})
1	0	0
2	1	4
3	2	7
4	3	13
5	4	18
6	6	14
7	9	9
8	12	6
9	24	0.5

[*Adapted From*: Garg KK,In:Pal TK, Ganesan M, (Eds): **Bioavailability and Bioequivalence in Pharmaceutical Technology,** CBS-Publishers & Distributors Pvt.Ltd New Delhi, India. 2009.

Based on the above data, one may calculate **AUC** by applying the **'Trapezoid Rule'** as given below:

$$AUC_{0-24} \text{ (mcg mL}^{-1}\text{ hr}^{-1}) = (0+4\times1-1)+(4+7\times2-1)+(7+13\times3-2)+(13+18\times4-3)$$
$$+(13+18\times4-3)+(18+14\times6-4)+(14+9\times9-6)$$
$$+(9+6\times12-9)+(6+0.5\times24-12)/2$$

$$AUC_{0-24} \text{ (mcg mL}^{-1}\text{ hr}^{-1}) = 4+11+20+31+64+69+45+78/2$$
$$ACU_{0-24} \text{ (mcg mL}^{-1}\text{ hr}^{-1}) = 322/2 = 161$$

Now, $AUC_{24-\infty}$, *i.e.,* the **remaining area under the curve,** can be easily calculated by dividing the **'Last Plasma-Level Point'** by using the **Elimination Rate Constant (K_E)** under the assumption that the aforesaid point is beyond the following *two phases*; namely:

- **absorptive phase,** and
- **distributive phase,**

---

[*] *Trapezoid*: It refers to a **four-sided figure having two parallel sides and two divergent sides.**

on the **Terminal Slope of the Plasma Level Curve.**

Hence,

$$AUC_{0-\infty} = AUC_{0-24} + AUC_{24-\infty}$$

1. **Estimation of AUC from Blood/Plasma Level Equations**: Thus, in a situation when the blood/plasma level-time curve of a specific drug substance in a certain dose-size is obtainable duly, the AUC may be calculated as per the following two relationships:

   - **Intravascular Route of Administration:** we have,

$$AUC_{0-\infty} = \frac{D}{K_E \times V_d} \; (mcg \times mL^{-1} \times hr^{-1})$$

or

$$AUC_{0-\infty} = \frac{D}{CL_{t_0-t}}$$

where,

D	= Drug dose (mcg),
K_E	= Elimination rate constant,
V_d	= Apparent volume of distribution and
$CL_{t0-\tau}$	= Total clearance.

   - **Extravascular Route of Administration:** we have

$$AUC_{0-\infty} = \frac{D \cdot f}{K_E \cdot V_d}$$

or

$$AUC_{0-\infty} = \frac{D \cdot f}{CL_{t_0-t}}$$

where,

f = fraction of drug absorbed.

Based on **AUC**, it may be possible to arrive at the following *two* **functionalities**, namely:

   - **Bioavailability (*f*) of a drug substance,** and
   - **Relative Bioavailability (RBA).**

Thus, we have:

$$f = \frac{AUC_{0-\infty} \; 'Oral' \, [mg \; mL^{-1} \; hr^{-1}] \cdot D \; IV \; (mg)}{AUC_{0-\infty} \; 'IV' \, [mg \; mL^{-1} hr^{-1}] \cdot D \; oral \; (mg)}$$

$$RBA = \frac{AUC_{0-\infty} \; 'Oral' \; TD \, [mg \; mL^{-1} \; hr^{-1}] \cdot D_{SD} \; (mg)}{AUC_{0-\infty} \; SD \, [mg \; mL^{-1} hr^{-1}] \cdot D_{TD} \; (mg)}$$

where,

  D is the dose of the 'drug',

  TD is the test drug and

  SD is the standard drug.

3. **Mean Absorption Time (MAT):** The mean absorption time (**MAT**) is normally calculated by using the following formula:

$$\boxed{\text{MAT} = \text{MRT (Oral)} \cdot \text{MT (IV)}}$$

4. **Plateau Time (PT):** The **Plateau Time (PT)** usually designates the time span of either **One Dosing Interval or One Dosing Cycle**, *e.g.,* **24 hrs** in the course of which the **observed serum/plasma-drug concentration critically deviate from the maximum concentration by an amount less than a clinically stipulated differences or percentage.** Importantly, in a particular instance related to-'**the controlled-release theophylline dosage forms, the observed PT represents the duration where the concentration exceeds 75% of the maximum concentration.**

It may be adequately denoted by '$T\,75\%\,C_{max}$', as illustrated in *Figure 4.9*.

Explanation

  Various important aspects include:

1. C_{max}' is attainable after **5 hrs** from the administration of the drug at an observed value of C_{max} = **19.25 mcg mL^{-1}**,

2. C_{min} is accomplished after **12 hrs** from the administration of the drug at a recorded value of C_{min} = **5 mcg mL$_{-1}$.**

3. **PT**-the plateau time comes out to be 5.6 hrs.

4. C_{avg}-the average concentration level of the drug in serum/plasma stands at 6.5 hrs.

5. **HVD**-the estimated half-value duration is found to be 9.3 hrs.

5. **Half-Value Duration (HVD):** The **Half-Value Duration (HVD)** duly refers to-'**the time span of one dosing-interval or one dosing-cycle of 24 hrs during which the serum/plasma-drug concentration-level critically deviates by 50% from the maximum concentration** (C_{max})'-as shown in *Figure 4.9*.

NOTE	In some specific instances, the HVD of certain drugs may almost correspond to the 'plateau time' (PT).

6. **Time Above the Average Concentration** $(T_{above}\,C_{avg})$**:** The time above the average concentration $(T_{above}\,C_{avg})$ relates to –'time-span of one dosing cycle or one dosing interval **24 hrs during which the serum/plasma-drug concentration almost stands above the average concentration** (C_{avg})' of one dosing cycle or dosing interval', as depicted in *Figure 4.9*. In fact, C_{avg} is duly calculated by dividing the **AUC of one dosing interval or dosing cycle by the dose time interval.**

7. **Percentage Swing (%S):** In reality,' swing' refers to-'**the peak-trough concentration difference of the drug substance in the course of one-dosing interval to the average concentration** (C_{avg})'. thus, we may have,

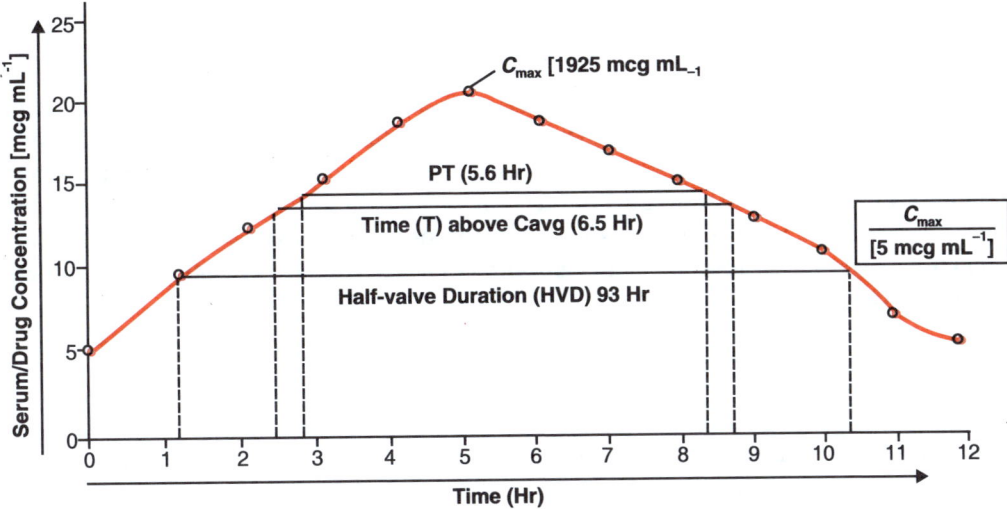

Fig. 4..9: Serum/plasmaDrug Concentration *vs.* Time Curve Showing C_{max}, C_{min}, PT and HVD.

$$\%S = \frac{100\,(C_{max} - C_{min})}{C_{min}}$$

8. **Area Under Curve Fluctuation (AUCF):** In true sense, AUCF is based upon the *partial AUCs over one-dosing interval*. Therefore, **AUCF** represents the difference between **AUC** both:

- **Above average range,** and
- **Below average range,**

specifically extended up to **AUC** in the course of **One-Dosing Interval.** It may be expressed by the following expression:

$$\text{AUCF }\% = \frac{100\,(\text{above } C_{avg}) - \text{AUC (below } C_{avg})}{\text{AUC}}$$

General Remarks: On the basis of the above-stated 'Additional Parameters' expatiated from (a) through (j), we may conclude the following overall general remarks:

1. PT the plateau time, $T_{above}\,C_{avg}$- the time above average concentration, and the plasma trough fluctuation (%) are solemnly regarded to be **Rate Characteristic of the Drug.**

2. **Percentage Swing (%S)** and the **area under curve fluctuation (AUCF)** distinctly measure the degree of fluctuation of the ensuing **serum/plasma-drug concentration at a predominantly steady state.**

3. Bearing in mind the glaring fact that both 'Fast-Releasing' and 'Conventional-Releasing' Drug Products do release 'drug' at a steady state, there exists an *appreciable degree of fluctuations observed generally in %S and AUCF.*

Explanation

Perhaps these critical findings could be better explained due to the fact that these '**Dosage Forms**' get absorbed rather rapidly when they are administered orally so as to cause **rapid elimination of drug** *via* the **First-Order Kinetics** ultimately leading to reasonably **Lower Trough Concentration.** Besides, it causes significant fluctuations in comparison to the corresponding **Sustained/Controlled Release Drug Products,** in which case the **rate of absorption of drug substance may appear to be much slower and extending over to a longer-duration, ultimately leading to a Lower Plasma/Serum Peak Concentration,** and **Higher Concentration Producing Less Fluctuations.**

4.3.3. *Bioequivalence Study Protocol*

In a broader perspective, any elaborate '**Bioequivalence Study**' is invariably geared by a well-planned **Study Protocol**. Importantly, the **Bioequivalence Study Protocol** must comprise the following **essential aspects,** namely:

1. **Title**-it specifically includes:
   - **Principal investigator or study director,** and
   - **Nomenclature of project, protocol number and date of commencement.**
2. **Study Objective**-it consists of major aspects pertaining to the engaged study objectives.
3. **Study Design**-it is most critical aspect of the entire study undertaken, and consists of
   - **Design**
   - **Dosage Forms (or Drug Products)**
     - ➤ **Test Product**
     - ➤ **Reference Product**
   - **Dosage Regimen**
   - **Sample Collection Scheme**
   - **Housing of Volunteers**
   - **Fasting and Meal Schedule**
   - **Analytical Method Selected**
4. **Study Population**-it forms an important aspect as well:
   - **Subjects (or Volunteers)**
   - **Selection of Subject:**
     - ➤ **Medical history of subject (S)**
     - ➤ **Physical check-up**
     - ➤ **Clinical laboratory tests**
   - **Inclusion and Exclusion Criteria**
   - **Limitations During Investigative Study**
5. **Clinical Methodologies**-to provide valuable information:
   - **Drug and Dosage Administration Profile**
   - **Biological Sampling Modes**
   - **Handling of Biological Samples**

6. **Ethical Considerations**-to cater for sufficient preventive measures
   - **Institutional Review Board**
   - **Informed Consent of Subject**
   - **Critical Indications for Withdrawal of Subjects**
   - **Adverse Drug Reactions (ADRs)**
   - **Emergency Procedures**
7. **Facilities Provided**-to include enough required facilities at the 'testing centre' as per laid norms.
8. **Analysis Presentation of Data**-to give authentic and dependable results
   - **Validation of Adopted Analytical Method**
   - **Statistical Methods Used**
   - **Statistical Treatment of Data Analysis of Vriance (ANOVA)**
   - **Format of Data**
9. **Appendix**-to provide all other allied information required.

4.3.4. *Bioequivalence Study Design*

It is so meticulously designated that it essentially decodes/interprets the observed '**Treatment Effects**' that are invariably produced soon after the administration of **Dosage Forms** (or **Drug Products**).

In usual practice, the **Bioequivalence Study Design** is of *two types,* namely:

- **Parallel Design,** and
- **Cross-Over Design,**

which will be discussed briefly in the following.

4.3.4.1. *Parallel Design*

The main objective of the **Parallel Design** is to-"**reduce the so-called 'experimental variables' to the lowest ebb so as to completely avoid any possible scope of 'bias'**".

Modus Operandi: In this particular instance, usually *two* **different formulations** (or **Dosage Forms**) are duly administered to '*two* **Groups of Volunteers**'. In order to avoid a bias, the **formulations are administered to the respective volunteers randomly.**

Merit: *The **major advantage** of the **Parallel Design** is that the **noticeable inter-volunteer variation need not be corrected.***

> **NOTE**   **Mostly, the inter-volunteer variation is observed to be distinctly more than the actual variation between *two* of the dosage forms being studied.**

4.3.4.2. *Cross-Over Design*

Generally, the **Cross-Over Design** has acclaimed a wide acceptance. In this particular instance, importantly both

- **the 'Test Product',** and
- **the 'Reference Product',**

are *usually compared in each subject,* i.e., **each subject serves as his/her own individual control.** Obviously, the **overall incidence of inter-subject variables (or inter-volunteer variables),** *viz.* **age, weight, metabolism, excretion** *etc.,* **are observed to be a bare minimal.** On the basis of the glaring fact that the **'Cross-Over Design'** exhibits the minimal degree of inter-subject variability, it is the most preferred method for carrying out the routine **Bioequivalence Studies.**

Modus Operandi: Various steps involved are as follows:

1. First and foremost, the volunteers (subjects) are divided randomly into *two* groups; and subsequently, the **'actual sequence'** of drug is assigned randomly.

2. When there are two altogether different **'Drug Products'** (or **Formulations),** *viz.* **Test Formulation (T)** and **Reference Formulation (R), Period I-Group I shall first receive T, followed by R.**[*]

3. The time-gap between the **actual administrations of the** *two* **selected drug products** must be wide enough so as to provide sufficient **'Washout Period'.**[**]

4. In actual practice, approximately **10 Plasma Half-Lives** legitimately ensures more than 99% of elimination phenomenon; and, therefore, the considered **'Washout Period'** must be at least 10 plasma half-lives.

5. Consequently, **Period II** shall commence soon after the completion of the respective **'Washout Period'.** Besides, in the span of Period II, Group I shall duly receive R followed by T.

Example

Let us consider a typical example when a drug substance requires a **Washout Period of 7 days (having a Plasma Half-Life of approximately 10 hrs),** the sequence adopted for the administration of the *two* **Drug Products** may be illustrated explicitly as given in Table 4.6.

Explanation

The various steps involved in the **Cross-Over Design** are as follows:

1. The observed sequence of administration (or treatment) for **Group I is T-R,** and for **Group II is R-T.** Thus, any two drug product trial is usually known as the **'*two*-sequence trial'.**

2. Based on Table 4.6. one may regard a **'2-Formulation Trial'** as a **'2-Period Trial'.** Thus, in Period I almost 50% volunteers (subjects) of Group I do receive T; whereas, the remaining 50% volunteers [Group II] receive R. In Period II, the order is just reversed.

Number of Volunteers Taken in a Study: In usual practice, the number of volunteers (subjects) taken in a **'Bioequivalence Study'** is solely based upon the **'Statistical Parameters'.** Nevertheless, 24 subjects are the most preferred number, but a **'Bioequivalence Study'** must never have less than 12 subjects.

---

[*] It is simply a hypothetical example, it may be the other way round, *i.e.,* first, Group I receiving R, followed by I.

[**] **Washout Period:** It critically ensures the complete elimination of a drug before the next administration.

Besides, I such an elaborated **'Bioequivalence Study'**, the critical blood sampling must be scheduled such that at least 80% of the **area under the drug-plasma concentration curve (AUC) is covered.**

Table 4.6. Suggested Sequence of Administration in an Elaborated Bioequivalence Study [Period I and Period II]

Group	Period I (Day 1)	Period II (Day 8)
I	T	T
II	R	T

T = Test Formulation; R = Reference Formulation.

Importantly, it is always advisable to schedule the blood sampling process in planned manner so as to give an appropriate determination of these *two* **vital estimations,** namely:

- C_{max}, and
- t_{max}.

4.3.5. Statistical Methods in Bioequivalence Study

In a broader perspective, the **Statistical Methods** involved for **Testing Bioequivalence** profile is exclusively based upon the following important criteria, such as:

- **attaining 90% confidence interval for the ratio of the means (Test/Reference) for a specific condition under an active investigative consideration,**
- **various Pharmacokinetics Parameters,** *viz.* C_{max}, **AUC are solely obtained from the statistical data, and these need to be analyzed using 'analysis of variance' (ANOVA),**
- **derived data requires to be duly transformed prior to statistical analysis by making use of a 'Logarithmic Transformation',** and
- **provision of adequate 'Summary Statistics',** *e.g.* , **median, minima and maxima.**

It is, however, pertinent to state here that **almost 90% confidence interval** as observed for a specific parameter under active consideration must fall within an acceptable range varying between **0.8 and 1.25,** viz. **80%-125%**. In other words, the **Drug Product** (or **Dosage Form**) is regarded to be **'Bioequivalent'**, provided the actual prevailing difference between the *two* **Drug Products** remains <±20%, *i.e.,* the average rate and the degree of a **Bioavailability** of the **Test Formulation (T)** lies very much within 20% *vis-a-vis* the corresponding **Reference Formulation (R).**

4.3.5.1. *Statistical Method Variants*

The **Statistical Methods** are usually of *two* **types,** namely:

- **Latin-Square Cross-Over Design,** and
- **Balanced Incomplete Block Design (BIBD),**

which will be discussed separately in the following sections.

Latin-Square Cross-Over Design: The Latin Square Cross-Over Design relates to a standard approach for carrying out a **Comparative Bioavailability Study** by using a **Randomized Balanced,** and **Open-label Cross-Over Design.** It essentially entails the following cardinal aspects:

- **each volunteer (subject) receives each formulation just once (drug product),** and
- **each formulation is duly administered just once in each study period.**

NOTE	Unlike the 'parallel design', all the volunteers do not receive the same formulation at the same time; they are administered with different formulations during a given study period.

The fundamental components of the **Latin-Square Cross-Over Design** are explicitly depicted in Table 4.7, wherein we have:

Table 4.7. A descriptive example of Latin-Square Design

Two-way Cross-Over Design

Group No.	Volunteers in Group	Treatment for Period No.	
		I	II
1	1, 2, 3, 4, 5, 6	A	B
2	7, 8, 9, 10, 11, 12	B	A

Three-way Cross-Over Design

Group No.	Volunteers in Group	Treatment for Period No.		
		I	II	III
1	1, 2, 3, 4, 5, 6	A	C	B
2	7, 8, 9, 10, 11, 12	B	A	C
3	13, 14, 15, 16, 17, 18	C	B	A

Four-way Cross-Over Design

Group No.	Volunteers in Group	Treatment for Period No.			
		I	II	III	IV
1	1, 2, 3, 4, 5, 6	A	B	C	D
2	7, 8, 9, 10, 11, 12	B	D	A	C
3	13, 14, 15, 16, 17, 18	C	A	D	B
4	19, 20, 21, 22, 23, 24	D	C	B	A

First Design: a 2-way cross-over design,

Second Design: a 3-way cross-over design, and

Third Design: a 4-way cross-over design,

that designates one of the many possible combinations invariably encountered in such a study.

Two-**Way Cross-Over Study:** In this particular instance, all **12 subjects** are taken to perform the bioequivalencies of *two* **Drug Products (Dosage Forms/Formulations),** *viz*. **Treatment A and Treatment B**. Thus, we have *two* **different segments** pertaining to the study period, for instance:

First Study Period: During this, **1-6 volunteers** receive treatment A, while volunteers 7-12 receive treatment B.

Second Study Period

Stage 1: It is initiated soon after the 'Washout Period' in the course of which

- **total elimination of drug occurs,** and
- **complete elimination of the drug metabolites takes place.**

Stage 2: Here, the volunteers 1-6 now receive treatment B, and volunteers 7-12 receive treatment A.

NOTE   **Thus, each volunteer (subject) serves as his own self-control.**

Advantages of Latin-Square Design: These essentially comprise:

1. It distinctly reduces the effect of inter-subject variability by means of employing each subject as his/her own self-control.
2. It minimizes grossly the so-called carry over effects that might come into play when a given **Drug Product (or Dosage Forms)** exerts its critical influence upon the bioavailability of a follow-up dosage form, due to the fact that each drug product is duly preceded and succeeded by other **Dosage Forms**.
3. It predominantly lowers the time-effect upon the observed bioavailability because each **Drug Product (Formulation)** is administered during **'each study-period'** carefully.
4. It definitely needs relatively a fewer number of subjects to obtain reasonably satisfactory results.

Disadvantages of Latin-Square Design: These essentially include:

1. The study usually takers a longer time because of the fact that an appropriate **'Washout Period'** between the *two* **drug-dose administrations is an absolute necessity that could be very long provided; the drug possesses a long plasma half-life ($t_{1/2}$).**
2. The total time required to complete the entire trial-study solely depends upon the exact **number of drug products (or formulations)** to be evaluated in the aforesaid study. It invariably takes a longer duration to complete the on-going study due to the increased number of drug products being investigated.
3. Obviously, an enhanced number of study periods frequently results into a relatively higher degree of **'Subject Dropouts'** and, therefore, the entire trial-study rather becomes difficult.
4. Imposed **'Medical Ethics'** does not permit too many trial-studies to be carried out on a particular volunteer almost at a stretch for a longer period.

Balanced Incomplete Block Design (BIBD): In true sense, **BIBD** helps to *eliminate a substantial amount of difficulties usually encountered* with **Latin-Square Design.**

Salient Features: The following are the predominant features:

- **Each volunteer never receives more than two drug products,**
- **Each drug product is administered the same number of times,** and
- **Each pair of drug products invariably occurs together in the same number of volunteers (subjects).**

Table 4.8 records **BIBD** of *four* **altogether different Formulations** (or Dosage Forms), *viz.,* A,B,C and D. importantly, in this design, each volunteer (subject) specifically is administered with *two* **Drug Products** in the following manner:

- **each drug product is given 6 times,** and
- **each pair of drug products occurs together in two volunteers** (*viz.* **dosage form pairs AB, BC, BD, AC, AD and CD).**

4.3.6. Bioequivalence Data: Statistical Interpretation

After having collected the data based upon an array of known statistical methods from the **Bioequivalence Studies**, the same may be applied judiciously to:

- **determine the degree of significance of any noticeable differences in the ensuing rate of absorption and/or**
- **estimate the extent of absorption,**

Table 4.8. Balanced Incomplete Block Design (BIBD) of four Different Drug Products

Volunteer	Treatment		For Period No.
	I		II
1	A		B
2	B		A
3	A		C
4	C		A
5	A		D
6	D		A
7	B		C
8	C		B
9	B		D
10.	D		B
11	C		D
12	D		C

so as to establish appropriately the '**Bioequivalence**' specifically prevailing between *two* **or more Dosage Forms** (Formulations).

Analysis of Variance [ANOVA]: Interestingly **Analysis of Variance [ANOVA] technique** is largely applicable to estimate accurately the '**Statistical Differences**'.

Therefore, in a critical situation when one observes a '**Statistical Difference**' significantly, it may become an absolute, necessity to establish and determine whether the '**Bioequivalence Data**' are significantly clinically or not.

Examples

Following are a **few typical example:**

1. A statistically significant difference of ~**10%** existing between *two* **Drug Products** is found to be '**Insignificant Clinically**'.

2. A simple and broadly accepted rule ascertains that in a situation when the so-called '**Relative Bioavailability**' of the **Test Formulation (T)** falls very much within the range

of **80%-120%** with respect to the **Reference Standard (R)**, it is considered to be **Bioequivalent** predominantly.1

3. The observed difference between the ensuing **Bioavailabilities** of the test formulation (**T**) must not, in any case, be greater than ±20% of the average values of the **Reference Standard (R)**.

4.3.7. US-FDA/EMEA Regulatory Requirements for Bioequivalence Studies

The various guidelines pertaining to the regulatory requirements for an elaborated **Bioequivalence Study** are now easily accessible over the '**Internet**'. Various *websites* related to such regulatory authorities as

US-FDA: United States-Food and Drug Administration, and

EMEA: European Agency for the Evaluation of Medicinal Products,

provide relevant details of the '**Regulatory Requirements**'.

Table 4.9 records the vivid comparison of the various aspects of the regulatory requirements of **US-FDA** and **EMEA**.

S.No	*Characteristic Features*	*EMEA*	*US-FDA*
	Table 4.9. US-FDA and EMEA: Comparison of the Regulatory Requirements		
1	Conditionalities to prove 'bioequivalence'.	C_{mas}; AUC_{0-i}; AUC_{ai}	C_{mas}; AUC_{0-t}; AUC_a;
2.	Confidence interval for Cmax.	Yes. Ranges between 80% and 125% (but if larger it can be justified easily).	Yes. Range between 80% and125%.
3	Need for 'steady-state'.	Yes. If the drug product is of sustained-release type.	Not required.
4	Need for a food-related	For immediate release, it is effect study. Required whether there exists a reported food effect associated with 'innovator product'. It is applicable to the sustained-release dosage forms.	Yes. Applicable only if the effect of food is clearly specified/pronounced on the labeling itself explicitly.
5	Need for reasonable, 'metabolic data profile'.	Yes. Provided the 'drug' is a 'prodrug' or if the metabolite contributes appreciably to the efficacy for the 'drug product'.	Supportive evidence required.
6	AUC percentage needs to be observed precisely *viz.* Ratio of $AUC_{0-t}/AUC_{0-\infty}$.	More than 80%.	More than 80%

Remarks: The overall '**Regulatory Requirements**' as stipulated under the **US-FDA** appears to be more stringent and safer.

4.3.8. *Good Clinical Practices (GCPs) in Bioequivalence*

Good Clinical Practices[GCPs] designates articulately an **international**, **ethical**, and *mandatory quality standard* pertaining to various '**Clinical Trails**' with respect to:

- **designing**,
- **conducting**,
- **recording**, and
- reporting,

which essentially involves the '**Active Participation**' of the healthy human volunteers (or subjects). Efforts should be geared to adopt only the '**Appropriate Guidelines**', *e.g.*, **ICH, GCP**, while generating **meaningful, reliable** and **authentic data** for the required submission to the respective '**Regulatory Authorities**'.

Modus Operandi: In usual practice, the relevant and appropriate '**GCP-Guidelines**' must be properly drawn out for carrying out each and every phase of the study. Furthermore, the '**Standard Operating Procedures [SOPs]**' must be outlined explicitly. Ultimately, the '**specific documents**' related to data collection must be so designed to maintain a very high standard of **GCP**.

Formulation of Clinical SOPs: In a broader perspective, the clinical **SOPs** must be so designed that it must entirely cover the following laid down aspects critically related to the '**Bioequivalence Study**' right from the initial step to the **final step** (*i.e., storage of samples properly*), namely:

- **Study protocol,**
- **Approval of ethical committee,**
- **Proper selection of 'trained staff' and available facilities,**
- **Recruitment of volunteers (or subjects)**
- **Retrieving trial samples,**
- **Carrying out actual 'Bioequivalence Study' (*i.e.*, collection and recoding of data),** and
- **Handling and proper storage of samples.**

Highlights of SOPs: The following are *three* accepted highlights:

- **SOPs must fully establish the 'clinical aspect of the bioequivalence study'**
- **SOPs should aid in carrying out most of the routine tasks,** and
- **SOPs must ascertain that a Standard Stipulated Procedures' be followed throughout the 'Bioequivalence Study'.**

Information Included in SOPs: These essentially comprise:

- **Name of Sop, Sop-number and effective date;**
- **Main aims and objectives of the SOP;**
- **Detailed stepwise instructions to perform the procedure;**
- **Entire list of materials/equipments required for the procedure,** and
- **Endorsement (with signature) of authorized person(s) including principal investigator.**

Systematic Collection of SOP-Data: The **SOP-Data** duly collected from a specific study method need to be arranged systematically. It ensures not only accuracy and consistency, but also provides integrity. There are several '**Data-Collection Documents**' which are put into **practice commonly**, *e.g.*, **Printed Forms, Logbooks, Case Reports, Clinical Reports** *etc.*, and these documents must be adequately maintained and archived.

NOTE It is absolutely necessary that a 'Comprehensive Blood Analysis' must be carried out in the course of complete screening of all volunteers (subjects) and such data must be duly stored in the 'Subject Bank' before the commencement of a 'bioequivalence study' and after completion of the study.

Parameters of Blood Analysis: These essentially include:

1. WBC count,
2. Haematocrit value[*],
3. Haemoglobin %,
4. Sedimentation,
5. Blood sugar,
6. Serum creatinine,
7. Serum Na^+ concentration level,
8. Serum K^+ concentration level,
9. Serum Ca^{2+} concentration level,
10. Serum bilirubin level,
11. SGOT [Serum Glutamate Oxaloacetate Amino transferase],
12. SGPT [Serum Glutamate Pyruvate Amino transferase],
13. Total cholesterol,
14. Total protein, and
15. Alkaline phosphatase

NOTE In addition, all the volunteers (subjects) must be thoroughly screened for HIV, hepatitis and syphilis infections and recorded duly in the 'Subject Bank'.

4.3.8.1. *Commonly Observed Non-Compliance in Bioequivalence Study*

Following are some of the **Observed Non-Compliance in Bioequivalence Study;** and, therefore, essentially need a special attention, such as:

- Subjects (volunteers) not receiving the drug products (dosage forms) either as the **Test Sample (T)** or the **Reference Sample (R)** strictly according to the randomized drug schedule.
- Collected '**Biological Samples**' compromised heavily under undue identification, and improper handling or storage.
- Ill-maintained '**Drug Accountability Records**'.
- Inadequate reporting of '**Adverse Drug Reactions' (ADRs)**' *viz.* diarrhoea, excessive vomiting, that are largely recognized to affect both absorption and elimination of drug substances significantly.
- Grossly inadequate medical supervision and proper coverage of all subjects.
- Protocol deviations, if any, not reported to the sponsor.

---

* **Haematocrit Value:** It refers to the percentage of erythrocytes in a specific volume of whole blood.

- Complete ignorance/failure to adhere strictly towards the respective inclusion or exclusion criteria.
- Consent of subject not recorded properly.
- Other miscellaneous aspects related to the improper/inadequately health and welfare management of the subjects that are ignored for one reason or the other.

Overall Remarks: In short, it may be concluded that the respective **'Bioequivalence Studies'** do occupy a 'coveted status' in the ever-expanding sphere of the scientific studies. It essentially implies and assures the entire health-care professionals across the globe that *two* **Drug Products** (or **Dosage Forms**) of the same drug molecule (may be produced by different manufacturers) shall undoubtedly possess the similar degree of:

- **efficaciousness,**
- **toxicity profile,** and
- **adverse effects.**

4.3.9. Exemptions in Bioequivalence Study

Certain exemptions are effectively implemented in **'Bioequivalence Study'** which essentialy comprise:

1. The **'Drug Product'** differs exclusively in the strength (or dose level); however, in such a situation the following laid down conditionalities must be satisfied and adhered to:
   - **Drug Pharmacokinetic profile must be 'linear',**
   - **Both in lower and higher strength drug products, the prevailing 'ratio' between the active substance (drug) and the excipients must remain the same,**
   - **Premises of manufacturing the drug product for both lower and higher strengths should be the same,** and
   - **Two 'Drug Products' under study should have the same (or ~ same) 'dissolution rate'.**

3. If minor necessary alterations have been duly carried out in the **Drug Product** (or Formulation) or method of manufacturing process, and based on the supportive fact that these affected alterations may be proved convincingly as quite reasonably irrelevant for the **Bioavailability of the drug substance.**

4. The **Drug Product** (or **Formulation**) needs to be administered parenterally in the form of a solution. Besides, such dosage forms must be available commercially.

5. The **Dosage Form** (or **Drug Product**) may be an oral liquid available in the form of a solution, *viz.* oral suspensions elixirs, syrups etc.

4.3.10. Bioequivalence Studies: Not Necessary

There are quite a few glaring situations wherein the **Bioequivalence Studies** are not necessary at all. The typical instances are as follows:

- **Drug product happens to be in a gaseous state meant for inhalation, *e.g.*, chloroform, nitrous oxide etc, and**

- Drug products are meant for 'local application' which are intended to exhibit the desired therapeutic effect without any systemic absorption whatsoever.

4.3.11. *Absolute Bioavailable Dosage*

Bioequivalency may be explained when *two* **Drug Products** prevalently differ in **Bioavailability** with regard to:

- **rate of absorption of the drug,** or
- **quantum of drug absorbed.**

It is, therefore, pertinent to state here that in a situation when *two* **Drug Products** are to be considered as **Bioequivalent**, they should never, under any circumstances, exhibit variance significantly in their:

- **Bioavailable Dose,** or
- **Rate of Supply.**

Based on the above facts, one may duly explain the '**Absolute Bioavailable Dose**' as the '**dose which a patient absorbs actually, in contrast to the dose that the patient takes**'.

In reality, the '**Bioavailable Dose**' could be calculated easily from the value of '*f*' (*i.e., the fraction of the administered dose*) by rearranging the following expression:

$$f = \frac{\text{Bioavailable dose}}{\text{Administered dose}} \qquad \text{(aj)}$$

From **Equation (aj)** we may derive (by rearranging):

$$\text{Bioavailable dose} = f \times \text{administrated dose} \qquad \text{(ak)}$$

Now, for a drug substance being described by the '**Linear Pharmacokinetics**', one may critically observe that the '**Total Body Clearance (CL)**' remains absolutely independent of both the '**dosage**' and '**route of administration**'. Thus, we may have:

$$CL = \frac{FD}{AUC} \qquad \text{(al)}$$

Equation (al), defines the '**Bioavailable Dose**' immediately followed by an **Extravascular (EV)** administration as stated under:

$$f\,D_{EV} = AUC_{EV} \cdot CL \qquad \text{(am)}$$

From **Equation (am)**, it may be inferred that the respective '**Bioavailable Dose ($f\,D_{EV}$)**' is directly proportional to '**area under the curve (AUC$_{EV}$)**', by virtue of the fact that the '**Total Body Clearance (CL)** remains constant.

In another situation, when the drug substance is duly administered via the **IV route,** $f = 1$ (*by definition*), because most of the administered dose of the drug substance gains entry to the blood. Now, as **CL remains constant, AUC$_{EV}$ is found to be directly proportional to the administered dose of the drug.** Thus, we have the following expression:

$$D_{IV} = AUC_{IV} \cdot CL \qquad \text{(an)}$$

Figure 4.10 illustrates the **Blood Concentration Time Paths** for a drug substance being administered by **fast and rapid IV dose of 2, 5 and 10 mg kg⁻¹ body weight.**

Explanation

As we know that the '**Total Body Clearance (CL)**' is a constant, the ratio of Equation (an) is given by the following expression:

$$\frac{f\, D_{EV}}{D_{IV}} = \frac{AUC_{EV}}{AUC_{IV}} \qquad \text{(ao)}$$

Interestingly, when '**equal doses of drugs**' are duly administered by both **Extravascular (EV)** and **Intravascular (IV) routes**, *i.e.,* $D_{EV} = D_{IV}$, we may have the following expression:

$$f = \frac{AUC_{EV}}{AUC_{IV}} \qquad \text{(ap)}$$

Equation (ap), evidently shows that in a situation when an '**equal doses are**' administered, the resulting '**Bioavailable Fraction**' designates simply the ratio of the *observed* AUC values. Now, when the administered 'doses are not the same', we may have the following *modified version of* Equation (ao) being used predominantly:

$$f = \frac{AUC_{EV}/D_{EV}}{AUC_{IV}/D_{IV}} \qquad \text{(aq)}$$

Thus, **Equation (aq)** exhibits that the ensuing '**Bioavailable Fraction**' represents the ratio of the respective '**Dose-Adjusted AUC-Values**; and, therefore, may be expressed as the **AUC dose⁻¹** for each individual routes, *viz.* **EV** and **IV**.

Variants in AUC Value: In actual practice, the **AUC-Values** are of *three* **distinct types**, such as:

- **AUC Value for Extravascular Route,**
- **AUC Value Estimated from Reference Plot,** and
- **AUC Value for an Exponential Concentration Time Course.**

which would be discussed individually in the following:

1. **AUC Value for Extravascular Route**: There are several means and ways to calculate the AUC value for the **Extravascular Route**, where we have already seen earlier:

$$AUC = \int_0^c C \,.dt \qquad \text{(ap)}$$

Importantly, the total **AUC** can be determined conveniently by making use of the well-known '**Trapezoidal Rule**', as may be observed in the particular instance related to an intravenous administration of a drug.

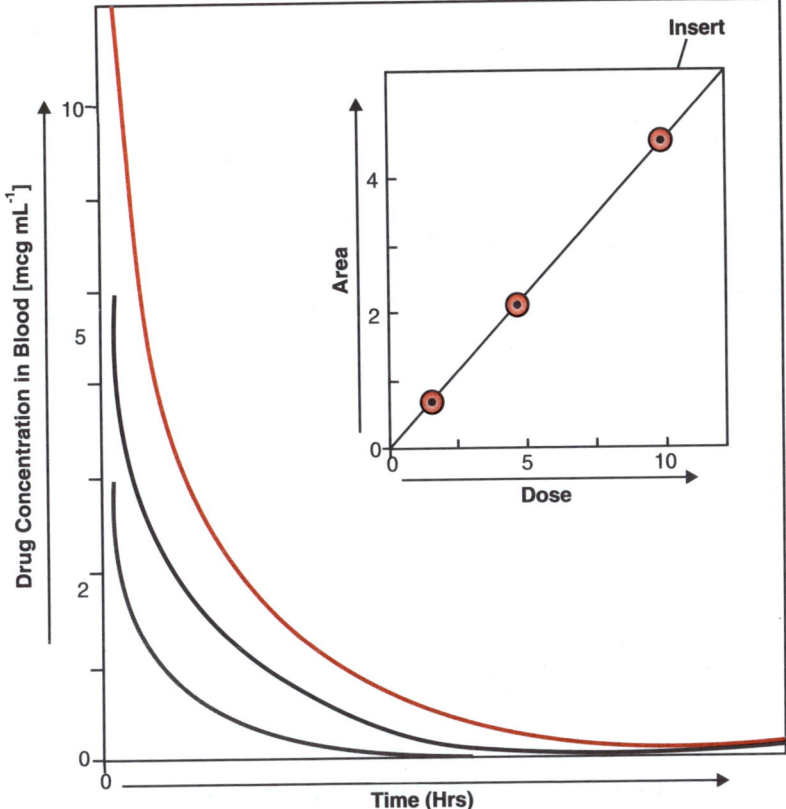

Fig. 4.10: A Plot Showing Blood Concentration-Time Course for a Drug Substance *via* Fast and Rapid IV Doses of 2, 5 and 10 mcg kg^{-1}.

Figure 4.11 illustrates the **total area under the typical concentration time-course following the extravscular administration,** which could be logically determined by summing up the areas pertaining to the respective **Trapezoids** and **Triangles** that nearly comprise it.

Explanation

The various steps involved are as follows:

1. The curve in Figure 4.11 is critically divided into a series of **'Trapezoids'** and ending with a 'triangle' in each of them.

2. Each individual areas of the **'Trapezoids'**, 1/2a (c+d); and also of the **'Triangle'**, 1/2ab, are invariably added up to determine the 'total AUC'.

3. With a view to compare the attained **AUC values** for different curves, it is absolutely necessary and important to make use of the:
   - **same drug concentrations** and
   - **same time units** (*viz.* hrs).

4. However, it is not quite mandatory to make use of the same scales in plotting the data.

5. Importantly, both **Trapezoids** and **Triangles** may even be allowed to be expanded on a 'full-sheet of graph paper'.

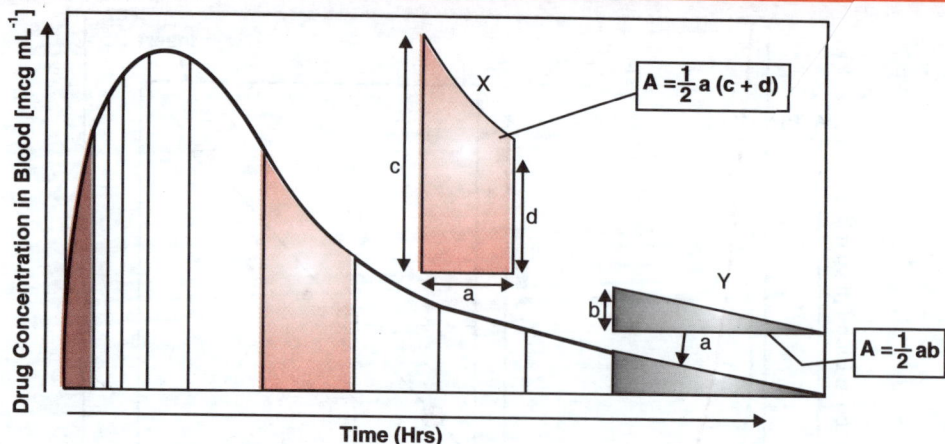

Fig. 4.11: Graphic Representation of Total Area Under the Concentration Time Course Immediately Following Extravascular Administration duly Determined by Simply Totalling up the Areas of the Trapezoids [X] and Triangles [Y] which Nearly Comprise it.

1. **AUC Value Estimated from Reference Plot:** In this particular instance, one may easily prepare the **'Calibration plot'** by

- **cutting carefully a number of squares from the graph paper, and**
- **plotting their respective weights *vs.* their areas which can be calculated quite conveniently with sufficient accuracy.**

Subsequently, the curve to be determined may be estimated precisely:

> ➤ **first, by cutting them out and weighing accurately,** and
> ➤ **secondly, by estimating the AUC value from the corresponding reference plot.**

NOTE	1. **One major advantage being that the irregularly shaped curves can also be assessed without any difficulty.** 2. **Necessary care must be taken for plotting the 'squares' and 'curves', which should be carried out preferentially on the same concentration-time scale.**

2. **AUC value for an Exponential Concentration Time Course:** Importantly, the observed **'drug blood concentration time profiles'** immediately following an oral administration may be invariably expressed by the **Bioexponential Equation** as given under:

$$C = C_{ie}^{-sz.t} - C_{ie}^{-si.t}$$ **(as)**

where,

S_z is the negative slopes of the first-order plots for the terminal data,

S_i is the negative slopes of the first-order plots for the feathered data,

C_i is the common intercept.

NOTE	S_z **designates the slower of the two exponentials**

Figure 4.12 represents the both of a **Bioexponential Drug-Plasma Concentration-time Course** as described by **Equation (as).**

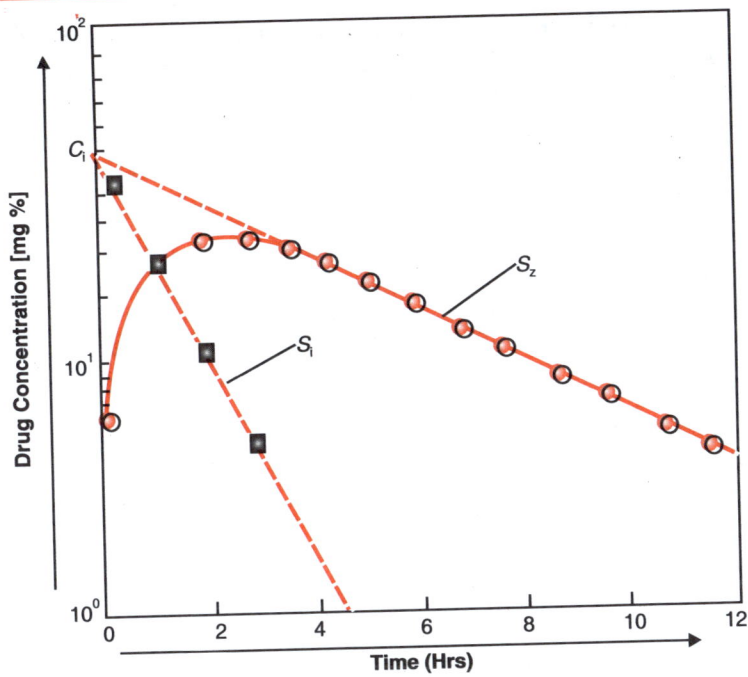

Fig. 4.12: Designates Feathering of a Biexponential Drug-Plasma Concentration-Time Course as Described by Equation (at).

Important Points: These essentially include:

1. The '**Negative Slope**' of the terminal log-linear plot is shown by S_Z.
2. The difference between the ensuing 'S_Z **line**' and the prevalent data points (•) are duly plotted (•) so as to determine S_i, i.e., the negative slope of the respective 'log-linear difference plot'.

Figure 4.12 may be further expatiated as follows

1. The appearance of an appreciable '**Lag Time**' before the absorption actually comes into play, one may observe these lines to meet at a negative time.
2. **Lag Period** is given by the difference between the **aforesaid time and zero time**. Thus, the observed intercepts for the two lines shall never be equal.

NOTE **1 At this stage, it is absolutely not possible to assign an '_absorption_' and an '_elimination_' phase to an '_oral curve_' unless and until additional informations are available.**

3. Thus, S_Z represents the slower phase; and hence, shall duly correspond to the slower step accordingly. **Byron and Notari** (1976)* and called this as the **Flip-Flip Phenomenon** based on the fact that either S_i or S_z may eventually relate to the ensuing absorption process.

---

* Byron PR and Notari RE: *J. Pharm. Sci.*, **65**: 1140, 1976.

1. The competing *gastrointestinal (GI) hydrolysis* rates shall critically appear along with the ensuing absorption rate constant, whereas the corresponding disposition rates may be an integral component of the so-called *elimination phase.*

2. Importantly, for such a treatment, it may not be quite necessary to assign any specific rate processes to the observed *two slopes* (viz S_i and S_z), instead what we need is to describe the data by the help of *Equation (as).*

AUC for a Mono-Exponential Concentration Time Course: As the **AUC** for an observed **Mono-exponential Concentration Time Course** could be expressed as

$$AUC = \frac{Intercept}{-Slope}$$

(at)

From **Equation (at)** it follows that the actual area of a given by **Equation (as)** denotes the prevailing difference between *two* **such terminologies:**

$$AUC = \frac{C_i}{S_z} - \frac{C_i}{S_i}$$

(au)

Interestingly, the aforesaid principle can be successfully used to supplement the prevailing 'Trapezoid Rule' in a situation when such data are ended abruptly.

In Figure 4.12, when the **'Final-Data Point'** is strategically located on the respective, 'S_z-line' (*i.e.,* $OC_{ie}^{-Si.t;=0}$), one may determine the **'Missing Area'** from the following expression:

$$AUC(t - \alpha) = \frac{C_i}{S_z}$$

(av)

4.3.12. Practice Problems

Problem I: A 70 kg patient is administered with a 500 mg oral dose of a drug that behaves as per the linear pharmacokinetics as described by the biexponential equation, $C = C_{ie}^{-Sz.t} - C_{ie}^{-Si.t}$, where $S_z = 0.087$ hr^{-1}, $S_i = 0.72$ hr^{-1} and $C_i = 23$ mcg mL^{-1}. When a 250 dose was administered via rapid IV route to the same patient, the corresponding concentration time course was duly described by $C = (16.7$ mcg mL$^{-1}) e^{-(0.087hr-1)t}$. what is the bioavailable dose?

Solution We know the following relationship:

$$\frac{f\ D_{EV}}{D_{IV}} = \frac{AUC_{EV}}{AUC_{IV}}$$

(aw)

Rearranging the above equation, we have

$$f\ D_{EV} = \frac{D_{IV} \cdot AUC_{EV}}{AUC_{\pm V}}$$

(ax)

Now,

$$AUC_{EV} = \frac{C_i}{S_z} - \frac{C_i}{S_i}$$ (ay)

Putting the given values of C_i, S_z, and S_i in Equation (ay), we have:

$$AUC_{EV} = \frac{23}{0.087} - \frac{23}{0.72}$$
$$= 264.36 - 31.94$$
$$= 232.42$$

But, $AUC_{IV} = 193.68$, and putting these values in Equation (aw):

$$f\,D_{EV} = \frac{250 \times 232.42}{193.68}$$
$$= 299.81$$
$$= 300 \text{ mg}$$

Hence, the **'Bioavailable Dose'** $f\,D_{EV}$ id 300 mg.

***Problem 2:* What does the 'S_z value' stand for?**

Solution Because 'S_z' represents a value equivalent to the mono-exponential rate constant duly accomplished by IV administration of a drug substance, it grossly designates the elimination constant (K_E) intimately associated with the biological half-life ($t_{1/2}$) which is equivalent to 0.693/ S_z = 8 hrs.

***Problem 3:* How would you determine the value of AUC from the data provided in Figure 4.12?**

Solution: Based on the following equation:

$$AUC = \frac{C_i}{S_z} - \frac{C_i}{S_i}$$ (az)

Let us insert the values of $C_i = 15$ mcg mL^{-1}, $S_{-z} = 0.082$ hr^{-1} and $S_i = 4.2$ hr^{-1} (as obtained from Figure 4.12) in **Equation (az):**

$$AUC = \frac{15}{0.082} - \frac{15}{4.20}$$

$$= 188.27 - 3.58$$
$$= 179.31 \text{ mg\% hr}$$
$$AUC = 180 \text{ mg\% hr.}$$

or

4.4. Pharmacokinetics Drug Interaction: Significance in Combination Therapy

Drug Interaction usually refers to the pharmacological influence of one drug on another, which may either prove to be beneficial or harmful.

Pharmacists do have a major role to play in such critical and important activities, namely:

- **examining for interactions.**
- **providing requisite advice to management when any interactions come into play, and**
- **closely monitor such interactions at:**
  - ➤ **patients bedside,**
  - ➤ **segment of 'dispensing process'** or
  - ➤ **sale of medicine at the pharmacists counter.**

Mechanism of Interactions: An array of mechanisms are solely responsible for the ensuing **Pharmacokinetic Drug Interactions,** that may be classified into *two* **major categories,** namely:

- **Pharmacokinetic Interactions,** and
- **Pharmacodynamic Interactions:**

which will be treated individually in the following sections.

4.4.1. *Pharmacokinetic Interactions*

In general, the **Pharmacokinetic Interactions** are of *four* **distinct types**, namely:

- **drug absorption,**
- **interactions changing drug distribution,**
- **interactions affecting metabolism,** and
- **interactions affecting renal excretion,**

which would be discussed briefly in the following sections:

4.4.1.1. *Drug Absorption*

Critically *important* and *specific* **Pharmacokinetic Interactions** which ultimately lead to the meaningful modification of **Drug Absorption Pattern** appear to be intimately associated with the **GI tract.**

Advantageous Interactions: There are quite a few advantageous interactions specifically with the **Parenteral Dosage Forms,** *viz.* **IV, Im, SC.**

Example

Adrenaline-a *vasoconstrictor*-on being used in conjunction with a *local anaesthetic, viz.* **Xylocaine**, retards the absorption characteristics of the latter thereby **prolonging the overall analgesic feature.**

Remarks: Instead of administering *two* **drugs** (*e.g.*, **Xylocaine + Adrenaline**), it is advisable to use a **Single Long-Acting Molecule,** *e.g.,* **Bupivacaine**, which eventually rules out the practice of using '*two*-drug-combo' to a patient.

Interactions in GI Tract: In true sense, such typical interactions may appreciably minimize the quantum of a drug substance which gets absorbed into the body; and, therefore, cause reduction or prevention in the overall **'Clinical Action Profile'** duly exhibited by a host of medicines. These are usually expatiated by such critically observed phenomena:

1. **Chelation:** Chelation is-'**a phenomenon whereby a 'claw' type of metallic complex is formed in which a 'multi-ligand molecule' produces a stable ring with a central metallic ion thereby rendering the ion inactive ultimately'.**

In particular, the **Heavy Metal Ions,** *viz.* Fe^{2+}, Ca^{2+}, Mg^{2+}, Zn^{2+}, may get bound to the **Anionic Drugs,** *e.g.,* **Tetracycline, Ciprofloxacin,** to yield poorly soluble salts which do not undergo dissolution; and, hence, are not absorbed into the body.

Case Study I

Mrs. SL is a young pregnant woman, who duly presents a prescription for 'Tetracycline HCL' to a pharmacy to be filled. When handling over the medicine, the pharmacist checks whether Mrs. SL is taking any other medicines. She clearly explains to the pharmacist that she regularly takes calcium and iron tablets each morning under the advice of a physician.

Pharmacists Advice: The following was advised by the physician:

1. To take **Tetracycline HCL (Capsule)** in the morning and at night, avoid milk and milk products at these times; and must take iron at lunch time only.

Reason: Since the **heavy metal ions,** *viz.,* Ca^{2+} and Fe^{2+}, **may bind with tetracycline (to form Chelates) to yield an insoluble salt which will neither**

- **Get dissolved,** nor
- **Be absorbed**

from the GI tract.

A word of caution suggests that such an **'interaction'** might cause absolute therapeutic failure of the recommended antibiotic.

2. The above anomaly may be intelligently circumvented by taking **Tetracycline HCL at least 2 hrs either before or after ingestion of Calcium or Iron.**

3. The aforesaid **'interaction'** by taking the **Iron Tablets** at lunch time, avoiding milk because that contains Ca^{2+}.

Avoiding Ion-Exchange Resins: The **Ion-Exchange Resins** invariably get bound to certain typical drug substances and thereby cause **huge obstacle in their absorption.**

Example

Cholestyramine, an anionic resin, is recommended profusely to bind the respective bile salts (*viz.* alkali salts of bile **sodium glycocholate** and **sodium taurocholate**); however, they can bind certain drugs, *e.g.,* **Digoxin, Thyroxine** and **Warfarin.**

Changes in GI Motility: It has been duly established that there are quite a few drugs that may enhance or reduce the rate of passage of drugs *via* the **GI tract.** Importantly, such critical discourses may obviously afford

- **rate of absorption of a drug,** and
- **degree of drug absorbed.**

Example

Metoclopramide, an *anti-emetic drug,* helps in **relaxing the Pyloric Sphincter**[*] at the base of the stomach and enhances the **GI motility** appreciably. It critically minimizes the time for a drug, **Paracetamol (acetaminophen)** to gain access in the small intestine. It predominantly possesses an enormous 'Clinical Importance' in migraine, in which case *two* processes occur sequentially:

- **delayed gastric emptying phenomena,** and
- **slowed action of paracetamol in reaching the requisite site of absorption (*i.e.,* small intestine).**

Remarks: Administering Metoclopramide together with Paracetamol reduces significantly the required on-set time for Analgesia.

Bowel Flora Effects: There are certain drugs which may particularly change the normal bowel flora, *i.e.,* normal microbial population present in the **colon (large intestine)** that usually may possess a major role to play in actual handling of a drug. Importantly, a number of broad-spectrum antibiotics, *viz.,* **Ciprofloxacin, Penicillin Tetracycline**s etc., do kill (destroy) a broad spectrum of microorganisms. Thus, ultimately it may permit only a few selected unsuspectible bowel bacterial species to dominate predominantly.

Example

The administration of the '**Combined Oral Contraceptives' (COCs)'** may critically help the bowel microorganism to split literally the so-called '**conjugated metabolic products of oestrogen (a hormone)'** to permit the release profile of '**free oestrogen'** for being reabsorbed into the human body.

Remarks: Therefore, in a situation when the population of bond Clearing organisms gets reduced appreciably due to the low intake of oestrogen-containing COCs, the prevalent '**low levels of hormones'** may not be sufficient enough to:

- **cause inhibition of ovulation phenomenon,** and
- **prevent contraceptive effectively.**

4.4.1.2. *Interactions Changing Drug Distribution*

Importantly, certain typical interactions which specifically affect the distribution pattern of a drug substance are invariably related to such drugs which are bound more intimately to the plasma proteins and, therefore, are being constantly displaced by another drug entity which gets bound rather more avidly.

Protein-Binding Displacement: As to date, the protein-binding displacement phenomena serves as the realistic and acceptable mechanism for '**drug interactions'** and appears to be scarcely having any significant clinical importance. Perhaps this could be duly explained by citing the example when a drug is displaced by another drug. thus, the ensuing concentration of the '**free drug'** present in the plasma shall rise appreciably while exposing the drug substance:

- **to normal elimination phenomena,** and
- **to lower the levels swiftly.**

---

[*] **Pyloric Sphincter:** it refers to a ring-like muscle which closes a natural passage pertaining to the pyloric part of the stomach.

Examples

Methotrexate (an anti-neoplastic drug) and Warfarin (an anti-coagulant agent) get duly displaced from proteins by 'Aspirin' (acetylsalicylic acid) and other **non-steroidal anti-inflammatory drugs (NSAIDs)**, *viz.* 'Ibuprofen', which was primarily described as the probable mechanism for drug interactions for these aforesaid displacements.

NOTE

Recently, it has been amply demonstrated that such 'protein binding displacements' comes into plays as
- **an alteration in the actual metabolism of Warfarin, and**
- **observed renal excretion profile with methotrexate, that are definitely significant in nature.**

4.4.1.3. *Interactions Affecting Metabolism*

In the recent past, the most vital and overwhelmingly critical interactions do take place *via* the following two modalities, namely:

- **enhancement in the drug metabolism, and**
- **blockade in drug metabolism.**

Importance of Cytochrome Isoenzymes: The vigorous intensive and extensive research being carried out on 'Cytochrome P-450* (CYP 450)'-'Isoenzymes**'-has more or less paved the way in:

- **accurate identification, and**
- **augmenting the explicit understanding of mechanism with regard to several on-going interactions**.

Example

CYP2D6 and **CYP3A4** designate the-'**major drug metabolizing isoenzyme systems; whereas, certain drugs are duly metabolizing by other cytochrome systems, for instance,**

CYP1A2, CYP2C9, CYP2C19 and CYP2E1.

Isoenzyme-Based Mechanisms: Importantly, for several **metabolic inter-reactions** the logical **Isoenzymes-Based Mechanisms** have not yet been fully established.

Example

A number of deaths have been reported from **the *critical* 'Inhibition of the Azallinoprine Metabolism'** caused by **Allopurionol**; however, the underlying probable mechanism still remains a mystery.

---

* **Cytochrome P-450:** It refers to cytochrome of liver microsomes responsible for the non-specific oxidation of drug substances and endogeneous steroids.

** **Isoenzymes**: An enzyme catalyzing the same biochemical reaction as another enzyme, but possesses an altogether different electrophoretic mobility.

Three situations may arise with regard to the various interactions affecting metabolism, such as;

- **metabolic enhancement,**
- **genetic polymorphism and drug interactions,** and
- **metabolic inhibition,**

which will be treated briefly in the following sections.

Metabolic Enhancement: It has been amply proven that when a *particular* **Drug (D_1)** [an '**inducer**'] enhances the overall metabolism of *another* **Drug (D_2)** [a '**substrate**'], it inherits a tendency to reduce the level of that **Drug (D_2),** *i.e.,* **the substrate in vivo, and in turn increases the levels of the ensuring metabolism adequately.**

Example

Various **Anti-Epileptic Medicaments,** *e.g.,* **Phenobarbitone, Carbamazepine** and **Phenytoin** do serve as potent '**inducers**' of the **Cytochrome [CYP3A4]**; and, therefore, shall interact with **(COCs) Combined Oral Contraceptives** to minimize the existing levels of both '**Active Oestrogen**' and '**Progestrogens**' (*i.e.,* **Progestational Agents**).

Another glaring example may be seen when the **action or toxicity of a Drug Substance** is critically produced by the help of an **active metabolite. In such a situation, if one enhances the rate of metabolism of the Parent Drug, it could significantly enhance the yield of the resulting metabolite.**

The above instance may be further expatiated by the typical example of **Paracetamol (acetaminophen)** being duly metabolized *via* **CYP2E1 (a Cytochrome Isoenzyme)** to a corresponding '**Hepatotoxic Metabolite**', **that gets eventually conjugated with** *Glutathione*[*]**into** an '**active form**'. Now, with the careful **metabolic induction of Paracetamol** *via* **CYP2E1-inducer,** *viz.* **Isoniazid** or **Ethanol,** one may achieve high levels of the toxic metabolite which may ultimately surpass the quantum of **Glutathione** duly stored in liver. Thus, it would be responsible for affording a **hepatic damage from the everlasting prolonged metabolite levels in vivo.**

Genetic Polymorphism and Drug Interactions: It has been reported widely that within altogether different populations and ethnic groupings, there exists several individuals who may distinctly possess a glaring '**deficiency**' in an **Isoenzymes,** and, therefore, shall not be able to handle efficiently the **metabolization of drugs by the aforesaid system** (also termed as the '**Poor metabolizers**').

Example

An individual when administered with **Flecainide**[**](a Class IC anti-arrhythmic Drug)** and serves as a **poor metabolite** *via* **CYP2D6**) shall critically experience reasonable therapeutic failure

---

* **Glutathione:** It shows a metabolic role in anti-neoplastic chemotherapy [Arriek BA and Nathan CF: Cancer Res., 44:4224-4232,1984].

** That is, a **CYP2D6 substrate.**

by means of a drug substance seeking conversion to a metabolite for exhibiting its desired activity, *e.g.*, **Codeine** (an **Opiate Analgesic**).

India has an array of '**ethnic groups**' who clearly display altogether different proportions of both **extensive and sluggish metabolizers,** for instance:

Indian population explicitly shows variant extent of poor metabolizer levels, *viz.*

- **2%-5%-Poor metabolizers of CYP2DC Substrates,** and
- **11%-North Indians as poor metabolizers of CYP2C19 Substrates.**

Metabolic Inhibition: In a most critical situation, when a subject is duly treated with a '**Parental Drug Substance**' that happens to be an '**active agent**', the respective metabolic inhibition of the 'drug' shall enhance the plasma levels of that drug possessing:

- **requisite potential for toxicity,** and
- **increased risk of adverse drug reactions.**

Salient Features: These essentially comprise:

1. **Prodrug** (*viz.* **Azathiopurine, Phenylbutazone, Sulindae**) must be metabolized for showing its activity and subsequently, the inhibited metabolism may
   - **retard the onset of action,** and
   - **prevent the activity of the drug.**
2. The '**Metabolic Inhibition**' may be preferentially employed to **lower the dose level** and **cost-effective measure for the highly expensive Medicaments.**

Example'

Dilitazepam (a Class IV 'Anti-arrhythmic Drug') specifically causes inhibition of the **Isoenzyme CYP3A4**; and, therefore, may be administered along with '**Cyclosporin**' (a **CYP3A4 Substrate**) in order to lower significantly the so-called:

- **marked reduction in the dose-level,** and
- **effective cost reduction of 'Cyclosporin' in organ transplantation** (*viz.* **kidney, liver, eyes etc.**)

3. Importantly, the **metabolic inhibition** also renders the subjects to a **High Risk of Toxicity level** profile. **Theophylline Toxicity** may be observed frequently in subjects administered with **Ciprofloxacin** thereby causing *immediate seizures*. **This untoward behavioural pattern of the drug could be explained logically due to the ability of inhibiting the metabolism of Theophylline in conjunction with Ciprofloxacin or some other Quinolone Antibiotics** (*viz.* **Cinoxacin, Norfloxacin, Enoxacin, Ofloxacin, Lomefloxacin**) *via* **critical inhibition of CYP1A2 and CYP3A4.**

4.4.1.4. *Interactions Affecting Renal Excretion*

It is particularly applicable to most of the *water-soluble drug molecules* that are duly eliminated via the following different means; namely:

- **kidneys,**
- **change in urinary pH profile,**

- **tubular secretion pattern,** and
- **glomerular filtration rate (GFR),**

and may appreciably alter the quantum of drug substance being excreted from the body.

The above **'Renal Excretion' phenomenon** may further be expatiated *with the help of some typical examples:*

1. **Lithium (Li) Excretion**: A good number of interactions that are intimately associated with the **Lithium-excretion** by the *kidney* give rise to a significant degree of interference being involved.

Thiazide Diureties (*e.g.*, Hydrochlorothiazide, Hydroflumethiazide, Bendroflumen-thiazide, Trichloromethiazide, Methyclothiazide Polythiazide, and Cyclothiazide) *distinctly enhances the renal-tubular reabsorption of Li;* and hence, may cause toxicity profusely. Besides, the **NSAIDs (*e.g.*, Paracetamol, Ibuprofen, Piroxicam etc.) are found to inhibit the Prostaglandins which are known to maintain the required blood flow right inside the renal glomeruli**. Obviously, at a reduced rate in blood flow, one may observe relatively lesser quantum of lithium being filtered *via* the glomeruli, which ultimately enhances the plasma levels.

2. **Sodium Citrate**: It serves as an **alkalinizing agent** employed invariably to **accomplish *two* main objectives:**

  - **enhancing the pH of urine,** and
  - .**minimizing the symptoms of an urinary tract (UI infection).**

In addition, it may exert its action upon the excretion of both *basic* **and** *acidic* **drug substances** as follows:

1. **Basic Drugs**, *e.g.*, **Amiloride, Cimetidine** and **Ranitidine**-the excretion gets reduced appreciably perhaps due to the *production of more unionized molecules,*

2. **Acidic Drugs**, *e.g.*, **Acyclovir, Cephalosporins, Penicillins** and **Thiazide Diuretic**-exertion gets increased by virtue of the quantum of *ionized drug molecules*, and corresponding depletion of *tubular reabsorption.*

4.4.2. Pharmacodynamic Interactions

The **Pharmacodynamic Interactions** usually take place whenever a drug exerts either an additive or antagonistic effect upon **pharmacological action** of another drug. Therefore, a sound and thorough knowledge in pharmacology actually renders it possible to anticipate/predict a plethora of such **pharmacodynamic interactions**. Therefore, in a specific situation when the patients are duly subjected to treatment with a relative number of **medicaments** (*drug products*), it would be rather be difficult to interpret the overall interactions justifiably.

Following are the *two* **cardinal aspects** pertaining to the **Pharmacodynamic Interactions**, namely:

- **Pharmacological Synergism,** and
- **Pharmacological Antagonism,**

which will be discussed briefly in the following.

4.4.2.1. *Pharmacological Synergism*

It may be expatiated by citing a typical example when one specific drug is being added to another drug to yield a definite and perceptible enhancement in the pharmacological activity observed ultimately.

As to date, an avalanche of so-called '**Drug Combinations**' are put in use abundantly for gainful therapeutic advantages.

Examples

1. **Combination of Trimethoprim and Sulfamethoxazole [Septron®]**-it shows a **synergistic effect against the bacterial infections.**
2. **Combination of Norfloxacin and Metronidazole [Norflox-MZ®], and Norfloxacin and Tinidazole [Norflox-TZ®]**-it exhibits a broad spectrum activity in *severe diarrhoea due to food poisoning.*
3. **Paracetamol and Ibuprofen [Combiflam®]**- It is used in *joint pain.*

4.4.2.2. *Pharmacological Antagonism*

This sort of action, *i.e.,* **pharmacological antagonism** could be seen when the effect of one drug prevents the action shown by another drug.

Examples

1. **Marked reduction in the anti-hypertensive activity of a drug by a Thiazide Diuretic, *e.g.,* Nebicard-H® (where H stands for hydrochlorothiazide).**
2. **A combination of Phenytoin and Amitriptyline, where former is an Anti-epileptic Drug and the latter is a Tricyclic Anti-depressant Drug.**

SUGGESTED READINGS

Hardman JG, Limbird LE : **Pharmacokinetics: The Dynamics of Drug Concentration, Distribution, and Elimination**. In: The Pharmacological Basis of Therapeutics, 10th edn. Mc Graw Hill, New York, 2001

Levine RJ : **Ethics and regulation of Clinical Research**: Urban and Schwarzenberg, Baltimore, ML), 1986.

Notari RE : **Biopharmaceutics and clinical Pharmacokinetics: An Introduction**, 4th ed: Marcell Dekker New York, 1986.

Pratts WB, Taylor P (Eds) : **Principles of Drug Action: The Basis of Pharmacology**, 3rd ed: Churchill Livingstone, New York, 1990.

Rowland M, Tozer TN : **Clinical Pharmacokinetics: Concepts and Applications**, 3rd ed. BJ Waverley Pvt. Ltd., New York, 1996.

Veatech RM : **The Patient as Partner: A Theory of Human Experimentation Ethics**, Indian University Press, Bloomington, UK, 1987.

Chapter

5

BIOAVAILABILITY AND BIOEQUIVALENCE

5.1. INTRODUCTION

Bioavailability refers to-**'the rate and extent at which a drug gets absorbed by the body when introduced in a given Dosage Form (or Drug Product)'.**

Bioavailability may also be defined as –**'the rate and extent to which an** *'Active Drug'* or *'Metabolite'* **enters the general circulation-thereby critically permitting an excess to the site of action. Besides, Bioavailability** is invariably determined either by:

- **accurate measurement of the actual concentration of the** *'Drug'* **in** *Blood Fluids viz.,* **Blood, Serum, Urine, Cerebrospinal Fluid (CSF), or**
- **by the precise magnitude of the** *Pharmacologic Response.*

It would be worthwhile to state at this point in time that-the so-called: **'Bioavailability of Drugs'** gets duly improved by minimizing the prevailing dimension (size) of the *suspension particulate matters* perceptively.

Importantly, the *'Drug Particles'* that are: **smaller than 20 mm do give rise to a definite lowering of:**

- **Pain-threshold and**
- **Tissue irritation,**

Specifically when injected parenterally. Nevertheless, the ensuing *Fine Particles* may apparently do exert:

"a typical deleterious effect upon the Chemical Stability Profile perhaps due to their High Dissolution Rate".

Another school of thought refers-**'Bioavailability'** **to the extent to which a 'drug' or other substance, becomes available to the respective 'Target Tissue' after its due administration.'**

The modern trend is gaining heat with regard to the tremendous quantum leap towards the development of highly improvised **'Drug Formulation'** (Drug Products or Dosage Forms) so that the active ingredients reaches the **'Targeted Tissue'** directly thereby giving prompt relief to the patient. Once this goal is achieved, the manufacturer assigns the **'Drug Product'** a **'Brand Name'**, *e.g.,*

- **Travatan®** : Travopost 0.004% (*w/v*) Ophthalmic Solution;
- **Allergan-P®** : Brimonidine Tartrate 0.15% (w/v) Ophthalmic Solution;
- **Lariago®** : Chloroquine Phosphate tablets (250 mg),

and sells it both within the country and abroad at a definitely higher 'price-level'[*].

In view of the above stark realities, the '**Formulation Selected**' and the '**critical manufacturing method**' of the dosage form may:

- **directly affect the 'bioavailability',** and
- **overall stability**

of the **active ingredient** (*i.e.,* **drug**). Therefore, it has become abundantly clear that the producer of **Generic Drug**[**] should mandatory demonstrate that the marketed '**Generic Drug Product**' proves to be both:

- **bioequivalent,** and
- **equivalent**

pertaining to their therapeutic efficaciousness to the corresponding '**Branded Drug Product**'. It is worthwhile to mention at this material time that the following *authorized professionally qualified personnels*, such as:

- **physicians,**
- **pharmacists,**
- **dispensers,** and
- **drug buyers,**

do share major responsibilities pertaining to:

- **selection of proper 'Dosage Form(s)' and**
- **perfect substituted 'Generic Drug Products'.**

United States-Food and Drug Administration (US-FDA) provides through annual published guidelines (both in print and on the internet) for the **Approved Drug Products with Therapeutic Equivalent Evaluations (also sometimes referred to as the 'Orange Book'.**[***] **Website: www.fda.gov/cder/ob/default.htm).**

5.1.1. *Definitions*

Following are some of the key terminologies related to '**Bioavailability**' and '**Bioequivalence**' as described under (1) through (18).

NOTE	For such drug products which are not meant to be absorbed into the bloodstream directly, the required 'Bioavailability' may be determined by such measurement modalities that are intended either to represent the rate or the degree to which the 'drug' is made available at the very site of action.

---

[*] Since the manufacturer has already spent a lot of money in its development in the Research and Development.

[**] Generic Drug: that is, denoting a drug name not protected by a 'Trademark'.

[***] Orange Book: It specifically identifies complete range of 'dosage forms' (*i.e.,* drug products) duly approved on the basis of safety and effectiveness by the US-FDA; and also comprises the 'therapeutic equivalence evaluations' for approved multi source for prescriptions.

1. **Bioavailability:** It may be defined as–'**the rate and extent to which the active substance or active moiety gets duly absorbed from a Dosage Form (or Drug Product) and becomes readily available at the site of action'**.

2. **Bioequivalence Requirement**: The **Bioequivalence Requirement** as imposed by the **US-FDA** for the critical testing of both *in vivo* and/or *in vitro* **Dosage Forms**, that should be satisfied satisfactorily as a pre-requisite condition for marketing.

3. **Bioequivalent Dosage Forms**: In a broader perspective, this terminology duly describes both:

   • **pharmaceutical equivalents,** and
   • **pharmaceutical equivalent products,**

which explicitly exhibit fairly comparable **Bioavailability** on being subjected to identical experimental parameters.

Systemically absorbed drug substances, such as: **test (generic) drug and reference (listed) drug** may also be regarded to the '**Bioequivalent**', if one may observe that:

   • Rate and degree of absorption of '**Test Drug**' fails to display an appreciable difference *vis-a-vis* rate and degree of absorption of '**Reference Drug**', only when given carefully at the same molar dosage of the therapeutic ingredient under identical experimental parameters in a single dose, or a multiple doses;

   • Degree of absorption of '**Test Drug**' does not exhibit a significant difference *vis-a-vis* degree of absorption of '**Reference Drug**' on being administered at the same molar dose of the therapeutic ingredient almost under identical experimental parameters in:

   ➢ **a single dose,** or
   ➢ **multiple doses**

whereby, the observed difference from '**Reference Drug**' with regard to the rate of absorption of the '**drug**' essentially remains to be:

   • **intentional,**
   • **shown in its proposed labelling,**
   • **must not attain effective body-drug-dose concentrations on chronic usage**, and
   • **regarded as medically insignificant for the drug substance**.

NOTE	It has been observed that the 'Bioequivalent Dosage Forms' may essentially comprise altogether different inactive ingredients provided the manufacturer clearly identities the actual differences, if any. Besides, the latter provides enough information to this effect that such inherent differences DO NOT affect either the efficaciousness or safety of the drug product.

4. **Chemical Nomenclature**: The chemical nomenclature used by the **International Union of Pure and Applied Chemistry (IUPAC)** to indicate the chemical structure of the drug.

Example

N-Acetyl-*p*-aminophenol or **Paracetamol**, or **Acetaminophen**.

Paracetamol

5. **Brand Name**: It refers to the 'trade name' of the **Drug Product** (or **Dosage Form**). In fact, this name is registered and privately owned by the pharmaceutical manufacturer in the country of origin; and is, therefore, used to make a clear-cut distinction of the specific drug product from other competitors products, *viz.*, **Tylenol**® **(Manufactured in USA by: McNeil Laboratories); Efudex**® **(Roche Laboratories, Switzerland); Pfizerpen A**® **(Pfizer, USA), Kelbeil**® **(Beecham, UK).**

6. **Drug Product**: It means the **finished dosage form** (*viz.* **Capsules, Tablets, Injectables, Elixirs, Suspensions, Inhalers** etc.) which solely contains the **active drug ingredient**, mostly, but not necessarily, in association with several other **inactive ingredients (adjuvants: starch, binders, emulsifiers** etc).

7. **Selection of Drug Product**: The critical phenomenon of selecting (or choosing) the most preferred drug product in a specified **'Dosage Form'** available commercially.

8. **Drug Substance**: A **Drug Substance** invariably refers to the **'Active Pharmaceutical Ingredients' (API)** or component present in the drug product which is solely responsible for providing the desired **Pharmacodynamic Activity** (*i.e.,* **pharmacologic activity**).

9. **Equivalence**: The term **'equivalence'** relates to the prevailing relationship with respect to the following aspects:

   • **Bioavailability,**
   • **Therapeutic response,** and
   • **A set of predetermined/established 'Standards' of one drug product to another.**

10. **Generic Nomenclature:** It largely refers to the established, recognized, nonproprietary or common name of an **'active drug'** in a **Drug Product**, *viz.* **Acetaminophen (USA)** or **Paracetamol (UK/India).**

11. **Generic Substitution:** The **generic substitution** usually means the typical process of

    • **dispensing an altogether different brand,** or
    • **an unbranded drug product**

instead of the originally prescribed **Dosage Form** (or **Drug Product**). Nevertheless, the **'substituted drug product'** mainly comprises:

   • **same active ingredients,**
   • **therapeutic moiety,** and
   • **present as same salt/ester**

usually present in the **same Drug Product** but is obviously made by an altogether different manufacturer.

Example

A prescription for *Glaxo Smith Kline Pharmaceutical Ltd. Brand* **[Calpol**®**] Paracetamol Tablets** might be dispensed by the pharmacist with either **Genmole**® by *Cadila Pharmaceuticals* or *Magadol*® by *Novocare Pharmaceuticals* or if the generic substitution is duly permitted and indicated by respective physician.

12. **Pharmaceutical Alternatives**: **Dosage Forms** which prominently consist of the same therapeutic moiety, but actually present as complexes, salts or esters.

Examples

Preparations available as '**Testosterone**' active drug:

- **Andractim®-Chemech Laboratories: Dihydrotestosterone:**
- **Nuvir®-Infar Laboratories: Testosterone Undercanoate:**
- **Sustanon-100®-Infar Laboratories; Testosterone Propionate,**

Remarks: Following *two* **important remarks** may be noted:

(a) **Drug Product Variants** having different strengths within a product line produced by a '**single manufacturer**' are usually considered as pharmaceutical alternatives, such as:

- **a sustained-release dosage form** and
- **a standard immediate-release drug product.**

(b) **US-FDA Requirement:** It critically examines and considers a '**Tablet**' or '**Capsule**' essentially comprising the '**same active ingredient**' present duly in the '**same dosage strength**' as in the **Alternative Pharmaceuticals** (or **Drug Products**).

13. **Pharmaceutical Equivalent:** It has been frequently observed that such drug products available in **Identical Dosage Forms** which consist of the **Same Active Ingredient(s)**, *i.e., the same salt or ester*, do designate the same dosage form; and hence:

- **may be administered *via* the same route, and**
- **show same strength or concentration.**

Examples

- **Chlordiazepoxide hydrochloride Capsules: 5 mg:**
- **Tobramycin-2 mL Vial: 80 mg:**
- **Dextromethorphan hydrobromide Syrup: 10 mg:**

Valid Requirements: These essentially include:

(a) **Pharmaceutically Equivalent Dosage Forms** are specifically formulated in such a way so as to:

- **comprise same quantum of 'active substance' in the same drug products, and**
- **fulfill the same or compendia or recognized applicable standards,** *e.g.,* **identity, purity, quality** and **strength**; however, they could be altogether different properties, for instance: shape; scoring profile; release mechanisms; packaging modalities; expiration time; labeling pattern and excipients (*viz.* **preservatives, colour, permissible flavours**).

(b) **Pharmaceutical Equivalents** should comply with the following characteristics features, such as:

- **uniformity,**
- **disintegration time,** and/or
- **dissolution rates.**

Modified-Release Drug Products: These essentially need such features as:

- **adequate overage,** and
- **reservoir of 'active principle'.**

Interestingly, there are certain **Dosage Forms,** *e.g.,* **'Prefilled Syringes'**

(Erythropoietin 4,00,000 IU SC-Injectables), wherein the ensuing residual volume may change and should be able to deliver identical quantum of the **'active drug ingredients'** over a certain stipulated **'identical dosing period'.**

14. **Pharmaceutical Substitution**: The **Pharmaceutical Substitution** refers to-'the **phenomenon of dispensing a pharmaceutical alternative for the prescribed dosage form':**

Examples

Following are a few typical examples:

- **Tetracycline hydrochloride-given instead of tetracycline phosphate;**
- **Testosterone undecanoate-dispensed in place of testosterone propionate;**
- **Amplicillin suspension-dispensed instead of amplicillin capsules.**

NOTE **The 'Pharmaceutical Substitution' invariably requires the physician's prior approval of recommendation.**

15. **Reference Listed Drug (RLD): FDA** *defines the reference listed drug* **(RLD) as-'the drug product (or dosage form) upon which an applicant relies at the time of seeking approval of an Abbreviated New Drug Application (NDA)'.**

RLD invariably designates the 'brand name drug' which has a fill **New Drug Application (NDA).**

FDA Guidelines: There are *two* **important aspects;** namely:

- **It represents a 'single reference listed drug' as the standard to which almost all generic versions should be proved to be bioequivalent,** and
- **FDA intends to circumvent any possible significant variations among the 'Generic Drugs' plus their contemporary brand name drugs. Evidently, such variations might come into being when the 'Generic Drugs' are compared with various listed 'Reference Drugs'.**

16. **Therapeutic Equivalents:** In general, the dosage forms are known to be **therapeutic equivalents** provided they happen to be **'Pharmaceutical Equivalents'. Besides, they may be expected to possess:**

- **same 'clinical efficaciousness',** and
- **same 'safety profile'**

on being given to the patients strictly as per the specified guidelines provided on the **'Label'** itself.

FDA-Classified Therapeutically Equivalent Dosage Forms: In reality, these '**Drug Products**' must comply with the following *five* **important criteria**, namely:

(a) They should be approved as **safe and effective.**

(b) They are **pharmaceutical equivalents**, whereby they specifically fulfill the following critical aspects:

- Consist of similar quantum of the same '**active drug component**' in the same *drug product* and essentially the *same route of administration,*

- Should comply with compendia or other approved standards related to: **strength, purity, quality** and **identity.**

(c) These are '**Bioequivalent**' in nature, and in that,

- They do not present either an already known or a potential '**Bioequivalence**' **problem;** however, they do comply with a stipulated acceptable in vitro standard and/or

- In case, they really pose a definite known or potential problem, they must afford a mutually suitable **Bioequivalence Standard.**

(d) They must be **labeled properly.**

(e) These '**Drug Products**' are normally manufactured in complete adherence to and compliance with the **Current Good Manufacturing Practice (cGMP) regulations and guidelines.**

NOTE	FDA reposes total confidence and belief that all such 'dosage forms' duly recognized and approved under the category of 'therapeutically Equivalents' may be substituted freely with the utmost expectation that the substituted product would certainly give rise to the same 'clinical effect' with required 'safety profile' in comparison to the 'Prescribed Product'.

17. **Therapeutic Alternatives:** The **Therapeutic Alternatives** invariably refers to the drug products (or dosage forms) comprising variant '**Active Components**' which are recommended for the same therapeutic or clinical objectives.

It is worthwhile to add here that the selected '**Active Ingredients**' duly incorporated in the therapeutic alternatives do normally belong to the same pharmacologic category; and, therefore, are obviously expected to display the same therapeutic effect on being administered to the patients by physicians (for all such conditions of usage).

Examples

Following are *two* **typical examples:**

- **Cimetidine is administered in place of 'Ranitidine', and**
- **Ibuprofen is recommended instead of 'Aspirin'.**

18. **Therapeutic Substitution**: The therapeutic substitution relates to the careful phenomenon of dispensing a therapeutic alternative instead of the prescribed **Drug Product (or Dosage Form).**

Examples

Following are *two* typical examples:

(a) **Ibuprofen may be dispensed in place of 'Naproxen', and**

(b) **Amoxicillin may be given instead of 'Impicillin'.**

Importantly, one may also come across the *therapeutic substitution in the event when one NDA-approved drug substance is being substituted for the same drug that has been duly approved by a different NDA.*

Example

Nicoderm®-a Nicotine Transdermal Product may be judiciously substituted by another drug product, *viz.* Nicotrol® (also a Nicotine transdermal System).

5.2. Bioavailability

5.2.1. *Preamble*

In true sense, '**Bioavailability**' designates the precise quantum of the '**Active Drug**' duly administered in a pharmacologic dose that eventually penetrates the systemic circulation soon after the oral administration. One may observe the fundamental underlying fact that different **Dosage Forms** (**Formulations**) of the same active drug may not be equivalent therapeutically for the simple reason that their **Bioavailability** differs grossly.

In other words, the present-day physicians do understand and appreciate the enormous importance of.

- **underlying concept of Bioavailability,** and
- **wide Practical Applications.**

Mechanism: The '**Bioavailability**', also sometimes known as '**Systemic Availability**', of an orally given **Drug Product (Dosage Form)** depends exclusively on the following *two* **cardinal aspects**:

- **Systemic Absorption Profile,** and
- **Degree of 'Hepatic Metabolism'.**

These are exerted upon its '**First-pass** *via* **the Liver**'-over and above its due action at the level of the receptors.

Important Points These essentially include:

1. **Bioavailability** is duly estimated by assessing either the plasma concentration or the wide concentration stretched over a stipulated time following the oral administration of drug product.

2. For being therapeutically equivalent, it is necessary that various available dosage forms of the same active drug must be **Bioequivalent**, suggesting thereby that *they should possess almost similar systemic availability.*

Observation: The **Drug Products** from different manufactures, and even different batches of '**Drugs**' from the same pharmaceutical enterprise, do exhibit:

- **non-compliance of bioeqivalency**, and
- **dissimilar systemic availability:**

Major differences in **Bioavailability** represent clinical relevance;

Minor differences in **Bioavailability** also seem to be important for such **'Active Ingredients'** that show:

- **steep dose-response curve** and/or
- **narrow margin of safety.**

3. Amazingly, a large volume of marketed **'Drug Products'** or **'Dosage Forms'** invariably possess prominent **'flat dose-reponse curves'**, in order that exclusively marked and pronounced observed differences in **'Bioequivalence'** shall eventually give rise to the ultimate difference in the therapeutic equivalence.

5.2.2. *Absolute Bioavailability*

The **Absolute Bioavailability** of an **active ingredient (drug)** present in a dosage form duly administered by an **Extra Vascular (EV) Route**, including the oral route penetrating the systemic circulation is designated by the fraction of the same dose of the drug being administered *via* the **IV route**. Thus, we have *two* **distinct situations;**

IV route-the entire administered **'Active Drug Dosage'** gets directly introduced right inside the systemic circulation; and, therefore, regarded to be **Bioavailable** even up to 100%;

EV route-the **'active ingredient' (drug)** needs to be absorbed so as to make its way right into the **'systemic circulation'.**

In this manner, one may calculate the **'Absolute Bioavailability'** by the following expression:

$$\text{Absolute Bioavailability} \frac{(AUC)_{abs}}{(AUC)_{iv}}$$

where,

$(AUC)_{abs}$ = **Total area under the curve following administration of 'single dose of the drug' *via* a given absorption site,** and

$(AUC)_{iv}$ = **Total area under the curve following administration of 'single dose of the drug' *via* rapid IV injection.**

Obviously, **Equation (a)** holds good in a situation when the same doses are usually employed for both the rotes, *i.e.,* **EV-and IV-Routes.** Importantly, when these doses are actually different from one another, a necessary correction for the definite dose size (strength) is required to be made as given by the following **'modified expression':**

$$\text{Absolute Bioavailability} \frac{(AUC)_{abs} \times D_{iv}}{(AUC)_{iv} \times D_{abs}}$$

where,

D_{iv} = **Dose size being administered via IV-route,** and

D_{abs} = **Dose size of the single-dose being given via the absorption site.**

5.2.3. *Relative Bioavailability*

The **Relative Bioavailability** designates explicitly a measure of a '**fraction**' of a given '**active drug**' which gets adequately absorbed right into the systemic circulation duly emanated from a specific dose level in comparison to a clinically established and proven standard dose of the same drug substance.

Evidently, it may be determined for the specific drugs which cannot be administered and an **IV Bolus Injection**. Therefore, to circumvent such a typical difficult situation, both products- '**Test Dose**' and '**Standard Dose**'- comprising equal quantum of the drug need to be given via the same route of administration to the same subject at different occasions; and ultimately, the necessary calculations is carried out based upon the previously discussed '**Plasma-Concentration Time Curves**'. Thus, we may have the following modified expression for the '**Relative Bioavailability**':

$$\text{Absolute Bioavailability} \frac{(\text{AUC})_{\text{test}}}{(\text{AUC})_{\text{standard}}}$$

where,

$(\text{AUC})_{\text{test}}$ = **Total area under the curve following administration of a 'Single Test Dose',** and

$(\text{AUC})_{\text{standard}}$ = **Total area under the curve following administration of a 'single Standard Dose'.**

Nevertheless, in a situation when different '**Test Dose**' and '**Standard Dose**' are duly administered, it is absolutely mandatory and necessary that a '**correction**' has to be made for the size of the dose. Thus, we may have the following modified version of the '**Relative Bioavailability**'.

$$\text{Absolute Bioavailability} \frac{(\text{AUC})_{\text{test}} \times D_{\text{standard}}}{(\text{AUC})_{\text{standard}} \times D_{\text{test}}}$$

where,

D_{standard} = **Size of the single dose of 'Standard Dose Form',** and

D_{test} = **Size òf the single dose of 'Test Dose Form'.**

 NOTE In general, the 'Absolute or Relative Bioavailability' can be logically expressed in terms of either a 'fraction' or 'percentage' of the 'test Drug' relative to the 'Standard Drug' dosage forms (or formulations).

5.2.4. *Bioequivalence Assessment and Data Evaluation (or Importance of Bioequivalence)*

Vigorous research in pharmaceutical sciences have ascertained that an array of parameters are invariably used to provide a general evaluation of:

- **the overall rate,** and
- **degree of absorption of an active drug substance.**

Importantly, a comprehensive analysis of almost all characteristic features is essentially needed before it could be rendered possible implicate either a '**Single Factor**' or '**Parameter**' showing:

- **prevalence of 'Bioequivalence' and**
- **absence of 'Bioequivalence'.**

5.2.4.1. *Bioequivalence Assessment*

The focal point of the '**Bioequivalence Assessment**' is given by the **Plasma Concentration-Time Curve** (*see Section 4(3.2): Fig 4.9*), which is duly obtained when sequential blood samples are taken after drug administration and are subjected to assay of drug by standard method.

Obviously, when a **Dosage Form** (or **Drug Product**) is administered orally at time '**zero**', the prevalent drug concentration at this material time must also be '**zero**'. From this point onwards, the fateful '**Drug Product**' takes the course via the **GI Tract** (*i.e., stomach, small intestine, colon*); and it should pass through a '**sequence of events**' as illustrated clearly in Figure 5.1.

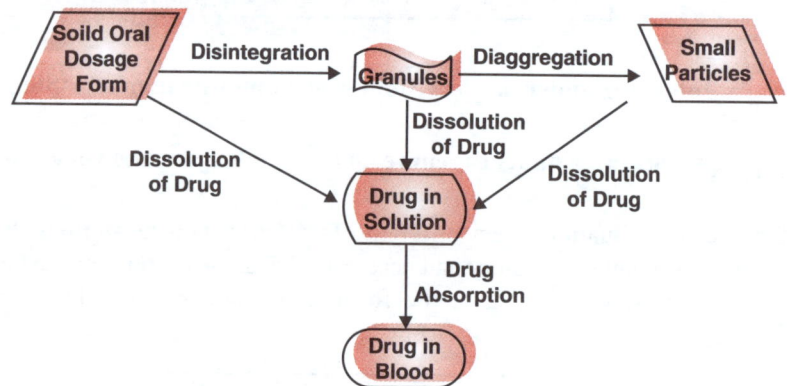

Fig. 5.1: Diagrammatic Representation of Sequence of Events Involved in the Dissolution and Absorption of a Drug from a Solid Oral Dosage Form.

Explanation

The '**Drug Product**' (or **Dosage Form**), *viz.* **solid oral dosage form** (Tablets), granules (in Capsules) and small particles (**microcrystalline drug**, *e.g.,* **microcrystalline Aspirin**) all undergo dissolution to result in the formation of '**drug in solution**' form, which upon systemic drug absorption reaches the circulating blood system.

5.2.4.2. *Urinary Drug Amount-Time Profiles*

It would be worthwhile to state at this point in time that one may not be solely confined to the usual drug blood-level profiles, but in a similar manner, can also be accomplished *via* the cumulative urinary drug amount-time profiles.

Modus Operandi: The following are the various steps involved:

1. **Determination of 'Drug Concentration' in discharged urine at specified time intervals.**
2. **The quantum of 'drug' excreted per interval is duly estimated by multiplying the concentration of drug by the volume of urine collected in that time interval.**

3. The quantities of drug collected in each interval are now combined, and finally the 'total amount' excreted in the urine is arrived at.

4. The resulting value is almost analogous to the area under the curve (AUC).

Example

An elaborated '**Cumulative Urinary Drug Amount-Time Profile**' for many marketed 'nitrofurantoin formulations' is duly represented in Figure 5.2.[*]

NOTE	It is almost total and unquestioning that the analytical methodology employed for the analysis of drug in the samples is not only precise and accurate, but also specific and sensitive.

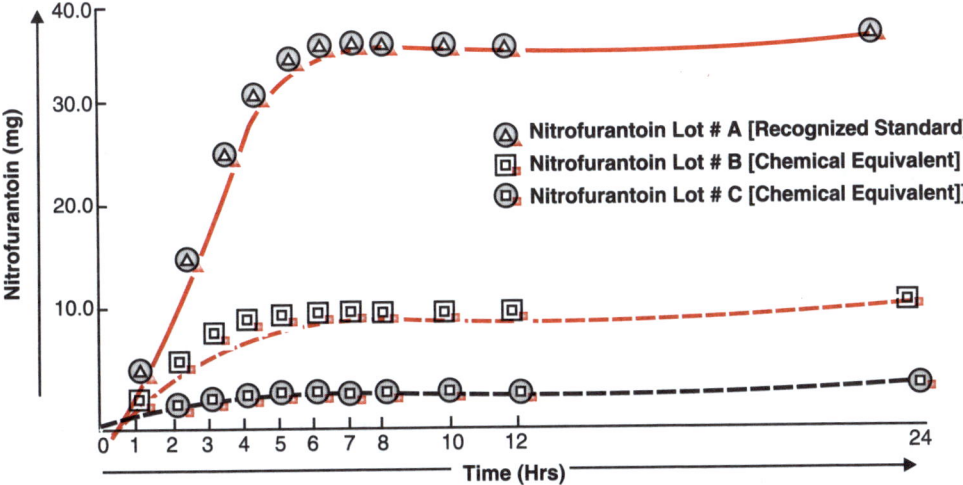

Fig. 5.2: Diagrammatic Representation of Average Cumulative Quantum of Nitrofurantoin Excreted from Three Different Lots (A,B and C) of Two Marketed Dosage Forms after a Single Oral Dose of 100 mg of Nitrofurantoin.

5.2.4.3. *Peak-Height Concentration*

The '**Peak-Height Concentration**' actually refers to the observed height of the peak of the **Blood Level-Time Curve** that critically represents the highest drug concentration accomplished after the oral administration. In usual practice, it is reported invariably as a quantity per volume measurement, such as:

mcg mL^{-1}: microgrammes per milliliter or

G 100 mL^{-1}: grammes per 100 milliliter

Importance: The most decisive importance of the '**Peak-Height Concentration**' is depicted in an elaborate fashion in Figure 5.3, wherein the **Blood Concentration-Time Curves** of *two* altogether different Dosage Forms of a Drug Substance are duly represented.

---

* **Adapted From: Gennaro AR: Remington: The Science and Practice of Pharmacy, Vol. I, 21st. e.d.,** Lippincott Williams & Wilkins, New York, 2005.

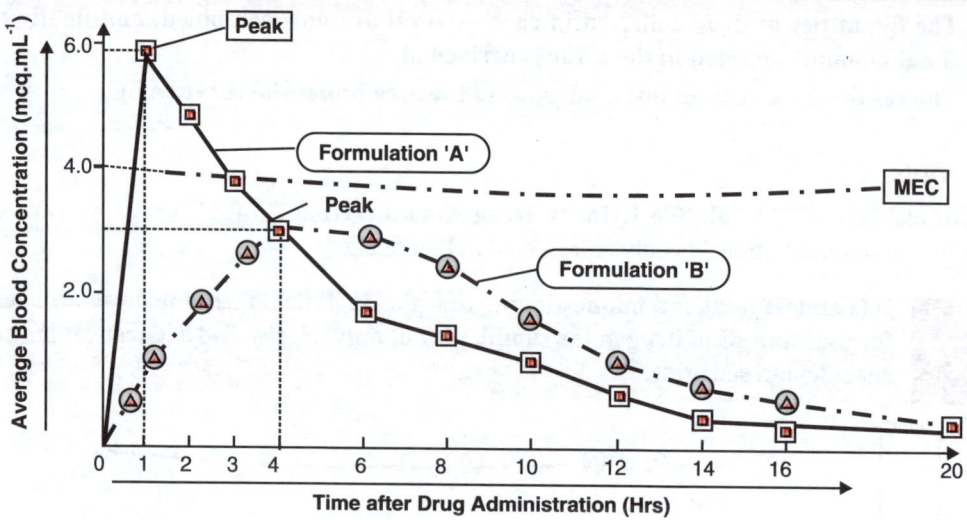

Fig. 5.3: Graphic Representation of Blood Concentration-Time Curves for Two Different Dosage Forms of the Same Drug Substance Showing Explicit Relationship of the Profiles to the Minimum Effective Concentration (MEC).

Explanation

The following is the explanation of the various aspects of Figure 5.3:

1. A horizontal line, parallel to X-axis, has been drawn across the **'average blood concentration'** (on Y-axis) at 4 mcg mL^{-1}.

2. Assuming that the 'drug' happens to be an 'analgesic', and **4 mcg mL^{-1} designates the MEC of the 'drug' present in the circulating blood.**

3. Here, the **Blood Concentration-Time Curves** in Figure 5.3 do distinctly signify the accomplished blood levels after due administration of 'equal doses' of the *two* formulations **(or Dosage Forms)** of the drug, and it is also supported by the fact that 'analgesia' will never come into effect unless and until the **MEC** was either duly obtained or exceeded. It obviously becomes explicit and clear that "**Formulation-'A'"** would be expected to give required 'pain relief' to the patient; whereas, "**Formulation-'B'"**, even though exhibits adequate degree of systemic absorption, may prove to be totally ineffective in causing 'analgesic effect'.

Example of a Cardiac Glycoside (*e.g.*, Digoxin and Digitoxin)

Let us assume that the two curves do designate the observed blood concentration after administration of '**Equal Doses**' of *two* entirely different drug products (or dosage forms) of the same **Cardiac Glycoside** (*viz.* **Digoxin** or **Digitoxin**). Thus, at a dose level of **4 mcg mL^{-1}**, this particular instance duly represents the **Minimum Toxic Concentration (MTC),** and at **2 mcg mL^{-1}** it designates the **MEC**, as illustrated in Figure 5.4. However, it never gives rise to any sort of toxicity levels *in vivo*.

5.2.5. *Bioavailability Studies in Human: Pharmacokinetic Profiles*

Largely, the observed inter-individual variations in the pharmacological response in subjects following administration of the **same Active Drug Product** (or **Dosage Form**) may be duly attributed to a host of factors:

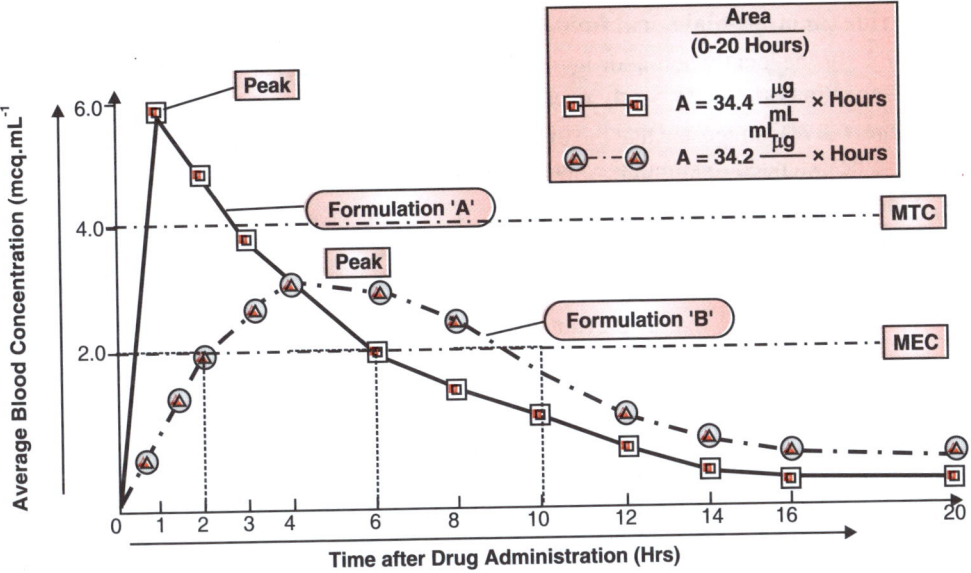

Fig. 5.4: Graphic Representation of the Blood Concentration Time-Curves Obtained for Two Different Dosage Forms of the Same Drug (Digoxin or Digitoxin), Clearly Showing the Relationship of the Profiles to the MTC and to the MEC.

Nevertheless, of these divergent factors, '**Bioavailability**' could hold the gum for an important role that in normal course may even be totally unrecognized. In true sense, there are *two* **vital conditionalities**, namely:

- **time required for the absorption of an 'Active Drug'**, and
- **exact amount of the drug being absorbed**,

that do exert their direct influence upon the speed of acquired onset of action, and the observed intensity of **pharmacological effects of drug**. Therefore, the aforesaid *two* **critical parameters** should by all means be precisely '**quantified**' by making use of an *exhaustive* 'Bioavailability Studies' that would determine the so-called:

- **rate of drug availability**, and
- **degree of drug availability**.

in the systemic circulation after the ingestion of '**Drug Product**'.

5.2.5.1. *Comparison with a Reference Drug/Formulation*

In usual practice, a comparison either with a '**Reference Drug**' or a '**Reference Formulation**' is determined preferably in the solution form or an altogether separate brand of the Drug Product (or **Dosage Form**), which is known to be well absorbed on being administered *via* the oral route.

In this regard, the '**samples**' drawn for carrying out the necessary **Bioavailability of Drugs** must be taken from a location wherein the '**drugs**' shows its maximum therapeutic effect, because it would be rather difficult to '**draw sample**' from the site of action. Therefore, the desired '**sample**' for such a study is generally taken from the respective:

* **venous or arterial blood (*i.e.,* circulating blood), and**
* **urine (another biological fluid).**

Importantly, for the locally acting drug products and those that act specifically upon **GI-Lumen**, the necessary **Bioavailability Study** need to be performed at other levels.

Ritschel (1974)[*] suggested that the bioavailability studies being carried out on healthy subjects should also be extended to simultaneous testing using in vitro tests, such as:

* **disintegration,**
* **degradation, and**
* · **speed of dissolution**

to establish critically that a relevant correlation do exist particularly between the **in vitro Tests** and **Bioavailability studies in humans.**

5.2.5.2. *Bioavailability Studies as per the Helsinki Declaration**[**]

It is, however, pertinent to state here that the **Bioavailability Studies** are required to be performed strictly as per the **Helsinki declaration.**

Modus Operandi: The following are the various sequential recommended steps by the **Helsinki declaration:**

1. Each **Bioavailability Study** has got to be approved duly by an '**Expert Committee**'/**Ethics Committee**', whose prime objectives and responsibilities would be to:

    (a) **verify that the method strictly conforms to the permitted moral standards for experiments with 'Human Volunteers',** and

    (b) all experimental studies must be carried out with perfect guidelines duly approved.

2. All '**Human Volunteers**'[***] must be thoroughly briefed with regard to the aims and objectives of the on-going bioavailability studies. For this, a properly signed consent need to be taken unreservedly; and the **Human Volunteers** or **Patients** must be duly informed about the necessary protective procedures to be followed so as to ensure their good health and well-being.

Recommended/ Approved Methods: These essentially include:

1. Comparative '**Bioavailability Studies**' in humans.
2. Comparative '**Pharmacodynamic Studies**' in humans.
3. Comparative '**Clinical Investigative Trials**'.
4. Exhaustive '**in vitro Studies**' for dissolution and disintegration tests.

---

[*] Ritschel WA: **Bioavailability Testing and Clinical Significance** *Pharma. Acta Helv.*, **49**: 77-83, 1974.

[**] Azarnoff DL: *Clin. Pharmacol. Ther.*, 13: 796-802, 1972; Moris RC: *Ibid*, **13**: 782-795, 1972.

[***] They refer to all healthy human volunteers and patients as well.

Evidently, the aforesaid *four* **recommended/approved methods** are frequently used to access and determine whether the '**Pharmaceutically Equivalent Products**' are found to be also '**Therapeutically Equivalent**' to one another so that the '**physician**' could interchange them appropriately for the patients.[*]

5.2.5.3. *Drug Dissolution Rate and Bioavailability*

It has been proved beyond any reasonable doubt that the inherent physiochemical characteristics features of several drug molecules do exert the greatest influence upon their 'absorption properties' from the **gastrointestinal tract (GIT).** It relates ultimately to the **actual dissolution rate of the drug product.**

Importantly, the most preferred means of assessing the therapeutic efficacy of drugs depends solely on the '**Slow dissolution Rate**', which is duly given by the in vivo estimation of their respective bioavailability profile. Therefore, it forms the essential pre-requisite mandatory for a '**New Dosage-Form**' intended to be launched into the commercial market successfully.

NOTE

The most preferred monitoring of the 'batch-to-batch uniformity' via the stipulated in vivo tests (on humans) is not only exorbitantly costly, but also tedious, time consuming and subjecting normal healthy volunteers to possible hazards of newer drug entities (molecules).

Bearing in mind the above ground realities, it is always desirable to replace reasonably the in vivo bioavailability tests with relatively cheaper (cost-effective) in vitro methods. Evidently, depending on the corresponding in vitro disintegration test may not always prove to be 100% trustworthy and reliable.

In reality, therefore, the **"best reliable, dependable and repeatable analytical equivalent 'tool' that may promise quantitatively the pharmacologic availability of the 'active drug' from its respective dosage form represents dosage form represents clearly its in vitro dissolution test".**

Testing Models: For In Vitro Dissolution Technique: A useful, effective and trustworthy **in vitro Dissolution Technique should be able to predict the in *vivo* Therapeutic Profile** (or pharmacological behavioural pattern) to such a degree that the need for an **in vivo Bioavailability Test may be ruled out completely.**

Although the results duly obtained from the so-called standardized test performance stands by no means a nearest perfect/comparable approach to the *in vitro* Dissolution Technique; the ultimate efforts are only focused to the point of mimicking the closest environment as found in the '**Biologic system**'.

Important Factors Governing the In Vitro Dissolution Technique: There as *three* **important experimental parameters which predominantly govern the *In-Vitro* Dissolution Technique,** namely:

---

[*] It should be noted clearly that even the '**Pharmacist**' attached to a '**Hospital Pharmacy**' is not empowered to change the '**Drug Product**' of a specific brand with another, unless he receives the substituted dosage form by the physician.

1. **The Dissolution Equipment:** The **dissolution equipment** is duly based on six important characteristic features, such as:
   - size of the vessel (ranging between several milliliters capacity to several litres),
   - design,
   - shape of the vessel (flat or round bottomed),
   - agitation modality (oscillating, rotation, stirring, vortex mixing),
   - variable speed of rotation,
   - convenient and ease of performance and
   - accuracy and precision of the **'Official Equipment'**.

2. **Dissolution Fluids**: There are many variants of the **'Dissolution Fluids'** that are used abundantly *in vitro* **Dissolution Assay Methods,** for instance:
   - demineralized (DM) water,
   - 0.1 M hydrochloric acid (freshly prepared),
   - phosphate buffer (as per IP, BP, USP),
   - simulated gastric fluid (or **'artificial gastric juice'**),[*]
   - viscosity of the medium,
   - operational **'volume'**,[**]
   - operational temperature (**37 ± 2°C**),
   - maintaining the **'sink parameters'**[***] and
   - maintaining the **'non–sink conditions'**[****].

   Importantly, most of these aforesaid criteria pertaining to the nature and properties of the dissolution fluids do play a vital role in the assay of drugs (dissolution test).

3. **Process Parameters**: The **Process Parameters** are solely responsible for the accurate determination in the *in vitro* **Dissolution Technique**, such as:
   - timely incorporation of **'drug product'** (or dosage form),
   - typical **Sampling Procedure** (and replacing the requisite volume of fluid with the dissolution fluid being used) and
   - changing the **'dissolution fluid'** periodically.

   The Drug Dissolution Estimation Apparatus: With the increase in need and advent of skilled technique and wisdom, the **'Drug Dissolution Estimation Apparatus'** has undergone a tremendous evolution gradually from a simple beaker-type assembly to a **Completely Automated and Extremely Versatile Models.**

---

[*]   That is, prepared strictly according to official method in **IP, BP, USP.**

[**]   **Volume:** It is usually greater than that needed actually to complete the dissolution of the active drug under investigation.

[***] **Sink Parameters:** It refers to the drug concentration in solution constantly maintained at low level.

[****] **Non-sink Conditions:** It means a gradual steady increase in the active drug concentration in the respective medium.

Furthermore, these available devices may be duly categorized into several manners that are eventually based upon the

- **absence of sink conditions,** or
- **presence of sink conditions,**

wherein the specific dissolution apparatus has been designed on the following two different principles:

1. **Open-Compartment Dissolution Apparatus:** It specifically represents the '**Perfect Sink Conditions**'. In this particular instance, the '**Drug Product**' is carefully contained in a column that is continuously brought in direct contact with a fresh flowing dissolution medium.

The aforesaid flow-through cell technique was initially developed by **Dr. F. Langenbücher at the Ciba-Geigy Laboratories (Switzerland).**[*] The Column-Type Dissolution Method has been explicitly illustrated in Figure 5.5(a) and (b).

Demerits of Open Flow through System: Importantly, the open flow through system found in an **Open-Compartment Dissolution Apparatus** [Figure 5.5(a) and (b)] possesses certain obvious demerits of its own as given below:

1. The **Sieves (Filters)** S_1 and S_2 do have a tendency to get clogged because of the unidirectional flow of the '**dissolution fluid**'.

2. Besides, there is a great scope of pressure build-up almost near the end of the run. Therefore, in majority of cases, it is absolutely necessary and importance to have:

   - **a build-in pressure transducers,** and
   - **an explicit feedback mechanism to enhance the pressure slowly so as to maintain a constant flow rate.**

3. '**Pump' Effect**: It represents one of the most vital limitations of an open flow through system. It has been duly demonstrated that different kinds of '**pumps**' used, *e.g.*,

   - **peristaltic pump** and
   - **centrifugal type pump variants,**

   invariably give rise to altogether **dissimilar dissolution results.**

4. Finally, one requires relatively large volumes of the **Dissolution Media** (or *fluid*) essentially required to perform **Long-Duration Testing Procedures.**

   (a) **Closed-Compartment Dissolution Apparatus**: The **Closed-Compartment Dissolution Apparatus** is fundamentally *a limited-volume apparatus usually working under the* '**Non-Sink Parameters**'. Interestingly, in this particular instance, the respective 'dissolution fluid' is strictly restrained to the size of the container, such as:

   - **rotating basket-type dissolution apparatus, and**
   - **rotating paddle-type dissolution apparatus,**

which shall be discussed briefly, with appropriate diagrammatic presentation, in the following sections.

---

[*] **Langenbücher F:** *J.Pharm. Sci.*, **58**: 1265, 1969; USP23/NF 18, 5th Supplement, p.3470

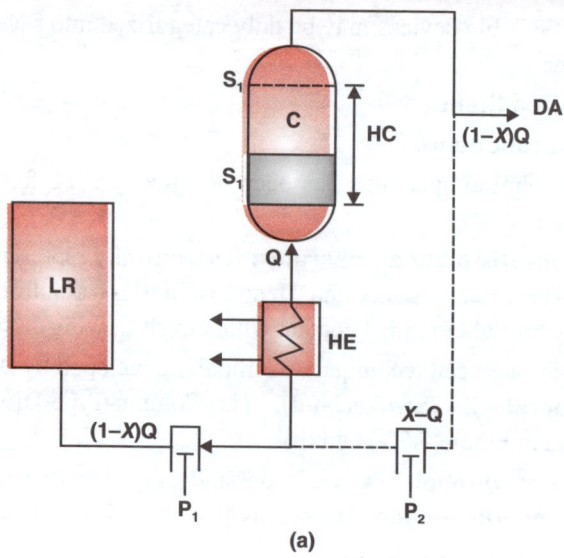

(a)

PB: Partiell Bed;	**P_1, P_2: Volumetric Pumps;**
C: Cell;	**LR: Liquid Reservoir**
S_1, S_2: Screens;	**x: Circulation Factor;**
HE: Heat Exchanger;	**Q, x, Q, (1-x)Q: Volumetric Flow Rates;**
HC: Height of Cell;	

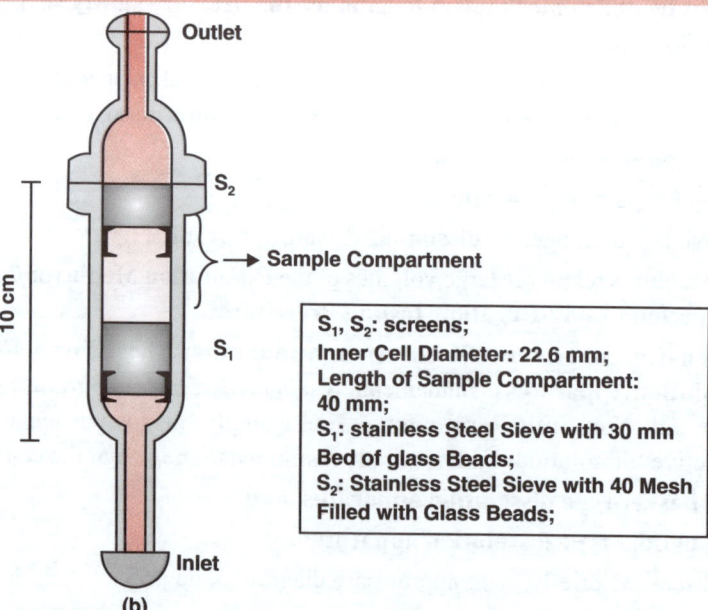

S₁, S₂: screens;
Inner Cell Diameter: 22.6 mm;
Length of Sample Compartment:
40 mm;
S₁: stainless Steel Sieve with 30 mm
Bed of glass Beads;
S₂: Stainless Steel Sieve with 40 Mesh
Filled with Glass Beads;

(b)

Fig. 5.5: (a) Column Type Dissolution Method: Representing the Sketch of the Column. Dissolution Apparatus (Schematic). (b) Specifications for the 4 cm² Dissolutions Cell (drawn to scale).

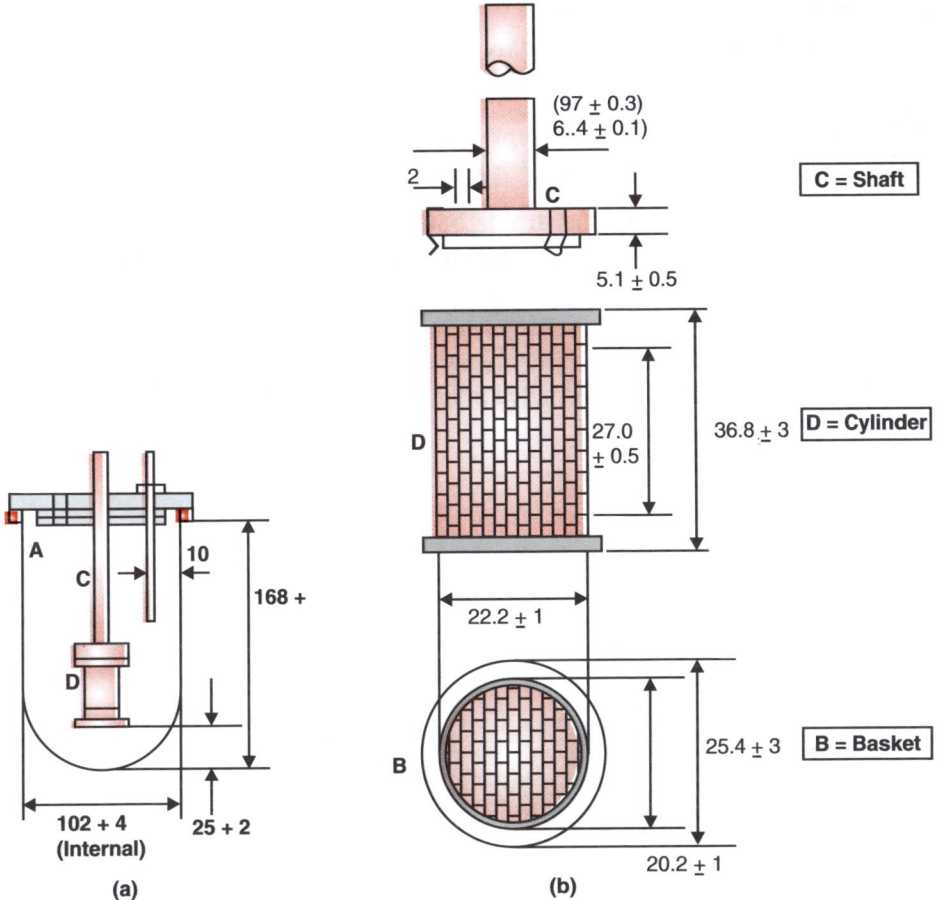

Fig. 5.6: (a) Diagram of Basket-Type Dissolution Apparatus. (b) The Detailed Cross-Section of the Stirring Basket Element.

(b) **Rotating Basket-Type Dissolution Apparatus:** in the **Rotating Basket-Type Dissolution Apparatus** [Figure 5.6(a) and (b)],[*] the stirring element is a '**Basket**'.

Modus Operandi: The various steps involved are as follows:

1. The metallic shaft rotates with a constant smooth motion and without causing any significant wobbling.

2. '**Basket**' has *two* distinct segments:

    ● **Top part with a vint is duly attached to the Shaft 'C'** and is fitted with three spring clips or other suitable means which would allow the lower part being removed, as and when required for needful introduction of the '**sample**' under investigation; and also holds the lower part of the basket concentric firmly with the axis of the vessel during rotation.

    ● **Lower part is a detachable component of the 'Basket (B)'** and is usually made up of welded-steam cloth having:

- ➢ wire thickness of 0.254 nm diameter, and
- ➢ 0.381 mm square openings, duly formed into a 'Cylinder (D)' with a narrow rim of sheet metal around the top and bottom.

NOTE	The entire *'basket'* may be appropriately *gold plated* with a 2.5 mm coating for its use in an acidic environment freely.

3. The actual distance between the '**inside bottom**' of the vessel and the '**Basket**' is duly maintained between 23 and 27 mm during the performance of the '**Dissolution Test**'.

4. **Rotating Paddle-Type Dissolution Apparatus**: The **Rotating Paddle-Type Dissolution Apparatus**[*] is crafted and designed in such a manner so as to determine the compliance with the **requisite dissolution requirements** for the solid **Drug Products** (or **Dosage Forms,** *viz.* **Tablets** or **Capsules**), as illustrated in **Figure 5.7(a) and (b)**:

    A = **Cylindrical Vessel**

    B = **Blade (Forming a Paddle)**

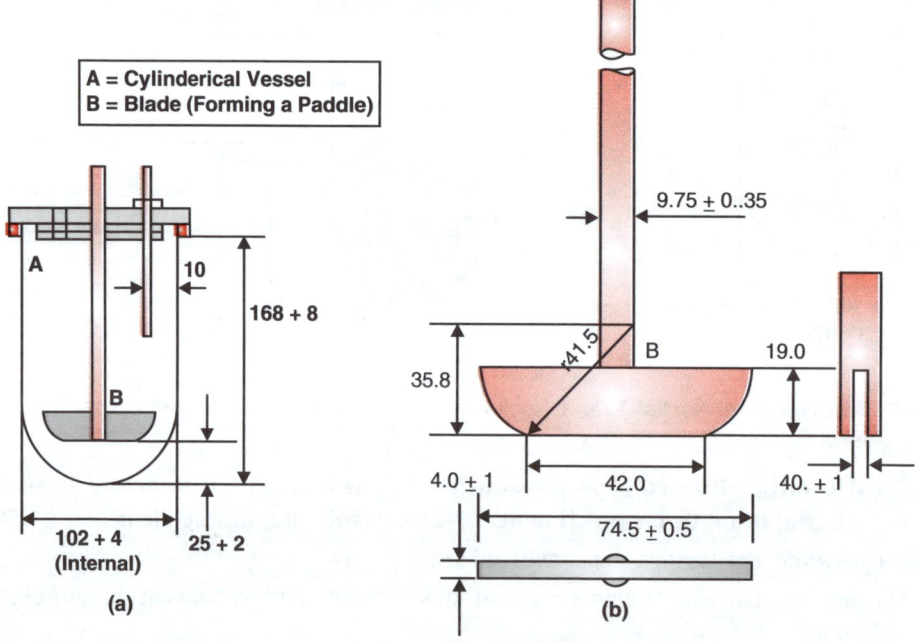

Fig. 5.7: (a) Diagram of a Paddle-Type Dissolution Apparatus. (b) The Detailed Cross-Section of the Paddle Stirring Element.

Descriptions of the Apparatus: The following are the various aspects of the apparatus:

1. All contact parts of the **Dissolution Apparatus with the Formulation (Drug Product)** under examination or with the dissolution fluid (medium) must be:

- • **chemically inert,**
- • **non-absorbable,**

---

[*] **Indian Pharmacopoeia, Vol. 2.** 6th ed., The Indian Pharmacopoeia Commission, Ghaziabad, India, 2010

- **non-reactive,** and/or
- **non-interfering with the 'Formulation' being examined.**

2. All metallic contact parts of the dissolution apparatus either with the formulation (or dosage form) or with the respective dissolution fluid (or medium) should always be made from **Stainless Steel (SS)** type 316 or equivalent or coated with an appropriate substance to ensure that such components do not interfere or react with the formulation being studied or the ensuing **Dissolution Fluid**.

3. Invariably, a **Dissolution Apparatus** that critically allows observation of the **Formulation** (or **Dosage Form**) under examination and the stirring process during the **Entire Dissolution Test** is indeed most preferable.

4. A **Cylindrical Vessel (A),** made up of either borosilicate glass or any other suitable transparent polymeric material (*e.g.,* polyacrylic sheet), has a hemispherical bottom. It should have a normal capacity of 1 L and an internal diameter of 98-106 mm, as shown in Figure 5.7(a). Besides, the **Cylindrical Vessel (A)** has a flanged upper rim duly fitted, with a lid which essentially possesses a **'number of openings'**, the main one of which is strategically located in the centre.

5. A separate electric motor is provided with a 'speed regulatory' duly capable of maintaining the speed of rotation (rpm) of the paddle within a limit 4% of the stipulated speed mentioned in the individual **monograph (IP, 2010)**. The aforesaid electric motor is carefully fitted with a 'stirring element' that essentially comprises [see Figure 5.7(b)]

- **a 'drive shaft',** and
- **a 'blade forming a paddle (B)'.**

6. The **'blade'** passes *via* the diameter of the 'drive shaft' in order that the bottom of the blade is flush with the bottom of the shaft. Now, the 'drive shaft' is positioned strategically so that its axis falls very much within 2 mm of the axis of the vessel; whereas, the **lower-edge of the blade (B)** is nearly 23-27 mm away from the inside bottom of the cylindrical vessel.

Finally, the **Rotating Paddle-Type Dissolution Apparatus** functions in such a manner that the paddle rotates smoothly and without significant noticeable wobbling.

7. **Electric Water Bath:** An electric water bath is set to **maintain the dissolution fluid between 36.5°C and 37.5°C.** However, the bath liquid is usually kept in constant and smooth motion during the test. The **Cylindrical Vessel (A)** is securely clamped in the water bath in such a fashion that the overall displacement vibration from the rest of the equipment, *viz.* water-circulating device, is minimized to the least extent.

Closed Column-Type System: Abdou *et al.* (1978)[*] developed an altogether newer technique based on a variation of the flow-through concept. It is essentially a closed column-type system that represents a combination of a miniaturized rotating basket having a closed flow-through dissolution apparatus to maintain and sustain the ensuing concentration of the drug substance at an acceptable and workable range for the required quantitative assay, as illustrated in **Figure 5.8(a) and (b).**

It may be worthwhile to state here that the aforesaid closed column-type happens to be

- **a semi-automated one in conjunction with HPLC[**], and**

---

[*] Abdou HM *et al.: J. Pharm. Sci.*, **67**: 1397, 1978.

[**] **HPLC: High Performance Liquid Chromatography**.

- employed for the accurate estimation of the dissolution rate of 0.1 mg fludrocortisones acetate tablets.

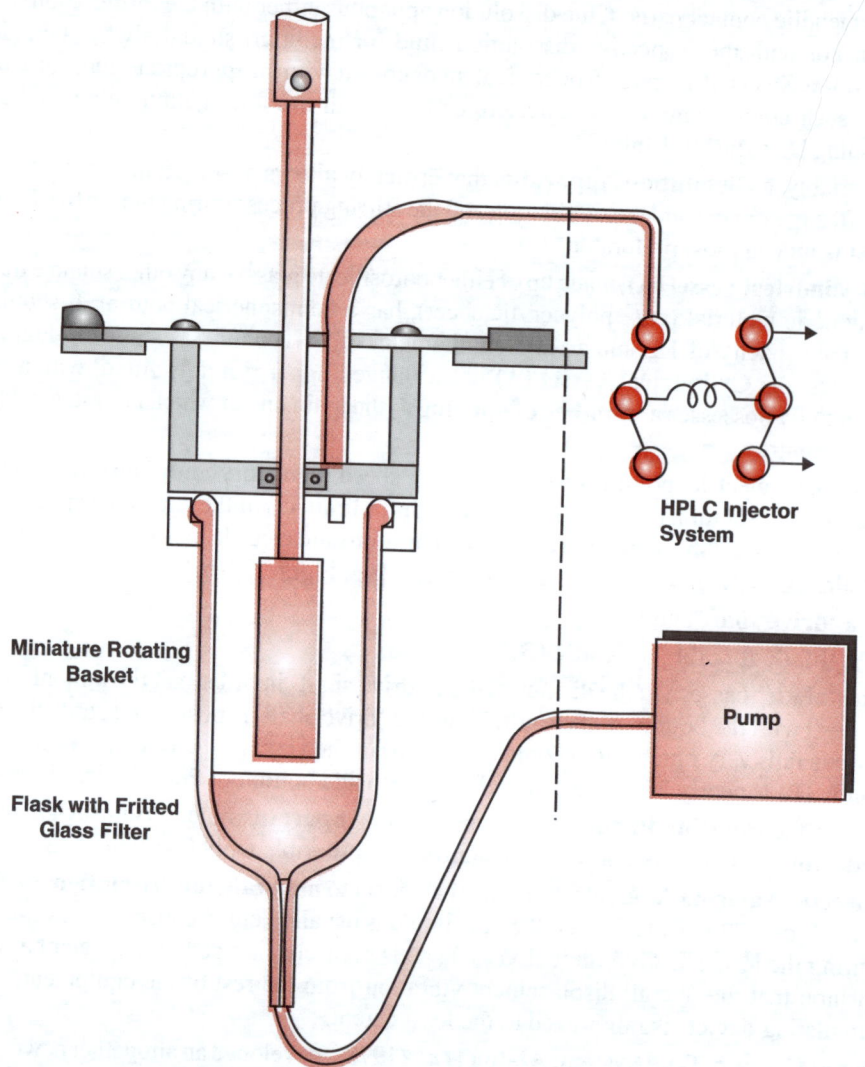

HPLC Injector System

Miniature Rotating Basket

Pump

Flask with Fritted Glass Filter

Fig. 5.8: (a) Diagram of a Closed Flow-Through Dissolution Apparatus for the Determination of Dissolution Rate of Dosages with Extremely Small Quantum of Active Ingredients.
[*Adapted from*: **Abdou HM** *et al.* **J. Pharm. Sci., 67, 1397, 1978).**]

Figure 5.8(a) explicitly depicts the **Miniaturized USP* Basket Apparatus**, duly combined with a *flow-through mechanism.*

Figure 5.8(b) shows a comparison between the observed **Dissolution Rate of Fludrocortisone Acetate** duly recorded at different rotation speeds of the miniature rotating basket [see **Figure 5.8(a)**]. Thus, each point is an average of *six* **drug tablets** taken carefully from the same lot:

---

* **USP 23/NF 18**, 5th Suppl. Pp. 3469, 3470; Ibid, 6th Suppl.p.3794.

O = at **50 rpm;**

□ = at **100 rpm;**

Δ = at **125 rpm;**

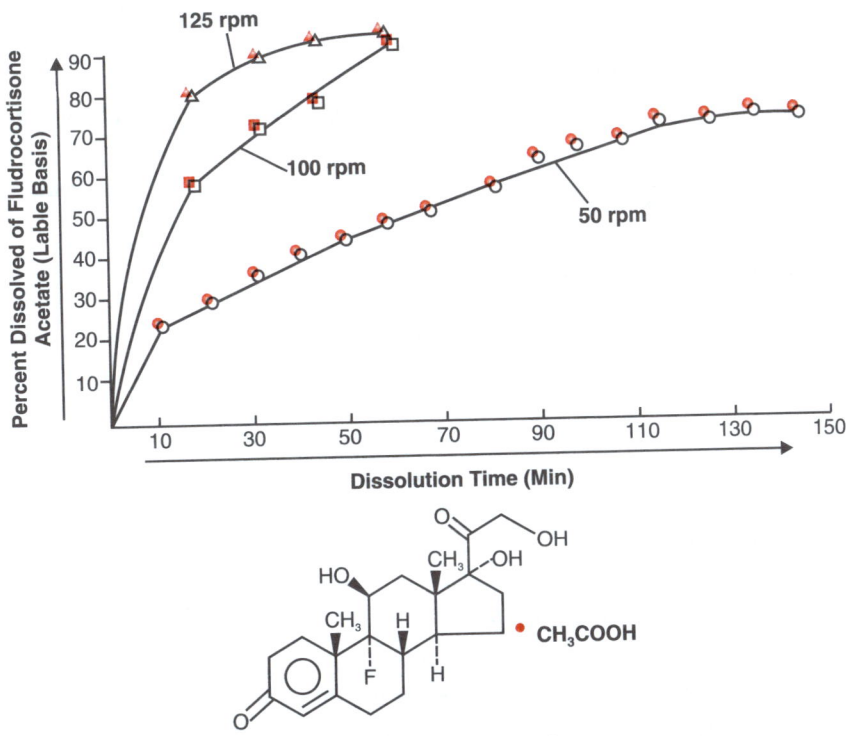

Fludrocortisone Acetate

Fig. 5.8(b): A comparison Between the Dissolution Rate of Fludrocortisone Acetate at Variable Rotation Sppeds, *viz*. 50, 100 and 125 rpm.

5.2.6. *Statistical Methods for Bioavailability Studies*

Preamble: It has been duly established that after having conducted

- **bioequivalence evaluation,** and
- **determining appropriate conditionalities,**

one should critically examine the obtained **Pharmacokinetic Data** as per the set of *predetermined characteristic features so as to either confirm to refute the relevant* '**Bioequivalency**' *of the* 'Test Sample', *and* 'Reference Drug Products'.

In other words, it is always necessary to determine whether the '**Test Sample**' and '**Reference Drug Products**' actually show a difference very much within a **predefined level of statistical significance**.

Importance of Statistical Methods: As the '**Statistical Results**' duly obtained from an elaborated '**Bioequivalence Study**' form the ultimate primary basis of the decision either for or against the so-called **Therapeutic Equivalence of two Dosage Forms**, it becomes absolutely important that the generated 'Experimental Data' may be analyzed with the help of a suitable **Statistical Test.**

Selection of Statistical Methods: The various available **Statistical Methods** intended to be employed in **Bioavailability Studies** must be selected with utmost care with respect to the following critical aspects:

- **Variations observed among individuals**
- **Variations seen among the batches of nominally identical produced 'dosage forms',** and
- **Skilful knowledge and wisdom duly solicited for planning, analysis and interpretations of these experimental results.**

5.2.6.1. *Methods of Data Analysis*

The duly planned and executed 'Bioequivalency Studies' invariably emerge with a copious volume of extremely useful experimental results that may be analyzed statistically in several available different means and ways.

Notari (1987)[*] and **Mcdonald** *et al.* **(1969)**[**] suggested and proved generously that the statistical methods of analysis solely depend on the **typical statistical model** of the 'Concentration-Time Curve'. Nevertheless, they observed various sources of *variation* in Statistical Model, such as:

- **person-to-person variations,**
- **non-independent measurements**[***], and
- **detailed experimental layout plans.**

Importantly, the most preferred and easiest way to make use of the **Concentration-Time Curves** generally for the **comparison of *two* Dosage Forms** may be precisely accomplished by:

- **not simply comparing the whole curves,** and/or
- **carrying out a comparison of the characteristic features of the 'Curves',**

with respect to such vital and important criteria, as:

- **Area under the curves (AUCs),**
- **Peak heights,** and
- **Rates of absorption.**

Paired Comparisons: In a specific situation when only a 'Single Characteristic Feature' is involved predominantly, one may use an appropriate technique of analysis referred to as 'Paired Comparisons'. Interestingly, here each and every individual gives rise to a typical 'paired difference'.

NOTE	Enough dependable 'statistical methods' that are usually employed for the critical comparison of *two* or more sets of variables may find their utility in the study involving more than two dosage forms.

---

[*]   Notari RE: ***Biopharmaceutics and Pharmacokinetics***: An Introduction, 4th ed., Marcell Dekker, New York, 1987.

[**]   McDonald H *et al.*: *Clin. Med.* (Dec): 30-33, 1969.

[***]   Barr WH *et al.*: *Clin. Pharmacol. Ther.* **13**(1): 97-108, 1972.

5.2.6.2. *Statistical Analysis*

The following important aspects related to the **Statistical Methods** used in '**Bioequivalence Study**' have been duly discussed in *Section 4(3.5)*. Besides, the corresponding statistical method variants, such as**: Latin-Square Cross-Over Design,** and **Balanced Incomplete Block-Design (BIBI),**have also been discussed under *Section 4(3.5.1).*

5.2.6.3. *Statistical Interpretation of Bioequivalence Data*

The '**Analysis of variance (ANOVA)**' refers to- '**a statistical procedure largely used to compare the means of two or more groups**'. Obviously, whenever a statistically significant difference is observed, it is absolutely necessary and important to establish whether it is '**really clinically significant**'. It has been found invariably that when the statistically significant difference stands at only 10%, it clearly indicates that the extent of absorption prevailing between the *two* **Dosage Forms** (or **Drug Products**) is almost insignificant clinically.

Universally Acceptable Generalized Rules: In usual practice, one may confidently make use of the universally acceptable generalized rule that if the observed **Relative Bioavailability of** the '**Test' Dosage Form** and '**Reference Standard**' falls within a range between **80% and 120% (of Reference Sample), it should be considered as 'Bioequivalent'.**

In addition to the above dictum, one may also rely upon the critical observation that the actual difference existing between the **Bioavailabilities** of the '**Test Drug Products' must appear to be greater than ±20% average of the 'Reference Standard'.**

5.2.7. *Factors that Decrease Bioavailability*

A survey of literature reveals that there exists *three* **crucial factors that decrease Bioavailability in a progressive manner,** namely:

- **Presystemic metabolism,**
- **Instability,** and
- **Complexation**.

which would be discussed separately in the following sections.

5.2.7.1. *Presystemic Metabolism*

Immediately after the oral administration of a **Solid Dosage Form,** the '**absorbed drug**' undergoes first pass metabolism which critically implies that the latter directly gains entry to the liver before ultimately reaching the systemic circulation. In fact, this kind of an approach definitely enhances the degree of metabolism with regard to an **IV dose**.

Example

Peripheral Vein *vs.* Portal Vein: In laboratory model '**dog**', the **AUC values** duly obtained for **Lidocaine (a local anaesthetic) and Aspirin (an analgesic)** *varies significantly, i.e.,* found to be

- **greater-when infused directly into a peripheral vein,** and
- **lower-when infused into the portal vein.**

However, the administration of drug(s) directly into the '**portal vein**' is very much similar to the '**oral absorption**'.

Cause of decrease **Bioavailability** may be expatiated due to the relevant exposure of drugs to the liver before approaching the circulating blood that eventually facilitates:

- **reasonable dilution,** and
- **effective distribution,**

of the available drugs to other sites.

Importantly, one may observe that a rapid IV dose, would at the same time enable the distribution through the whole body; whereas, the circulating blood will pass through the liver prominently. In this way, the drug being distributed in other functional organs is being blocked temporarily from undergoing the 'Hepatic Metabolism'.

Presystemic Metabolism may evidently come into play not only confined to the '**liver**' but also in the '**intestine**' itself or while passing *via* the intestinal wall. Amazingly, in all these cases, the net overall consequences are duly exhibited by a loss of '**intact drug**'. till such time a proper logical explanation is not available for its actual mechanism it may be:

- **explicitly identified as 'first-pass metabolism',** or
- **clearly understood as 'presystemic metabolism'.**

Table 5.1 records a comprehensive list of certain important drug substance for which the prevalence of the '**Presystemic Metabolism**' is considered to be quite significant.

Observations: Following are certain important observations:

1. The **Presystemic Metabolism** may exhibit a tendency to check and prohibit the oral administration of a drug substance.
2. **Lidocaine** (a *local anaesthetic*) shows a **variable and sluggish variable bioavailability** on account of the **high First-Metabolism** whereby between **21% and 46%** of orally given lidocaine ultimately reaches the circulating blood.
3. The observed **bioavailability of Nortryptyline** (a *tricyclic anti-depressant*) gets reduced upto **40%** (approximately) immediately followed by an oral dose relative to **IM administration**.
4. Low and variable **Bioavailability of Imipramine** ranging between **30% and 75%** has been duly caused due to the **First-pass Metabolism**.

Observed Positive Deviation from Linearity: It has been duly observed that when the **First-Pass Metabolism** is extended to saturation level, it is prone to the generation of a critical non-linear dependency for the

Table 5.1. List of Certain Selected Drug substances which may Undergo Presystemic Metabolism when Administered Orally			
S. No.	**Drugs**	**S. No.**	**Drugs**
1	**Paracetamol (acetaminophen)**	15	**Meperidine**
2	**Aldosterone**	16	**Methadone**
3	**Alprenolol**	17	**Methylphenidate**
4	**Aspirin (acetylsalicylic acid)**	18	**Morphine**

5	Chlorpromazine		19	Nitroglycerin
6	Cortisone		20	Nortriptyline
7	Desipramine		21	Papaverine
8	Dopamine		22	Pentazocine
9	Estrogens		23	Propoxyphene
10	Flurazepam		24	Propranolol
11	Hydralazine		25	Salicylamide
12	Imipramine		26	Terbutaline
13	Isoproterenol		27	Testosterone
14	Lidocaine			

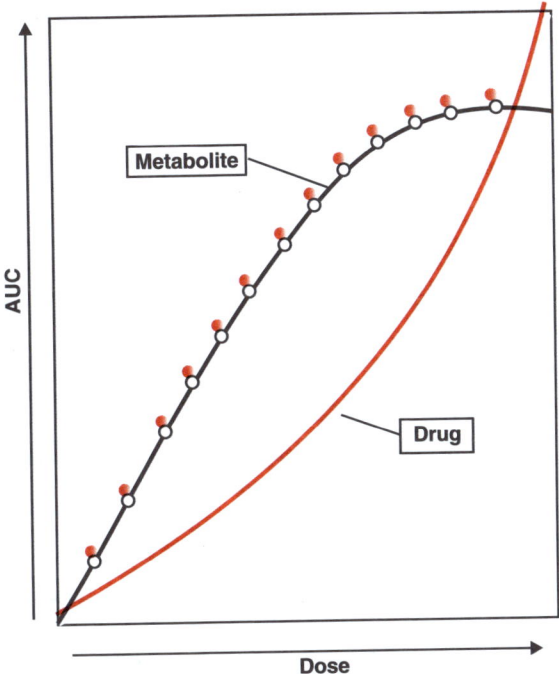

Fig. 5.9: Diagrammatic representation of area Under the Plasma Concentration-Time Curve (AUC) immediately Following the Oral Absorption of a Drug that Undergoes Saturable First-Pass Metabolism.

'**AUC**' **as a Function of Dose**. Besides, the exact quantum of the so-called '**Surviving Drug**' that eventually gains entry to the bloodstream gets enhanced by virtue of saturation phenomenon of the respective enzymes. In this way it produces positive deviation from linearity, as illustrated in Figure 5.9.

Explanation

In figure 5.9 it may be observed that:

1. **At lower dose levels, practically most of the absorbed drug invariably appears in the plasma as its respective metabolite.**

2. **Importantly, at a sufficient higher dose level nearing to almost saturate metabolism, the resulting metabolite critically approaches a constant value, and, therefore, the AUC values for the drug substance duly increase with the dose.**

Hollister (1972)* observed a similar phenomenon pertaining to the rate of presentation of the drug entity.

Example

The '**Intact Aspirin Ester**' reaching the circulating bloodstream gets reduced appreciably on being released gradually from a **Sustained-Release Dosage Form** (*e.g.*, **Enteric Coated Aspirin Tablets**) in comparison to a **Fast-released Aspirin Product** (*e.g.*, **microcrystalline soluble Aspirin Tablets**). Interestingly, in both these products, the actual *Bioavailability of total salicylate was more or less identical.*

NOTE	It is worthwhile to state here that the product which specifically presented aspirin at a faster rate (second product) showed eventually a greater AUC for aspirin per se by causing reduction in the presystemic metabolism.

5.2.7.2. Instability

Generally, a majority of drugs are found to be quite unstable to the following *two* **biological entities**, namely:

* **gastric juice (or acid)**, and/or
* **enzymes in GI tract.**

Nevertheless, the inevitable '**Hydrolysis of Drugs**' usually comes into play particularly in the stomach fluids (including gastric juice). Therefore, in such a critical situation when a drug substance undergoes hydrolysis in the GI tract, it eventually gets involved in the parallel rate processes, as duly expressed by

$$\text{Drug Present in Blood} \xleftarrow{K_a} \text{Drug Present in GI Fluids} \xrightarrow{K_b} \text{Hydrolysed Drug Products} \qquad \text{(a)}$$

Thus, the apparent **First-Order Rate Constant [k_{app}]** may be defined by:

$$\frac{k_h}{k_a} = \frac{\text{Hydrolyzed product}}{\text{Drug absorbed}} \qquad \text{(b)}$$

where,

k_a = Rate constant of '**absorbed drugs**', and

k_b = Rate constant of '**hydrolyzed product**'.

Therefore, the ultimate ratio of the observed rate constants shall define the ratio of the competing rate phenomena so that we may have the following expression:

---

* Holliseter LE: Measuring Problems in Oral Prolonged-Action Medications. *Clin. Pharmacol. Ther.,* **31**: 1, 1972.

In **Equation (c),** the numerator designates the actual quantum of the **degradation product** (*i.e.,* the **hydrolyzed product**), whereas the denominator represents the actual amount of drug being delivered into the bloodstream.

How does this phenomenon relate to 'absorption'? We may explain the underlying relationship of the aforesaid phenomenon to absorption by citing the following typical example: 'Let us assume that k_h/k_a stood at 2, *i.e.* the rate constant for degradation was 'twice' as fast as the corresponding rate for absorption. In other words, for each and every molecule of drug absorbed, two molecules will undergo degradation. This obviously indicates that the maximum observed absorption of the 'drug' would turn out to be only 33%.

Important Remarks: The overwhelming problem(s) associated intimately with the ensuing hydrolysis taking place in the **'Gastric Fluids'** are duly focused on two distinct **'groups of drug substances'** such as:

- **'drugs' intended for immediate absorption,** and
- **'drugs' whose absorption may be delayed critically till they enter the intestines.**[*]

Hydrolysis of Weak Acidic Drugs (Penicillins) in Gastric Fluids

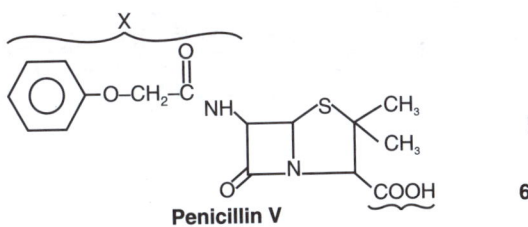

Penicillin V

6-Aminopenicillanic Acid
[6-APA] (pKa: 2-3)

In **Penicillin V_d** the carboxylic moiety of the patient structure, 6-Aminopenicillanic **Acid (6-APA),** shows a **pK_a value** in the range **2-3**. Thus, the rapid absorption that almost commences in the stomach is very much desired clinically. One way, however, observe the primary difference in the basic structure of the penicillins confined particularly to the substituents strategically located upon the **'amide group'** marked X. noticeably, this specific moiety is solely responsible for the most viable and important difference with respect to the following aspects:

- **gastric stability,**
- **enzymatic stability,**
- **drug-protein binding phenomena,** and
- **pharmacokinetics.**

Explanation

The following are the various aspects:

1. The presence of α-lactam structure (in penicillins) is found to be highly prone to hydrolysis thereby causing an overall loss in activity.

---

[*] This specific category of drugs need to be discussed separately, because it evidently poses the critical problem of getting the 'drug' *via* the stomach without undergoing degradation at all.

2. Another most crucial limitation exhibited in the 'systemic activity of the penicillins' is perhaps due to its instability to the enzyme 'penicillinase'.*

3. Obvious, instability in gastric juice designates another prominent limitation in the oral efficacy of the penicillins.

4. **Plasma Half-lives ($t_{1/2}$):** The $t_{1/2}$ values for the hydrolysis of the penicillins in an aqueous acidic environment at 35°C are provided duly in Table 5.2 in a summarized form.

Observations from **Table 5.2** essentially comprise the following:

- It is quite evident why **'Methicillin'** (1) is usually dispensed in the form of injectables.

- It could be less obvious why **'Penicillin G'** (2) should ever be selected for usual administration via the oral route. Besides, the **Bioavailability of Penicillin G** is found to be variable and not dependable, which is critically based on the fact that the drug is extremely labile (unstable) to stomach acid (HCI).

- **'Methicillin'** (1) possesses an added advantage for being comparatively stable to the enzyme 'pencilinase'. The same also holds good for **Other Penicillin Variants**, *e.g.*,
    - ➢ **Oxacillin (5)**
    - ➢ **Cloxacillin.**

Table 5.2. Plasma Half-Lives ($t_{1/2}$) for the Hydrolyzed Products of Various Penicillins at pH 1.3 and Temperature 35°C*

S. No.	Penicillin Variants	Plasma Half-Lives ($t_{1/2}$ in min)
1	Methicillin	2.3
2	Penicillin G	3.5
3	Phenethicillin	68.0
4	α-Methoxybenzyl Penicillin	77.0
5	Oxacillin	160.0
6	Penicillin V	160.0
7	α-Chlorobenzyl Penicillin	300.0
8	Amoxicillin	540.0
9	Ampicillin	660.0

*Hou JP and Poole JW: α-Lactam Antibiotics: Their Physiochemical Properties and Biological Activities in Relation to Structure, *J.* Pharm. Sci., **60**: 573, 1971; Sehwartz MA and Buckwalter FH: Pharmaceutics of Penicillin, *J.* Pharm. Sci., **51**: 1119, 1962.

- **Penicillin G (2)** is found to be the 'least stable' among all **the Penicillin Variants from (1) through (9).**

- The rest of the Penicillins, *viz.* 3, 4, 6, 7, 8 and 9 do actually fall between these extremes.

Delaying Absorption until Reaching Intestines Based on the basic 'pH Partition theory', the unaltered form of a drug is invariably absorbed much better in comparison to the charged species. In fact, this could eventually lead one to believe and expect that the **intestinal pH between 6 and 8** may ultimately allow the critical absorption of:

- **weakly basic drugs,** and
- **non-ionizable drugs.**

---

* Penicillinase: An enzyme duly produced by the Staphylococcus species of microorganisms

However, in actual practice, the absorption efficaciousness of the intestines largely predominates over the theory. Importantly, in a situation where the **'clinical utility'** of a drug substance does not demand an immediate onset of action (as seen with chronic dosing), it is definitely a viable alternative for promoting and intentional protection against the so-called **'Gastric Dissolution Phenomena'.**

Example of Erythromycin: It is an **acid–unstable drug** which is commercially available in various dosage forms. **Erythromycin** is found to be most stable between **pH 6 and 8**, and **gets quickly deteriorated at pH < 4**. Importantly, the **'Protonated Version of the Erythromycin Base'** (see below) exhibits a **pK_a value ~8.9**; and, therefore, the drug shall remain in its protonated status all through the **GI tract.**

Protonated Version of Erythromycin Base

The combination of the aforesaid **'charged species'** and **'gastric instability profile'** perhaps would render the oral absorption of the drug (**Erythromycin**) not only poor, but also irregular as well. Hence, the best way to circumvent such an ordeal is to cause an effective intestinal absorption rather than the stomach absorption. **Enhanced GI absorption** may be duly accomplished by specifically shielding erythromycin particles from getting exposed to the **'gastric juices'** (or *fluids*), which may be carried out by different well-known recognized modalities:

1. **Enteric Coating Preparations: Enteric coating** refers to-**'a specialized 'covering material' carefully applied to granules used in tablets, capsules and pellets (or pills) to protect them and prevent disintegration or dissolution particularly in the gastric fluids, thus, enabling the dissolution to be effective only in the small intestines.' Wagner *et al.* (1960)**[*] reported that the average times taken for the passage of the **enteric-coated tablet right from the stomach to the intestines found to be 3.53 and 2.53 hrs.**

2. **Using Salts of Erythromycin**: The various salts of the *tertiary* **aliphatic amine of Erythromycin,** such as:
   - **ethylsuccinate,**
   - **stearate, and**
   - **estolate,**

   are also available abundantly besides the **enteric coated tablets of Erythromycin Free Base'.**

It has been duly reported that the aforesaid **Salts of Erythromycin** do not get dissociated so rapidly *in vivo*; and, therefore, their **ultimate degradation retarded significantly.**

Important Points: Obviously, once present in the intestinal environment, the 'salt' undergoes critical dissociation thereby releasing **'Free Erythromycin Base'** that eventually gets absorbed at a pH more favourable to its desired stability.

---

[*] Wagner et al.: **Enteric Coatings IV** . *J. Pharm. Sci.*, **49:** 128, 1960.

NOTE	As the final disintegration of the 'dosage form' takes place in the stomach, one may critically predict the passage of the 'drug substance' more explicitly as a divided powder form.

3. **Product of Erythromycin**: The **lauryl sulphate salt of Erythromycin Propionate Ester** designates the prodrug of Erythromycin. Interestingly, the '**prodrug**' effectively promotes the phenomenon of absorption in *two* **different manners**'.

- **Salts of weak carboxylic acids/erythromycin base do show a tendency to get dissolved in the 'human gastric fluid' predominantly, and lose the antibiotic activity rapidly.**
- **Lauryl sulphric acid itself being a fairly strong acid prominently resists/prevents the ensuing displacement by the 'human-gastric fluid'.**

In this manner, the '**estolate ester**' not only remains in an '**undissolved status**', but also retains critically its desired potency for a longer span of time (**Stephens *et al.* 1959**)[*].

Complexation: **Complexation** may be defined as '**the physical binding of a chemical, entity with another substance resulting in a change in properties**'.

Scheiner and Altemeier (1962)[**] and **Remmers *et al.* (1965)**[**] studied exhaustively the underlying problem pertaining to the reduced absorption of drug substances due to the complexation with other '**agents**' in the respective **GI tract**, *e.g.,* **Complexation of the Tetracyclines and Heavy Metal Ions (Ca^{2+}, Mg^{2+}, Fe^{2+}, Al^{3+}).**

Salient Features: These essentially comprise the following:

1. The co-administration of aluminium hydroxide gels [$Al(OH)_3$], milk and milk products along with the tetracyclines apparently reduce nausea and vomiting.

Explanation

This could be explained by the fact that *Complexation* of '**Tetracyclines**' with Al^{3+}, Ca^{2+} etc., invariably occurs that might glaring minimize such symptoms (nausea/vomiting), because the generated 'complex' turns out to be quite inactive and hence unable to penetrate the surrounding **Biological Membrane.**

2. As the '**Tetracyclines**' quite **often imbalance the normal GI flora** since the complexation may cause a **decreased GI distress**; whereas, the source results could be accomplished by **replacing Tetracyclines with other antibiotics**'.

5.2.8. *Factors that Increase Bioavailability*

It has been established beyond any reasonable doubt that specifically enhancing the lipophilicity of a drug substance proves to be one of the most important and viable approaches to improve upon the drug's so-called '**Passive Transport**' [*Section 2(6.5)*]. Importantly, by virtue of the increased bioavailability it may now be possible and feasible to minimize the actual intended dose of drug. in other words, the overall therapeutic treatment eventually is rendered not only 'more economical', but also causes apparent minimization of the '**undesirable side effects**' intimately associated with the relatively high dose of drug.

---

[*] Stephens VC *et al.*: **Esters of Erythromycin IV**, *J. Pharm. Sci.*, **48**: 620, 1959.

[**] Scheiner J and Altemeier WA: *Surgery*, **114**: 9, 1962.

[***] Remmers RG *et al.*: *J. Pharm. Sci.*, **54**: 49, 1965.

An obvious poorly bioavailable drug product (or dosage form) should exhibit the following *four* **characteristic features**; namely:

- **Extremely low (poor) hydrophilicity (or aqueous solubility), and/or slow dissolution rate in the biological fluids.**
- **Significantly poor stability of the dissolved drug at the physiologic pH (*in vivo*).**
- **Insufficient partition coefficient of drug product thereby giving rise to sluggish permeation *via* the biomembranes.**
- **An overall extensive presystemic metabolism.**

5.2.8.1. *Overcoming Acute Bioavailability Issues*

In order to overcome various acute bioavailability issues, one may make use of any one of the following three *modus operandi:*

1. **Pharmacokinetic Means:** It essentially engages critical modification in the chemical structure of the drug molecule to afford a change in the **Pharmacokinetic Profile of Drug Product.**

Example

Following are some of the typical examples:

Acetonidation (or Esterification) of Corticosteroids: The prodrug approach to 'fluocinolone' remarkably **enhances the extremely low skin permeability of this steroidal drug, containing hydroxyl moieties is mainly attributed to its specific interaction with:**

- **skin (epidermis), and**
- **binding sites in keratin**[*]

Thus, **acetonidation** (or *esterification*) of **Corticosteroids (Fluocinolone)** enhances the permeability to skin perceptively. Interestingly, the **Fluocinolone Acetonide** (a '**prodrug**' *belonging to the corticosteroid class*) is abundantly useful in these *two* well-known skin manifestations, such as:

- **inflammatory conditions, and**
- **pruritic conditions.**

The '**prodrug**' gets duly activated *in vivo* by the enzyme esterase

R = H: Fluclorolone (or Flucocinolone Acetomide)

$R = C CH_3$: Fluclorolone (or Flucocinolone)

Prodrug of Fluclorolone (or Flucocinolone)

2. **Pharmaceutic Approach**: The *pharmaceutic approach* involves particularly the modification(s) of the '**drug entity**' with respect to the following aspects:

---

* **Keratin**: It refers to any of a family of scleroproteins that are the main constituents of epidermis, hair, nails and horny tissues.

- formulation fundamentals,
- manufacturing process, and
- physiochemical properties of the drug substance, without altering its basic chemical structure.

Example

Acyclovir (an *antiviral drug*) inherently possesses **poor bioavailability** on account of its three prominent properties, for instance:

- extremely low solubility,
- poor GI absorption rate, and
- biotransformation to an 'Inactive Metabolite'.

A precursor-type of prodrug, 6-deoxyacyclovir, gets duly oxidized by the help of the enzyme 'Xanthine Oxidase' to reproduce **Acyclovir.**[*] Amazingly, the **prodrug,** *i.e.,* **6-deoxyacyclovir,** is remarkably found to be showing:

- 18-fold greater water solubility, and
- 5-6-fold higher bioavailability after oral administration.

6-Deoxyacyclovir   Xanthine Oxidase (Enzyme)   **Acyclovir**

[A Precursor-Type Prodrug]

3. **Biological Method:** The biologic method essentially deals with the 'route of drug administration' which could be altered suitably to retain the maximum desired bioavailability of the drug released from the respective dosage form, *e.g.,* from '**Oral Route**' to the corresponding '**Parenteral Route**'.

Example

The following well-known '**General Anaesthetics**' are administered *via* the IV Route:

- Barbiturates-Thiopental sodium,
- Non-Barbiturates-Propofol, etomidate, ketamine.

5.2.8.2. Physiochemical Characteristics of a Drug

The host of diversified and judicious attempts dealing with such focused activities, such as:

- formulation optimization,
- manufacturing protocols, and
- physiochemical characteristic of a drug

are invariably carried out so as to accomplish an increase in the '**Dissolution Rate**', since it categorically represents the most critical and major '**Rate-limiting Step**' in the actual absorption

---

[*] **Acyclovir**: It is active against **Herpes Simplex Viruses (HSV) 1 and 2**, varicella zoster, Epstein-Barr viruses and cytomegalovirus.

of an array of drug substance. Based on the literature survey, it has been amply demonstrated that the ensuing 'Dissolution Rate of a Drug' may be increased appreciably through many well-known means and ways. Following are some of the predominant time-tested and tried procedures, a majority of which are usually aimed at enhancing the prevailing 'surface area of the drug substance', and will be discussed briefly in the following sections.

Micronization: **Micronization** actually refers to-'**the reduction of particles to micrometer diameter sizes specifically**'.

In actual practice, **Micronization** essentially involves the critical reduction of the solid drug particulate matter between **1-10 micrometer (μm)+ = 0.000,001 m].** This may be duly obtained by:

- 'spray-drying process',* or
- 'fluid-energy mill'**(or air-attrition techniques).

Examples

Following are certain **typical examples of drug substances:**

1. **Aspirin**- for getting relief from headache rapidly.
2. **Sulpha Drugs**- for rapid bioavailability.
3. **Griseofulvin**- for much faster, safer and rapid absorption in vivo.
4. **Steroidal Drugs**- being bulky, water immiscible nature need to be obtained in micronized for quick absorption *in vivo*.

The '**Micronization**' of a drug substance shall critically enhance the solubility profile in the small intestine, which happens to be a better absorption site but at the same time there would be a definite '**increased rate of drug degradation**' in the stomach perhaps due to the induced and increased '**surface area**'.

Surfactants (or Surface-Active Agents) The '**Surfactant**' invariably refers to a substance that minimizes:

- **surface tension,** and
- **interfacial tension,**

particularly in small concentrations. The most common examples of the '**Surfactants**' are: **emulsifiers, defloculants, suspending oils, dispersants, soaps and detergents.**

The **Surfactants specifically increase the dissolution rate primarily due to the dual functional phenomena,** namely:

- **augmentation of 'Wetting',** and
- **penetration of Dissolution Fluid',**

right inside the solid-drug particulate matter.

---

* **Spray-Dryer:** It refers to a machine that removes moisture from 'atomized particles', almost instantaneously, using a controlled 'solution feed' through a high rpm wheel (atomizer) and an upward flow of heated air. Particles are dried as they fall through the heated air (fluidized bed) in an enclosed SS chamber and are duly collected in a container at the bottom of the chamber. The moisture-laiden vapour is vented up and escapes out of the chamber.

** **Fluid-Energy Mill:** It is a device used to reduce particle size by rotating particles at high speeds in a bed of air against the sides of a chamber and against other particles. The particles get duly reduced in size by attrition and mostly obtained in spherical shape.

In usual practice, the surfactants are employed at a concentration level much below their **actual Critical Micelle Concentration (CMC)**[*] values, because above **CMC** the drug substance thus entrapped into the micelle structure does not undergo partition in the dissolution medium at all.

Non-ionic Surfactants-These designates such surface-active agent (or surfactants) that fails to get ionized solution. In fact, they do exhibit fewer chemical incompatibilities in comparison to other surfactants.

Examples

Tween 80, Polysorbate 80, Tween 20 etc.

 NOTE   **Spironolactone (an aldosterone diuretic) has its bioavailability increased significantly by making use of the surfactants in the drug formulation.**

Salts of drugs: In a broader perspective, the salts of drugs do exhibit an improved solubility profile and dissolution characteristics in comparison to the 'parent drug molecule'.

Example

Following are a few typical examples:
1. **Penicillins** (*acidic drugs*) form **salts with alkali metals**, *viz.* **Penicillin G/Potassium.**
2. **Atropine** (*basic drug*) forms **salts with strong acids**, *viz.* **Atropine Sulphate**.
3. **Chloroquine** (*basic drug)* forms **salts with phosphoric acid**, *viz.* **Chloroquine Phosphate.**

Metastable Polymorphs: The term **Metastable** refers to-'the slight margin of stability of a substance that changes into another substance as conditions change'.

Therefore, invariably a metastable polymorph is found to be more soluble in comparison to the stable polymorph of a drug substance which explicitly exhibits the **Phenomena of Polymorphism** (*i.e., existing in several forms*).

Example

Chloramphenicol Palmitate (*Syn*: **Chloramaban, Chloropal, Chlorolifarina**) usually occurs in three different forms-A, B and C-of which form '**B**' is found to be much more water soluble via-a-vis the '**A**' and '**C**' forms.

Change in pH Drugs Microenvironment: It has been duly established that a critical change in the '**pH of Drugs Microenvironment**' can be achieved in two different conspicuous ways:
* **In situ formation of salt,** and
* **Incorporation of buffers to drug products**

Example

Buffered 'Aspirin Tablets'.

Pseudopolymorphism (or Solute-Solvent Complexation): Importantly, the solvates of drug substances in organic solvents is usually termed as **Pseudopolymorphism** (or *solute-solvent*

---

[*] **Critical Micelle Concentration (CMC):** CMC refers to-'the concentration of an amphiphile (*i.e.*, a molecule having affinity for both aqueous and lipid media) above which micelles begin to generate'.

complexation). The resulting products invariably do possess a definite higher aqueous solubility in comparison to their respective '**Parent Drug**' or '**Hydrated Drugs**'.

In actual practice, one may even attain much higher degree of solubility by simply '**Freeze-Drying**' a drug with an appropriate solvent (*i.e.*, in solution form), which is known to form a desired 'solvate'. Nevertheless, pseudopolymorphism gives rise to the drug substance into a powder form having particulate matter of submicron size:

Example

Griseofulvin Hexane Solvate [1:2]

 NOTE Care must be taken that the solvent must be nontoxic in nature [*e.g.*, 'Benzene' being carcinogenic is not to be used].

Preferential Adsorption on Insoluble Carriers: The thoughtful utilization of '**Bentonite**', an *inorganic clay* with a highly active adsorbent characteristic features, may also increase the critical dissolution rate of poorly water-soluble drugs, *viz*:

- **Prednisolone- a Glucocoticoid (anti-inflammatory/immunosuppressive effects)**
- **Indomethacin-a NSAID**, and
- **Griseofulvin- an antifungal agent**

due to the remarkable maintenance of the ensuing concentration gradient at its maximum level.

Explanation

The *two* logical explanations put forward to explain the preferential absorption on the insoluble carriers thereby causing rapid release of medicament(s) are:

- **fairly week physical bondage existing between the adsorbate and adsorbent,** and
- **hydration followed by swelling of the 'Bentonite' in the aqueous environment.**

Solvent Deposition: In this particular instance, the *poorly water-soluble drug, e.g.,* **Nifedipine** (*a Ca^{2+} Antagonist*) is made to dissolve in a polar-organic solvent (ethanol), and subsequently deposited on an inert-hydrophillic solid matrix like either **microcrystalline cellulose** or **pure starch (IP/BP)** obtained by evaporation of the solvent.

Solid Solutions: In general, the solution designates a homogeneous mixture composed of one or more substances, known as 'solutes' dissolved in another substance termed as a '**solvent**'. There are *three* known modalities that may be employed whereby the respective particle size of a 'drug' could be minimized up to a **Submicron Level (0.000,001 m):**

- **Utilization of 'solid solutions',**
- **Utility of 'eutectic mixtures',** and
- **Usage of 'solid dispersions'**

Interestingly, in all the three aforesaid, the '**Drug**' (*i.e., solute*) is mostly a sparingly water-soluble drug critically acting as a '**Guest**'; whereas, the solvent is an extremely water-soluble compound or polymer acting a '**Host**' (or '**Carrier**').

Solid Solution-The solid solution is defined as 'a binary system consisting of a solid solute dispersed molecularly in a solid solvent'.

As the *two* **aforesaid components** usually crystallize out almost simultaneously in a perfect homogeneous one-phase system, the solid solutions are also termed as:

- **molecular dispersions,** or
- **mixed crystals.**

However, based on the accomplished reduction in the '**particle size'** right up to the molecular level, the solid solutions thus obtained do exhibit the following features:

- **enhanced aqueous solubility,**
- **rapid dissolution profile than eutectics,** and
- **faster dissolution pattern than solid dispersions.**

Preparation of Solid Solution: The following are the various methods involved:

1. It is usually prepared by '**Fusion Method'** whereby a simple physical mixture of both solute and solvent are melted together and subsequently cooled for '**Rapid Solidification'.**

In actual practice, such aforesaid procedures adopted through sheer fusion are invariably termed as 'melts', such as: **Griseofulvin-Succinic Acid (Solid Solution),** as depicted in *Figure 5.10.*

Importantly, the *dissolution profile of* 'Griseofulvin' from such a **solid-solution gets dissolved almost 6-7 folds faster in comparison to the untreated pure Griseofulvin Sample.**

Faster Dissolution Systems: The faster dissolution systems may be obtained when the following *two* criteria are duly fulfilled:

- **diameter of solute molecules <60% of diameter of solvent molecules,** and
- **volume of solute molecules <20% of the volume of solvent molecules,**

so that ultimately the solute molecule may be duly contained very much within the intermolecular spaces of the solvent molecules.

Examples

Digitoxin-PEG 6000 Solid Solution (*i.e.*, an admixture of digitoxin and polyethyleneglycol having its molecular weight ~6000).

Glass Solution: A 'solution' refers to a clear mixture of *two* or more substances wherein neither separates upon standing.

Thus, when the resultant solid solution is a homogeneous transparent and renders a brittle system, it is invariably termed as the '**Glass Solution'.**

Example

The most commonly used '**Carriers'** which predominantly give rise to the formation of a **glassy structure (*i.e.*, a glass-like structure)** are:

- **Sugars–Dextrose, Galactose and Sucrose,** and
- Chemicals–Polyvinylpyrrolidone (PVP), Critic Acid and Urea.

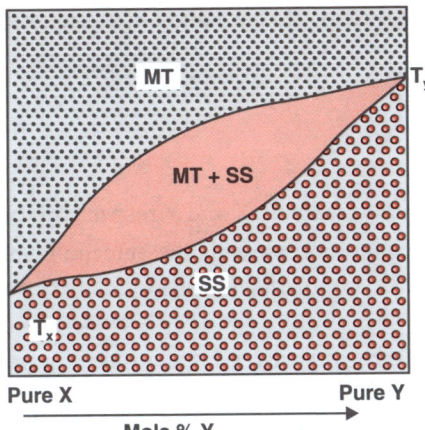

MT = Melt (....)
SS = Solid Solution (....)
MT + SS = Mixture of Melt + Solid Solution (IIII)
T_x = MP of Pure X
T_y = MP of Pure Y

Fig. 5.10: Diagrammatic Representation of a Binary Phase for Continuous Solid Solution of X and Y.

Mechanisms of Molecular Dispersions: The **Molecular Dispersion** relates to the mixing phenomena brought about by the kinetic motion of molecules of two or more entities duly present in the same system.

In a broader perspective, *two* **mechanisms** have been put forward to afford an **increased solubility**, and **fast dissolution of molecular dispersions,** namely:

- The **'Binary System'** on being exposed to an aqueous environment critically aids the soluble-carrier to dissolve rapidly thereby rendering the insoluble drug in a typical state of microcrystalline dispersion having very fine particulate matters.
- The **'Solid-Solution'**[*] is duly exposed to **dissolution medium**, whereby the soluble carrier undergoes dissolution rapidly with the respective '**Insoluble Drug**' almost stranded at the molecular levels.

Eutectic Mixtures: Eutectic Mixture refers to –'**a physical combination of two or more solids that softens or liquefies due to a depression of the melting point below that of each component taken separately'.**

Eutectic Point designates-'**the lowest temperature (at constant pressure) at which a frozen (solid) mixture begins to melt'.** It relates to-*the temperature and pressure at which solid and liquid states of a mixture of substances exist in equilibrium.*

It has also been proved that these eutectic systems can also be obtained by simple fusion method. In true sense, the eutectic mixtures do differ from solid solutions (see **Solid Solutions** *in this section*) wherein the fused melt of solute-solvent exhibit the following *two* **criteria:**

- **Almost complete miscibility,** and
- **Negligible solid-solid solubility.**

In other words, such typical systems truly **represent 'the fundamentally perfect blend of a physical mixture of *1* crystalline entities'.**

---

[*] **Solid Solution**: The physical state of matter in which the constituent molecules, atoms of ions have no translator motion although they are capable of vibrating about the fixed positions that they occupy in a crystal lattice.

Figure 5.11 represents a typical **Phase Diagram** depicting the formation of a simple eutectic system.

Explanation

The various steps involved are as stated under:

1. T_x and T_y designate the melting points of the pure ingredients X and Y respectively.
2. The **point 'C' on the line AB** of the aforesaid diagram represents the eutectic point, and, therefore, shows the bare minimum melting point in comparison to any other mixture in the series.
3. The actual composition at **point C** is the eutectic mixture composition; whereas, the temperature corresponding to **C is** the eutectic temperature.
4. Importantly, at **point C** an equilibrium gets established between
   - *two* **solid phases,** and
   - **one liquid phase.**

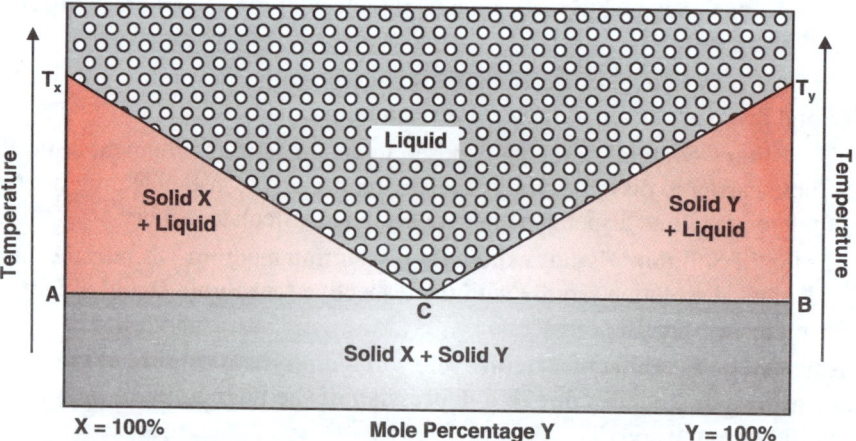

Fig. 5.11: Illustration of a Phase Diagram Depicting the Critical Formation of a Simple Eutectic System.

5. Therefore, for a condensed system, one of the variables present is rendered constant and hence, the **Phase Rule** becomes:

$$F = C - P + 1$$

6. Thus, as per the '**Phase Rule**' for a condensed system, we have:

$$F = C - P + 1 = 2 - 3 + 1 = 0$$

i.e., the **degree of freedom 'F'** becomes zero, and, therefore, the prevailing system is rendered 'invariant' at the **Eutectic Point C. Why does an 'eutectic mixture' not regarded as a 'compound'?** The **Eutectic Mixture** possesses not only a definite composition, but also a definite melting point. In spite of this, it is never regarded as a full-fledged '**compound**' because of the following reasons:

- **The ingredients present are not in a stoichiometric proportion,** and
- **It fails to provide any positive indication pertaining to formation of a compound by any experimental method.**

Important Points

1. Furthermore, in **Figure 5.11** along the line T_xC, one may critically observe the **separation of solid X from the melt.** The various points that are strategically located on this line do explicitly indicate the following *two* aspects:

   - **initiation of freezing process**, and
   - **evolution of the liquids course.**

   Thus, along the line T_xC, the **solid-liquid equilibrium** prevails, and as per the **Phase Rule** $(F = C - P + 1)$ we have $F = 1$, which clearly suggests that the ensuing system is univariant.

2. Likewise, the corresponding line T_YC designates the second liquidus curve; and hence, the various points falling on this line indicate *two* **cardinal aspects:**

   - **beginning of freezing phenomena**, and
   - **separation of solid Y from the melt.**

   In short, we may conclude that the aforesaid simple eutectic system essentially comprise *two* **Liquidus Curves,** *viz.* T_xC **and** T_yC.

3. One may critically observe that the 'end of freezing process' and 'beginning of melting process' with respect to the altogether different composition of the simple eutectic system is invariably given by the line **ACB**.

   Thaw-Melting Temperature: The temperature duly recorded along the **line ACB** is usually termed as the **thaw-melting temperature.**

   Table 5.3 records the various observed phases that are duly present in different areas of the phase diagram (*Figure 5.11*).

   Microstructures of Certain Eutectic Mixture: The **Eutectic Mixture** (or **Eutectics**) do have altogether different microstructures. Following are *two* **well-defined microstructures of Eutectics: (a) O-Phenylenediamine, and (b) Carbontetrabromide-hexachloroethane eutectic alloy** (*Figure 5.12*).

   Solid Dispersions The solid dispersion are usually prepared by the following *two* **common methods:**

   - **solvent method**, and
   - **co-precipitation method**

S.No.	Area	Phase(s)	Degrees of freedom $(F = 2 - P + 1)$
1	Above T_xCT_Y	Liquid phase only	2
2	T_xAC	Solid X and liquid	1
3	T_yBC	Solid Y and liquid	1
4	Below ACB	Solid X and solid Y	1

Table 5.3. Area, Phase(s) and Degrees of Freedom Observed in Simple Eutectic-Type Phase Diagram (Figure 5.11)

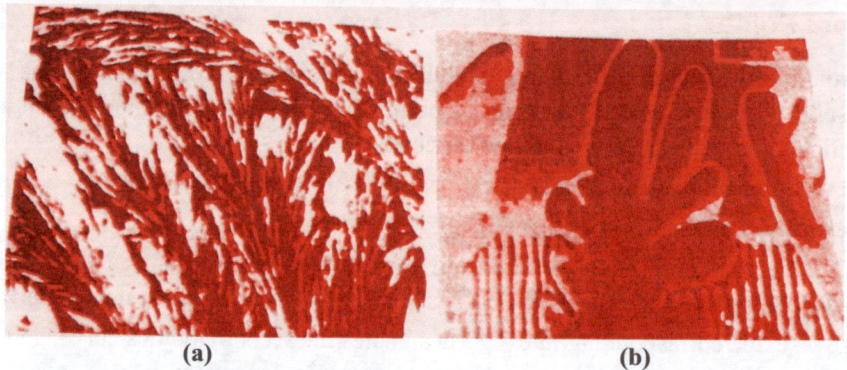

(a)   (b)

Fig. 5.12: The microstructures of eutectic mixtures: (a) O-phenylenediamine (feather-like structure); (b) Carbontetrabromide-hexachloroethane.

wherein both the components, *viz.,* **Solute** (as a **'Guest'**) and **Solid Carrier Solvent**, are duly dissolved carefully in a common *pure volatile organic solvent, e.g.,* **Ethanol**.

The next most critical step is to cause the effective precipitation of the **'Guest Solute'** in a crystalline carrier, which may be duly accomplished by:

- **evaporation of solvent (liquid) by evaporation under reduced pressure (in a rota-evaporator), and**
- **freeze-drying of the product.**

In this manner, the drug substance is precipitated duly in an **'amorphous state'**. Therefore, the fundamental differences prevailing between the *two* adopted phenomena, namely:

- **solid dispersions, and**
- **solid solution (or eutectics),**

are that in the former instance the drug is obtained in an amorphous state; whereas, in the latter instance as a crystalline state.

Example

A typical example is given by the following instance: **Sulphathiazole (amorphous state) + Urea (crystalline state)**.

Co-precipitates (or Co-evaporates): The above cited example of **Sulphathiazole** and **Urea** is invariably termed as **Co-precipitates (or Co-evaporates).**

Merits: The method of **Co-preciptates** is found to be appropriately suitable for a good number of **thermolabile substances**, *e.g.,* **Terpenoids, Alkaloids** etc.

Demerits: These essentially include such aspects as:

- **high-cost of processing,**
- **usage of large-quantum of solvent, and**
- **difficulty in removal of solvent.**

Glass Suspensions (or Glass Dispersions): Figure 5.13 explicitly depicts the various observed **Dissolution Rates of Griseofulvin from the matrix of Polyvinylpyrrolidone (PVP) dispersions.**

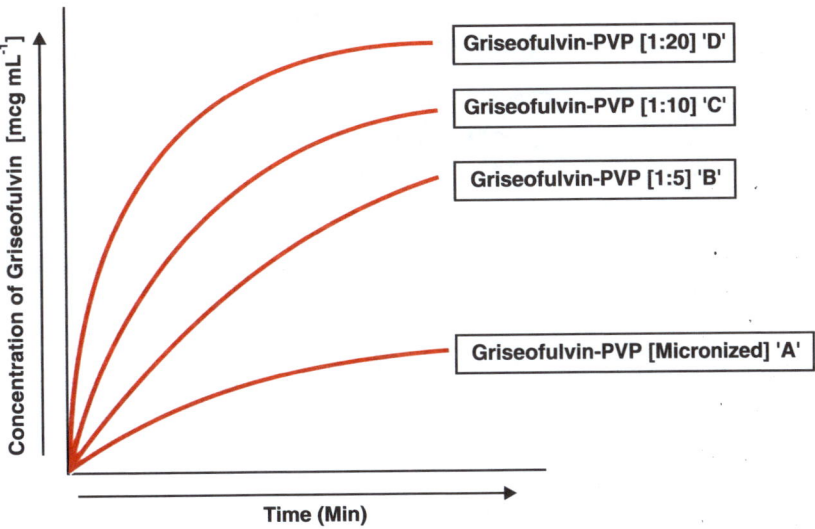

Fig. 5.13: Enhancement in Rate of Dissolution of Griseofulvin by Solid Dispersion Method.

Explanation

The *four* **distinct glass dispersion profiles** of **Griseofulvin** both alone and in combinations with **PVP** may be expatiated as following:

1. The concentration of **Griseofulvin** as such in micronized form seems to be the lowest (see 'A' above).

2. The combination of **Griseofulvin micronized** in different proportions of **PVP** clearly exhibit different profile of concentration of **Griseofulvin**, *viz.* **Maximum 'D' (1:20) Intermediate 'C' (1:10)** and **Minimum 'B' (1:5)**

Molecular Encapsulation (with Cyclodextrins): Encapsulation refers to-'the process of enclosing a substance in a capsule, *viz.* preparation of soft-gelatin capsules filled with vitamin A or vitamin E and sealed thereafter'.

Molecular Inclusion Complexes: It has been duly researched that α-and ψ-**Cyclodextrins** together with some of their structural analogues do have exceptional characteristic features in exhibiting the ability to produce the '**Molecular Inclusion Complexes**' with specifically the hydrophobic drugs bearing poor inherent water solubility.

Importantly, the various **Cyclodextrin Molecules** (*having a wide range Molecular Weights*) are exclusively found to be fairly versatile in possessing a '**Hydrophobic Cavity**' which can adequately accommodate the so-called **Lipophilic Drug Substances** as its '*Guests*'. Nevertheless, the outer-zone of the host molecule is relatively hydrophilic in native as illustrated in figure 5.14.

Salient Features: These essentially comprise the following:

1. The molecularly encapsulated drug, such as: **Chlorthiazide** (a *Thiazide Diuretic*), **Pentobarbitone** (a *Barbiturate*), **Ibuprofen** (*NSAIDs*), **Nitrazepam** (*Benzodiazepines*) *etc.,* invariably shows much improved characteristic features, namely:

   • **aqueous solubility,** and
   • **dissolution rate.**

2. In general, the **Bioavailability** of the molecularly encapsulated drug substances are progressively being adopted, tested and used commercially across the globe:

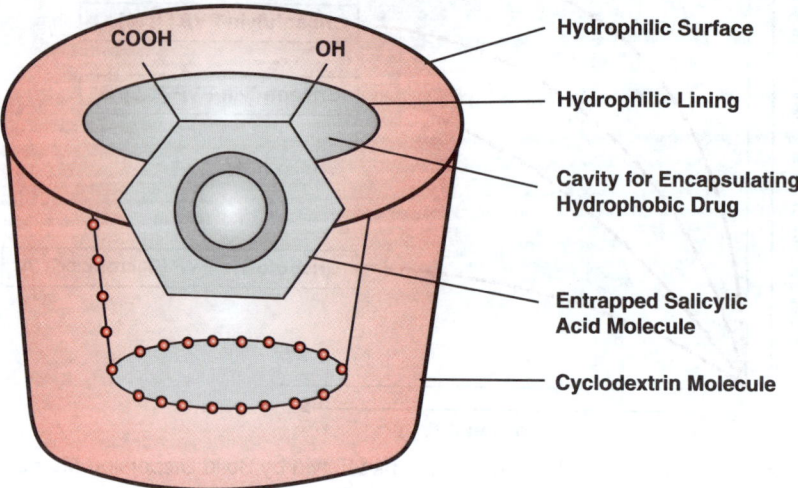

COOH OH

Hydrophilic Surface

Hydrophilic Lining

Cavity for Encapsulating
Hydrophobic Drug

Entrapped Salicylic
Acid Molecule

Cyclodextrin Molecule

Fig. 5.14: Structural and Functional Features of Cyclodextrin Molecule Depicting an Encapsulated Drug.

5.3. Bioequivalence

5.3.1. *Preamble*

Two 'Drug Products' (or 'Dosage Forms') are pronounced to be-'**Bioequivalent when they contain the same amount of an identical active drug substance; and when, their Bioavailability remains the same when administered in equal doses under similar conditions'.** Alternatively, **Bioequivalence** relates that a drug in two or more similar dosage forms critically gains entry into the general circulation almost at:

- **Same relative rate,** and
- **Same relative degree**.*

In a broader perspective, **Bioequivalence** entails an absolutely important consideration in an array of key situations that predominantly involve:

- **lot to lot consistency,**
- **innovator to 'Generic Product'** ** **therapeutic equivalence, and**
- **such circumstances when a marketed (commercial) product undergoes specific alterations with respect to formulation, manufacturing process technology and dosage strength of medicament.**

---

* That is, the plasma level patterns of the drug obtained by making use of the two dosage forms are the same (or identical)

** **Generic Product**: It refers to a '**dosage form**' prepared from **basic active drug substance** *e.g.,* **Chloro-quine Phosphate 250 mg Tablet.**

5.3.2. *Design and Conduct of Bioequivalence Studies*

The following *two* **epoch-making events** in the domain of **'Bioequivalence Testing Methods'**, such as:

- **Patent expiration on the 'Wonder Drugs' of the 1950s and 1960s,** and
- **Drug Price Competition (DPC) and Patent Term Restoration Act (PTRA) of 1984, eventually recognized and established the 'generic drug' approval methods which are very much in place as to date.**

The prevalent importance of the **'Bioequivalence Testing Procedures'** based upon the glaring awareness of several potential aspects for the various clinical differences between two chemically equivalent **'Dosage Forms'** has come into being *via* a host of cardinal factors, namely:

- improved methods for **'Clinical Efficacy Evaluation'.**
- development of methodologies to determine **mcg or ng quantum of drugs in biological fluids,**
- remarkable improvements in the ever-growing technology of **Drug Product formulation** and **Physical Testing,**
- knowledge of declared **Clinical Inequivalencies in the literature,**
- enhanced costs of **Classical Clinical evaluation,**
- objective and quantitative nature of various **Bioavailability Tests**, and
- an enormous enhancement in the number of **Chemically equivalent Products on the market.**

In the present-day scenario, the availability of an array of **'Dosage Forms'** from multiple sources invariably has placed the **'physicians'** really in a tight corner to choose and select one from among several commercially **Marketed Drug Products**. Obviously, the *Physician's Decision* will entirely rest upon the one for which more explicit and pertinent data are immediately available. Thus, the more **'comfortable** one' was certainly recommended in **Doctor's Final Decision.**

Important Points: These essentially comprise the following:

1. The greatest reliability and dependency upon the critical bioequivalence testing as an alternative measure to the need of clinical testing for:
   - **establishing the efficacy of 'Dosage Form',** and
   - **fixing the 'Dosage Regimen' in patients.**
2. It provides an authentic reliable means whereby the **'Generic Drugs'** are duly approved
   - **for 'Marketing',** and
   - **for the maintenance of 'Product Quality' of most drug products,**

particularly in such instances that predominantly involve either alternations of ingredients in **Formulation** or **Specific Manufacturing Process.**

3. The most critical requirements for the *generated* **Bioequivalence Data** pertaining to **Dosage Forms** must be applied cautiously and reasonably.
4. The fundamental **'Pharmacokinetic Evaluation'** of the **Bioavailability Data** perhaps does not serve as a necessary requirement to depict the **'Bioequivalence'** of *two* **Drug Products**.

5.3.2.1. *Criteria for the Design of Bioequivalence Study*

It has been established beyond any reasonable doubt that the '**Design**' must be focused entirely on the following *two* **important aspects**, namely:

- **Sufficient in-depth knowledge of Pharmacodynamics of the Drug Substance,** and/or
- **Information(s) pertaining to the Pharmacokinetics of the active substance in question (under investigation).**

In general, most likely, the so-called '**Single-dose Evaluation Studies**' shall be more than enough to carry out the **Bioequivalence Study**. However, there could be certain typical and crucial situations wherein the '**Steady-state Studies**'* may be needed urgently, such as:

1. When the arising problems of sensitivity preclude enough the exact *plasma concentration evaluation after a single dose.*
2. When the obscured intra-individual variability in either the *plasma concentrations* or the *disposition rate* remains noticeably large inherently.
3. Such instances in which either the *dose-dependent or time-dependent Pharmacokinetics* do occur.
4. Also applicable to the '**Extended Release Products**'.

NOTE   In this type of steady-state studies, the adopted drug-administration scheme must follow the usual dosage recommendations as closely as possible. From this critical observation one may safely conclude that the so-called 'multiple-dosing system' should prove to be the most preferred logical choice for drugs duly intended for a long-term usage. Perhaps it may interestingly result in a more realistic comparison in the manner the drug is given normally.

Multiple-Dose Study *vs.* Single-Dose Study   There are several significant advantages of conducting a **Multi-Dose Study *vs.* Single-Dose Study**:

1. The **Multiple-Dose Study** particularly excludes the long washout periods invariably needed in between the *single-dose administrations*. **Thus, it duly facilitates the smooth switch-over from one dosage form to another in a perfect steady state,**
2. The **Single-Dose Study** may usually cause serious problems pertaining to sufficiently long sampling periods so as to obtain *reliable estimates of the* **Terminal Plasma Half-Life**, that is required critically for the precise and exact calculation of the entire **Area Under the Curve (AUC).**
3. Obviously, the '**Multiple-Dose Studies**' give rise to relatively higher concentrations of drug in the circulating blood thereby making the various measurements both precise and easier.

NOTE   Besides the drug concentrations which require to be measured exclusively over a single-dosing interval at a steady state, the necessity to measure the same at lower concentrations in the course of a disposition phase gets eliminated almost completely.

---

* **Steady-State Studies**: They usually refer to the studies when during the course of a chemical reaction, the concentration of an intermediate remains constant, the intermediate is said to be in a '**Steady-State**'.

4. Importantly, the typical multiple-dosing studies may be adequately conducted in patients rather than healthy subjects, that could allow the usage of **Higher Dose Levels conveniently**.

5. Interestingly, one may come across 'Smaller Intersubject Variability' specifically in the steady-state studies quite often that may eventually allow the actual use of fewer subjects.

6. It is quite easy to detect the **Nonlinear Pharmacokinetics** more rapidly critically at steady-state dosing immediately followed by **Multiple-Dosing Profile.**

Demerits of Multiple-Dose Bioequivalence Studies: A few **demerits of the Multiple-Dose Bioequivalence Studies** are as follows:

1. The 'Healthy Volunteers' must not be administered with any investigative drug substance for a fairly long duration.

2. The **Multiple-Dose Bioequivalence Studies** are invariably found to be more cumbersome to perform effectively with particular reference to absolute compliance to subjects having **frequent dosing as well as dietary restrictions.**[*]

3. Preferentially, the **Multiple-Dose Studies** must be carefully carried out only in a situation when a **Single-Dose Study** does not serve as a 'Reliable Indicator' with respect to the **bioavailability aspects.**

5.3.2.2. *Design*

The design of dosage regimens has been discussed *under Section 4(2)*. In addition, the specific 'Bioequivalence Study Design' with particular reference to 'Parallel Design' and 'Cross-Over Design' has been duly dealt *under Section 4(3.4)*.

Two-Period Crossover Design: The various important features **of the Two-Period Crossover Design** are as follows:

1. First and foremost, the **N volunteers** selected for the study are duly separated into two treatment sequences or two categories. Now, the N_1 **subjects** usually take the dosage forms in the order **AB and N_2 subjects** in the order **BA**. Thus, the N subjects are given by the expression:

$$N = N_1 + N_2$$

From a total of 24(N) selected volunteers, 12(N_1) take first the 'Genetic Drug' followed by the 'Branded Product'; whereas, 12(N2) first take the 'Branded Product' followed by the 'Generic Drug' (*i.e.,* in a reverse sequence).

2. After the administration of drug product in the 'First Period', the blood concentrations of the respective 'Active Drug' are duly determined at appropriate intervals.

3. It is now adequately followed by a 'Wash-Out Period', which is of sufficient duration so as to ensure the 'Total Elimination' of the drug substance administered during the **First Period**. For this, one may safely use an 'Interval of at least Nine Drug Half-Lives' that would be just enough to ensure and justify the total elimination of the drug ultimately.

NOTE In usual practice, quite often a minimum of seven half-lives is duly recommended.

---

[*] This could perhaps be the actual reason why most of the **bioequivalence investigative studies are usually carried out as the single-dose studies**

4. The '**Second Product**' (or the 'alternative product') is duly administered in the '**Second Period (N_2)**'; and subsequently, the blood concentrations determined as during **Period 1.**

In short, it may be added that the '**Crossover Designs**' are planned such that each individual treatment is duly provided an equal number of times in each period. It is, in fact, regarded to be most efficient and gives rise to genuine and unbiased estimates of dosage form differences, in case there is a '**Period Effect**' prevails.

5.3.2.3. *Subjects (or Volunteers)*

In common practice, the Bioequivalence Studies are invariably carried out in different categories of human voluntcers (or subjects), such as:

Normal Healthy Adult Volunteers: The Normal Healthy Adult Volunteers are usually selected for carrying out '**Single-Dose Bioequivalence Studies**'.

In this specific instance, *two* glaring situations may crop up, such as:

- Reproduction Toxicological Studies may be rendered feasible by selection subjects of either sex between the **age group 18 to 55**. However, the same holds good in the particular instance of genetic polymorphism.
- Patients under critical supervision and precautions may really help to ascertain the toxic characteristic feature of the '**Active Ingredient**' (**drug**)[*]
- Inter-subject variants may not be useful as significant Determinants of Bioequivalence.

Salient Features: the various cardinal aspects pertaining to the selection and treatment of subjects are as follows:

1. A minimum of **12 subjects** is normally recommended; however between **18 to 24 subjects** seem to be '**Ideal**' and employed frequently to enhance reasonably the '**Data-Base for Statistical Analysis**'.
2. Both the '**Test Samples**' and '**Reference Products**' are invariably given to the selected subjects specifically in the **fasting state.**[**]
3. The time schedule and composition of meals taken soon after the administration of drug must be standardized appropriately.
4. Since the overall '**Fluid Intake**' could enormously exert its influence upon the '**gastric passage**', it must be specified and standardized rigidly.
5. All '**Selected Subjects**' must avoid taking any other medicament(s) for at least 1 week prior to such an investigative study and also during the study period.
6. Complete avoidance from '**Junk Foods**', '**Alcoholic Beverages**' and '**Spicy Preparations**' should be maintained in order to prevent and check the possible interaction with:
   - **circulatory functions.**
   - **GI functions,** and
   - **renal functions.**
7. Both '**Smokers**' and '**Non-Smokers**' must be identified separately.

---

[*]   That is, the applicant may have to justify his alternative approach reasonably.

[**]   **Fasting State:** That is overnight fast for at least 10 hrs together with 2-4 hrs after administration of the dose.

8. The critical investigative studies related to the **'High Clearance Substance'** need to be standardized suitably.

5.3.2.4. *Reference and Test Product*

In usual practice, all drug products under the investigation should, by all means, be manufactured strictly in accordance with:

- **GMP guidelines,** and
- **ISO-9000 certified procedures.**

Important Points: Following important points must be adhered to strictly:

1. The **'Batch-Control Results'** of the test product need to be reported as an essential component of quality assurance reports.

2. It must be practiced to compare the **'Generic Products'** with the corresponding form of

   - a **'Reference Product'**
   - a **'Branded Product'**, or
   - a well-known **'Innovator Medicinal Product'.**[*]

3. In general, the **'Test Product'** shall largely belong to a 'test batch'. Immediately, after the scale-up operation, the respective samples of the product from the production batches (A) must be critically compared with those of the corresponding **'Test Batch (B)'**. Hence, these *two* samples (A) and (B) must essentially show up the identical 'dissolution rate' in vitro performed duly in a discriminatory test.

However, it is pertinent to mention here that the **'Study Sponsor'** may have to retain a sufficient quantum of the product samples for the accepted shelf-life together with 1 year to enable repetition of both in vitro and in vivo investigative studies at the behest of the designated authority.

5.3.2.5. *Analytical Methods*

In a broader perspective, the actual conduct of the **Bioavailability Studies in Humans** critically needs a **'dosage form'** to be given to a group of individuals. Besides, the time-course (or duration) of the concentration of the drug substance in the circulating blood is determined:

- **directly,** or
- **indirectly.**

Obviously, to evaluate such vital information one should have the availability of suitable **Analytical Procedures**[**] for estimating the concentration of the active drug present duly in the **Body Fluids.**[***]

Barr *et al.* (1972)[****] proposed the following guidelines, such as:

---

[*] The **'Reference Product'** and its due selection should be justified by the applicant.

[**] Notari RE: **Biopharmaceutics and Pharmacokinetics: An Introduction**, 4th ed. Marcel Dekker, New York, 1987.

[***] McDonald H *et al.*: *Clin. Med.*, (Dec): 30-33, 1969.

[****] Barr WH *et al.*: *Clin. Pharmacol Ther.*, **13**(1): 97-108, 1972.

- Standardized methods for administering dosage form,
- Withdrawing suitable blood and/or urine samples, and
- Sufficient recognized methods for performing the statistical analysis well as interpretation of results obtained.

Bioanalytical Methods: The **Bioanalytical Methods** (or **Bioanalytics**) refer to-'the critical application of various analytical techniques to estimate either a drug substance or the metabolite concentration in a host of 'biological matrix samples' related to:

- plasma, serum or urine sample *viv-a-vis* bioavailability, and
- certain bioequivalence studies.

In true sense, it does play a role throughout the drug development right from 'drug discovery' to '**Drug Approval**'. Besides, the **Bioanalytics** are employed to determine the '**Active Drug Component**' and/or its '**Biotransformation Products**' that are adequately present in plasma, serum, blood, urine or any other appropriate matrix which must meet the requirements pertaining to specificity, accuracy, sensitivity and precision. Nevertheless, the perfect and sound knowledge with regard to:

- **active drug substance** and/or
- **biotransformation product(s)**

that are essentially present in the sample matrix seems to be an absolute pre-requisite for accomplishing good/reliable results.

Assay of Biotransformation Product: In general, one may crucially take cognizance of the fact that the **Evaluation of Bioequivalence** shall be solely based upon the measured concentrations of active substance. In case, the above line of action turns out to be quite impracticable, it is always advisable to make use of a *better and major* Biotransformation Product. Thus, its ultimate measurement is virtually rendered absolutely essential only when the chemical entity under investigation is a '**Prodrug**'.

Example

In a specific instance when the urinary excretion rate is measured, the drug determined must designates a major fraction of the dose; and, therefore, the excretion rate must be taken into consideration almost equivalent to the **Plasma Concentrations of the Active Drug Substance**. Presently, the advent of **recent technological breakthroughs, such as: GLC, MS, HPLC, Fluroscence Methods, AAS, Radioimmuno Assays**, and **Microbiological Assays**, have enormously enhanced the scope, capability and versatility of determining **the Active Drugs upto microgramme and nanogramme levels accurately**. In fact, quite a few of the aforesaid methods not only exhibit extreme sensitivity and precision, but also enough selectivity which will enable to quantify the '**drug**' in the presence of:

- its metabolites, and
- its endogenous compounds,

which may show a tendency to interfere with the assay of the compound present in '**Biological Fluids**' (*viz.,* Blood, Serum, Urine, CSF)

Use of Radioactive Labeled Molecules: Importantly, in some typical cases for which no sensitive enough chemical method is suitable to determine the '**Active Ingredient**' accurately, one may rely solely upon the *skillful utilization of* **Radioactive Labeled Molecules**. Hence, it should be verified accurately that the measured profile of **Radioactivity** is duly contained in the intact chemical entity (or compound) which has been separated/isolated from its respective 'Metabolites'.

In adopting the aforesaid **radio-labelled technique**, it may be absolutely necessary to be assured that the drug product embodying the 'radioactive drug' to be given to a patient should possess identical physical and chemical characteristics features resembling to those of the **Drug Product (*unlabelled product*).**

NOTE | A sincere and constant effort is always geared towards further simplification, authentication and improvement of the existing techniques and also to develop newer rapid, reliable and versatile 'bioanalytical methods'.

5.3.2.6. *Investigation of Characteristic Features*

It is, however, pertinent to state here that with a view to compare the bioequivalent aspects of different **Drug Products** (or **Dosage Forms**) of the some drug substance, they need to be absolutely equivalent with particular reference to the following *two* **cardinal features**, namely:

- **Rate of 'drug absorption', and**
- **Extent of 'drug absorption'.**

Importantly, the *two* **most prevalent and predominant aspects** that are intimately involved in the critical assessment of **Bioequivalence** are:

- **the Pharmacokinetic Parameters which most appropriately describe the characters of the rate and degree of absorption, and**
- **the most befitting technique of utilizing the 'Statistical Analysis' of the accomplished data.**

Based on the extensive research being made in the domain of the **Therapeutic Efficacy of a Drug**, the **AUC** is found to be directly proportional to the quantum of drug being absorbed in vivo. Therefore, the aforesaid **Pharmacokinetic Parameter** is found to be the most abundantly used one so as to duly characterize the actual degree of absorption:

- **in single-dose studies,** and
- **in multiple-dose studies.**

Furthermore, in case one makes use of the **Pharmacodynamic Effects** to serve as the characteristic features, the various measurements must give rise to an elaborated:

- **time course, and**
- **initial observed values,**

that tends to be the same, perceptively.

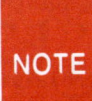

NOTE | 1. **The non-linear characteristic profile of the dose-response relationship must be given an important thought and consideration.**
2. **All measurements need to be essentially sufficient with respect to precision, reproductibility and specificity.**

5.3.2.7. *Generalized Approach: Single-Dose Pharmacokinetic Bioequivalence Studies*

A survey of literature would reveal *several generalized approaches* which are exclusively suggested and recommended for the **Single-Dose Pharmacokinetic Bioequivalence Studies.**

Study Conduct: Following are the *five* **most important aspects** with regard to an elaborated and meaningful study conduct, such as:

1. **Food-Effect Bioavailability (BA)/Bioequivalence (BE) Study:** In usual practice, the **Test Products** (*viz.* **Dosage Forms**) or the **Reference Products** (*viz.* **Branded Drug Products**) need to be given along with **240 mL water** to a suitable pre-determined number of subjects/ volunteers under the **'Fasting Conditions'**, unless the intended study refers to-**'a food-effect BA/BE study'**.

2. Usually the maximum available marketed strength of the **Drug Product** must be administered duly in the form of a single unit. Nevertheless, due to the requirement of the analytical reasons, **one may duly administer multiple units of the highest strength of Dosage Form thereby giving rise to the total single-dose falling very much within the labeled dose range.**

3. **Washout Duration**: An appropriate washout duration (*viz.* more than 5 half-lives of the drug molecule to be measured) must actually separate each individual treatment by all means.

4. **Retention of Test and reference Product**: the various vital information as mentioned on the **'label'**, *viz.* lot number, date of manufacture, date of expiry, strength *etc.*, of the **Dosage Form (Test Product)** and **Branded Drug Product (Reference Product)** must be recorded duly. Importantly, there should not be more than 5% variance in the drug content of the test product and reference product. Besides, the sponsor may also essentially include a careful comparison of:

   - **composition of 'test product',** and
   - **simultaneous comparison in the composition of the 'test product' and 'reference product'.**

NOTE   The original samples of the 'Test' and 'Reference' products should be retained at least up to five years from the date of manufacture.

5. **Water/Food Intake of subjects During Phase:** It is absolutely necessary that both prior to and during each and every study phase, the selected subjects must be allowed to take water, as and when required, except 1 hr before and **after the administration of dosage form.** [*] They must be provided with standard balanced meals usually after 4 hrs of the drug administration.[**] All subjects must refrain from consuming **'Alcoholic Drinks'** both 24 hrs, prior to each study-phase and till the 'last'. Sample is duly collected from each defined interval.

Collection of Sample and Sampling Times: The collection of sample and sampling times actually are regarded to be most critical aspects of a relevant Bioequivalence Study Protocol. The following guidelines are required to be followed as far as possible and feasible:

---

[*] Notari RE: **Biopharmaceutics and Clinical Pharmacokinetics: An Introduction**, 4th ed., Marcell Dekker Inc., New York, 1987.

[*] McDonald H: *Clin. Med.*, 30-33, 1969.

1. Invariably, under normal circumstances, it is always preferred to collect blood samples instead of urine or tissue.
2. In most instances, the 'drug' or 'metabolites' are duly determined either in serum or plasma.

NOTE In certain specific cases, the determination in the whole blood proves to be more reliable and suitable for carrying out the routine analysis.

3. It is absolutely important to draw the 'blood Samples' at appropriate time schedule to relate justifiably the absorption, distribution, metabolism and elimination (ADME) phases of the drug substance.
4. In usual practice, nearly 12-18 samples (including a predose sample) must be collected methodically per subject per dose.
5. The aforesaid 'Sampling Profile' must be continued for at least three to five terminal half-lives of the drug (under investigation).
6. Precise and exact timing for 'Sample Collection Schedule' safely depends upon the following two aspects:
   - nature of the drug substance, and
   - actual input from the administered 'Drug Product'.
7. Sample collection protocol must be spaced in a manner such that:
   - Maximum concentration of 'drug' in the circulating blood [C_{max}], and
   - Terminal log-linear phase in order to accomplish a precise estimate of K_{EL}* from the linear regression.
8. Actual Clock-Time/Elapsed Time: In reality, the actual clock time when the respective samples are duly drawn and the elapsed time intimately related to drug administration must be recorded carefully.

5.3.4. Bioanalytical Method Development and Validation for Bioavailability and Bioequivalence Studies

5.3.4.1. *Preamble*

The 'Bioanalytical Methods' predominantly embraces a broad cross-section of the domain of Modern Analytical Techniques, and Latest Sophisticated Analytical Equipments, *e.g.*, GLC, MS, AAS, H-NMR, ORD, FT-IR, HPLC** and the like. Indeed, it has become more or less an absolute prime requirement to decide to carry out the determination of:
- analyte(s) exclusively,
- metabolite(s) solely, and/or
- both analyte and metabolite simultaneously,

before connecting the meticulous exercise with regard to the Bioanalytic Method Development.

---

* K_{EL}: Elimination Rate Constant.
** www.ncbi.nlm.nih.gov/entrez.

An exhaustive literature survey together with thorough **internet exploration/book references** pertaining to such critical features as chemical structure, molecular weight, solubility profile, stability status, instruments, suggested techniques and kind and volume of matrix required.

Important Points: Following are some of the **important points,** namely:

1. Requirement of more quantum of matrix or even to enhance the dose of the formulation in a typical situation when the citied **Analytical Method** does not achieve the desired level of sensitivity.

2. Certain of blood samples and its subsequent steps:
   - **Collection of blood samples and its subsequent steps:**
     - ➤ **protection from UV light,**
     - ➤ **incorporation of a stabilizing agent** (*e.g.,* **sodium citrate**),
     - ➤ **addition of an anti-oxidant** (*e.g.,* **vitamins A, C and E**), and/or
     - ➤ **suitable derivatization of the analyte itself**
   - **Proper validation and calibration of the aforesaid sophisticated analytical instruments, glass wares, centrifuges, Millid water plant etc.**

before going ahead with the development of a newer method.

3. *Environmental conditionalities* also play a critical role in the development of a **New Method Assay:**

Examples

Following are some typical examples, such as:

LC-MS or GC-MS: Temperature should be **22 ± 1°C;** Other Instruments: Temperature should be **25 ± 2°C.**

Relative Humidity for the above instruments must range between **50 and 75.**

4. All '**standards**' intended to be used for **Bioanalytical Methods** should be obtained from genuine authentic sources only.

5. **Water** which is mostly employed for the **Bioanalytical Purpose must be of USP Grade.**

NOTE

It is worthwhile to state here that it is equally important to have a proper 'Certificate of Analysis monitoring the extent of purity, storage condition, name and address of manufacturer, and expiry date for all the 'Standards' used in the bioanalytical method.

5.3.4.1.1. Bioanalytical Instruments

The **Bioanalytical Instruments** may be categorized into *two* **types,** namely:

1. **Important Sophisticated Instruments:** These essentially consist of the following instruments:
   - Electronic balance
   - Deep freezer

- Refrigerator centrifuges
- Biological oxygen demand (BOD) incubators
- UV visible double-beam spectrophotometer
- Atomic absorption spectrophotometer (AAS)
- High Performance liquid chromatograph (HPLC)
- Gas liquid chromatograph (GLC)
- Hyphenated analytical instruments:
    - Gas chromatograph with mass spectroscopy (GC-MS)
    - Liquid chromatograph with mass spectroscopy (LC-MS)
- Mass spectrometer (MS)
- X-ray diffraction (XRD)
- Optical rotary dispersion (ORD)
- Circular dichroism (CD)
- Fluorescence spectrometer

All these instruments need to be standardized/calibrated before carrying out the analysis.

2. **Supplementary Analytical Instruments:** Following are the most commonly used supplementary analytical instruments, namely:

- pH metre
- Potentiometer
- Evaporates (rotary type)
- Vortex mixers
- Sonicators
- Sample shakers
- Refrigerators
- Vaccum manifolds
- Electric water baths
- Magnetic stirrer-cum-hot plate
- Top loading electric (digital type).

5.3.4.2. Factors Governing Retention Time-Sensitivity-Selectivity

There are an array of vital and important factors governing retention time, sensitivity and selectivity with regard to the **determination of Analyte Sample in Biological Fluids** by various sophisticated analytical procedures, such as:

- **Instrument to be used,**
- **Selection of GC/HPLC column,**
- **pH of mobile-phase buffer,**
- **Specific composition of 'Mobile Phase',**
- **Column-oven temperature,**

- **Sample injection volume,** and
- **Extra column volume.**

All the above-mentioned aspects pertaining to the retention time, sensitivity and selectivity shall now be treated individually in the following sections:

5.3.4.2.1. *Instrument to Be Used*

There are *three* **sophisticated instruments,** namely **HPLC, LC-MS** and **GC-MS,** that are mostly pressed into service for the assay of analytes as described in *Table 5.4*.

Table 5.4. Various Analytical Instruments- HPLC, LC-MS and GC-MS- and Their Salient Features with Specific Conditionalities

S. No.	HPLC	LC-MS	GC-MS
1.	Requires more time analytical method development.	Needs definitely less time to develop a new method	Essentially requires several derivatization Steps for the analyte sample.
2.	Total span of 'run-time' ranges between 8 and 20 min	'Run-times' extend between 1.8 and 2.5 min.	'Run-times' vary between 12 and 20 min.
3.	Can take up any sort mobile-phase buffers.	Only volatile mobile-phase buffers to be employed.	Helium to be used as a carrier-gas.
4.	UV visible, fluroscence or Electron capture Detector (ECD) may be used based on the nature of analyte molecule.	A unique combination of HPLC and mass spectroscopy (MS) detector.	A suitable combination of GC and MS detector.
5.	Both sensitivity and selectivity are achieved with great difficulty.	Easy to accomplish sensitivity and selectivity	Needs specific precautions to achieve easily both sensitivity and selectivity.
6.	All types of analyte samples may not be possible to perform efficiently.	Most suitable for handling all analyte samples.	Only suitable for volatile and thermally Unstable analytes.
7.	Column dimensions-Usually range between 4.6 × 150 and 360 mm.	Column dimensions-usually range between 2.1-4.6 × 50 and 75 mm.	Column dimensions-usually of 30 m in lengths.
8.	To develop a feasible method for combination of analytes in a single run in rather difficult.	It is a lot easier to accomplish.	It is found to be easier when the analytes do have the same nature.
9.	No specific gases are needed.	Gases like N_2, zero air, compressed air are required. He has is only required.	
10.	Sample injection volume ranges between 20 and 100 μL	Sample injection volume should be < 40 μL.	Sample injection volume must be <5 μL.

| 11. | Needs minimum skill and training. | Requires specialized expertise. | Needs a specisl expertise. |
| 12. | On-line sample processing and injection not that beneficial. | On-Line sample preparation and injection enhances throughput. | For certain specific molecules solid-phase microextraction is available adequately. |

5.3.4.3. *Selection of GC/HPLC Column*

It has been duly observed that based on the exact nature of the 'Analyte Samples', one may critically select

- **Normally-Phase Column (NP-Column),** and
- **Reverse-Phase Column (PP-Column)**

1. **Column Performance**: Preferentially, all **HPLC-columns** must be purchased from the authorized suppliers and their respective performances need to be carried out **according to the certificate provided by the manufacturer or as per the standard operating procedure (SOP) of the 'Bioanalytic laboratory'.**

Examples

These essentially comprise:

- **Normal Phase Columns** *e.g.,* **Silica, Amino, CN etc.**
- **Reverse Phase Columns** *e.g.,* **C-18, C-8, C-4 etc.**

The most commonly employed **columns** in **HPLC, LC-MS and GC-MS** are stated in Table 5.5 together with their **length, width, particle size** and **theoretical plates.**

S. No.	Instrument	Length (mm)	Width (mm)	Particle size (μ)	Theoretical plates (per m)
	Table 5.5. Column Dimensions of HPLC, LC-MS and GC-MS with Regard to Length, width, Particle Size				
1	**HPLC**	150-300	4-4.6	5-10	50,000
2	**LC-MS**	50-75	2-4.6	3	-
3	**GC**	50 m	0.25	0.25	3,000 (capillary)

5.3.4.3.1. *pH of Mobile-Phase Buffer*

It is now required to select a *proper buffer* for HPLC, since its **Molarity and pH** do play a prominent and critical role in terms of better selectivity, sensitivity and resolution. However, the **ideal pH range** essentially needed for the said **Mobile-Phase Buffers range between 2.5 and 7.5** solely depending upon the very inherent nature of the 'Analyte Sample' being investigated. Nevertheless, in most instances particularly in: **RP-HPLC,** *a decrease in pH invariably causes:*

- **decrease in 'Retention-Time' and,**
- **increase the 'Shape of Peak',**

whereas, it would affect simultaneously '**Selectivity**' and '**Resolution**'.

Important Points These include predominantly the following aspects:

1. It is always better to make use **of 1-20 milli-molar buffer.**
2. Evidently, an increase in the molarity of the buffer may no doubt afford a relatively good separation, but at the same time shall reduce:
   - **shape of the peak,**
   - **sensitivity,** and
   - **life of column.**
3. **Conventional Buffers for HPLC:** The most abundantly used **Conventional Buffers for HPLC** are as stated below:
   - **Sodium acetate,**
   - **Sodium dihydrogen phosphate,**
   - **Potassium dihydrogen phosphate,**
   - **Ammonium dihydrogen phosphate,** and
   - **Tris-Buffers.**
4. **Ion Pairing Agents**: Invariably, along with the aforesaid **Buffers** [in (3)] it is advisable to make use of the ion-pairing agents, such as '**Butane, Bentane, Heptane, Sulphonic Acids**, in different proportions so as to sustain and retain the **Ionizable Analyte Samples upon the typical RP-HPLC Columns.**
5. **LC-MS: The LC-MS Hyphenated Analytical Technique** a host of *volatile buffers* are used, such as:
   - **Acetic acid (0.1%),**
   - **Formic acid (0.1%),**
   - **Ammonium acetate,** and
   - **Ammonium formate.**

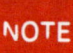 **NOTE**   It is pertinent state here that one may obtain better results by carefully adjusting the pH of the buffer with conjugated acid or base as per the necessary requirement.

6. **Preparation of Buffers for HPLC**: The various steps involved are as follows:
   - It is usually prepared by using '**Ultra-Sonicators**' *for rapid dissolution of inorganic salts.*
   - **Degassing of the resulting solution is a must.**
   - The **degassed buffer solution is filtered via 0.24 μ membrane filter.**
   - **Filtered HPLC-buffers** are normally stored in '**glass containers**' to avoid fungal growth.
   - **Prepared buffer solutions** must be used within 48 hrs.

5.3.4.3.2. Specific Composition of 'Mobile-Phase'

In actual practice, the exact composition of the '**Mobile-Phase**' exclusively rests upon the specific type of such criteria as;

- **matrix,**
- **instrument,**
- **column selected,** and
- **total number of 'Analyte Sample' being assayed.**

LC-MS vs. HPLC: Obviously, in the particular instance of **LC-MS**, the precise and exact proportion of the organic solvent needed usually remains very high as compared to the **HPLC Method**. Besides, it has been observed in many cases that the critical enhancement in the proportion of the organic solvent directly increases the corresponding peak height/shape as well as sensitivity, whereas, it may minimize the extent of both selectivity, and resolution criteria simultaneously.

Development of HPLC Method: In the course of developing a new **HPLC Method** it is always advisable to allow the proper mixing of the buffer and solvent together in large quantum unless one makes use of the quaternary **HPLC System** (which prevents wastage of solvent appreciably).

Use of Allegation Method: It has also been recommended to make use of the allegation method intelligently for the development of **HPLC Method**.

Example

In a situation, when one has duly prepared:

- **Solvent (50% v/v),** and
- **Buffer (50% v/v).**

and **one intends to enhance the solvent ratio 65% simply follow the underlying procedure of allegation:**

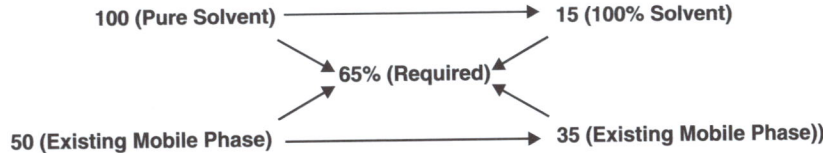

100 (Pure Solvent) → 15 (100% Solvent)
65% (Required)
50 (Existing Mobile Phase) → 35 (Existing Mobile Phase))

NOTE   **The aforesaid 'allegation method' is solely meant for quantitative purposes; however, during finalization of the method, the mobile phase has to be prepared afresh as and when needed.**

5.3.4.3.3. *Column-Oven Temperature*

The effective use of an **Optimized Column-Oven Temperature** is found to yield reasonably good reproducibility in the retention time of the **Analyte Sample:**

Salient Features: these essentially comprise:

1. Certain typical analyte samples do require higher temperature for the desired elution just above the ambient temperature.
2. Salient Features

These essentially include the following:

    (a) Mostly one may observe that the **retention time and length of column** are found to be inversely proportional.

(b) **Length of column** on being enhanced leads to improved

- **selectivity,** and
- **resolution,**

whereas, both **sensitivity and peak-shape may get reduced appreciably.**

(c) **Reduction in particle size** of the adsorbent may give rise to **better sharp peak shape,** but it may **lower the life-span of the HPLC column significantly.**

(d) To develop a reasonably **good HPLC method,** one should be selective in choosing

- **right type of column** (*viz.* **C-18, C-8 C-4**), and
- **appropriate dimensions,**

(e) Use of 'C-Loaded Columns' may be used rather than unnecessarily increasing the length of the column for handling the assays related to **Complicated Analyte Samples.**

(f) To prevent **damage caused to the main HPLC Analytical Column,** one should always make use of the 'Guard Columns'.

3. **Special Care of HPLC Columns**: These predominantly consist of the following:

(a) All **HPLC Columns must be stored after proper washing as recommended/certified by the manufacturer.**

(b) For the **Reverse Phase HPLC Columns** it is always advised to do the necessary thorough washings with 100% water so as to get rid of the buffers that are left behind in the column[*] and then with the requisite organic solvent(s) in the reverse order to remove the entrapped water, if not, it would lead to serious 'Fungal Growth' inside the column.

(c) When the **HPLC Columns** are not in use, it is required to be capped properly soon after the washing operation.

4. **Procedure of Regeneration of HPLC Column**: Obviously, the laid down procedure the regeneration of **HPLC Column** do vary from the exact type of column, such as:

(a) **Silica Columns**: For the regeneration of **Silica Columns in HPLC,** it is required to pump in nearly 50 mL of the following **HPLC Grade Solvents at the rate of 1-2 mL per min** sequentially:

- **Tetrahydrofuran (THF),**
- **Methanol,**
- **Aqueous acetic acid (2-4%),**
- **Aqueous pyridine (2-4%),**
- **Tetrahydrofuran,** and
- **tert-2-Butylmethyl ether**

(b) **Reverse Phase Columns**: For the regeneration of the **Reverse Phase Columns in HPLC,** it is most preferred to pump in approximately 50 mL of the following **HPLC Grade Solvents at the rate of 1-2 mL per min,** sequentially:

- **Water + 4 × 100 μL of DMSO (dimethyl sulphoxide) injected,**
- **Methanol,**

---

[*] Otherwise, the salts in 'Buffer' may crystallize and cause clogging of column.

- **Chloroform**, and
- **Methanol.**

2. An increase in column temperature may help in the definite reduction in the retention time of the analyte, but contrarily enhances the shape of the peak. Ultimately, it may affect upon both the selectivity and resolution.

3. A significant decrease in the viscosity of the mobile phase may be observed while increasing the column temperature. Therefore, it usually indulges in accomplishing *two* **glaring aspects**, namely:

- **permits enhanced flow rates,** and
- **increases the diffusibility.**

which predominantly reduces the critical resistance cause to the respective '**Mobile-Phase Mass Transfer' largely.***

Demerits of Increased Column Temperature: Following are the *two* **most vital demerits of increased column temperature in HPLC assays,** namely:

- **possibility of analyte components and solvent components to undergo decomposition, and**
- **changes of vapour pressure of solvent(s) to rise, thereby enhancing the high-risk of bubbles present in the detector that would ultimately give rise to the production of:**
  - ➤ **an uneven baseline,** and
  - ➤ **ghost (false) peaks.**

5..3.4.3.4. *Sample Injection Volume*

Based on various experimental data, it has been duly established that the precise sample injection volume fails to cause a noticeable effect upon the following aspects:

- **selectivity,**
- **sensitivity,**
- **shape of peak,** and
- **column life.**

Importantly, an increase in sample injection volume may also enhance the sensitivity ehereas, it would reduce the shape of peak and column life significantly. Therefore, it is mostly preferred to reduce the sample injection volume till a situation demands it urgently.

NOTE	In some instances, an increase in the sample injection volume shall tend to merge even the imputrities right into the 'analyte peak'.

5.3.4.3.5. *Extra Column Volume*

Interestingly, the ensuing volumes occurring within an **HPLC Equipment** that eventually causes the separation of the components present in the analyte sample are invariably termed as the **Extra Column Volumes.** It is worthwhile to state at this point in time that such '**Critical Volumes**' that are strategically located

---

* That is, the analyte molecules get diffused *via* the mobile phase faster at elevated temperatures.

- **Just prior to the injector,** or
- **Just behind the detector**

must not be regarded as the extra column volumes.

Necessarily, the ***extra column volumes*** must be maintained as low as feasible and possible, since they could finally affect noticeably:

- **separation of component,** and
- **shape of peak.**

In fact, the **extra column volume is solely responsible for affording:**

- **Band Broadening,** and
- **Band Tailing.**

5.3.4.4. *Method Validation*

After having developed an elaborated bioanalytical method it is very much desired and advisable to carry out a '**trial**' comprising a calibration curve. Besides, necessary 'quality control' checks has got to be done before commencing a **complete Validation Method.**

In a broader perspective, the bioanalytical method validation essentially includes practically all of the procedures which clearly prove and demonstrate that a specific method employed for the 'quantitative measurement of analyte samples' in a given matrix, for instance, serum, plasma, blood and wine, is established to be absolutely:

- **reliable,** and
- **reproducible,**

for all future intended usage.

In general, the fundamental experimental parameters required predominantly for this 'validation' necessarily must include the following cardinal aspects, namely:

- **selectivity,**
- **sensitivity,**
- **ruggedness and robustness,**
- **repeatability,**
- **accuracy,**
- **recovery,**
- **linearity,** and
- **stability.**[*]

---

[*]   It essentially comprises **in-injector or post-processing, bench-top, freeze-thaw, short-term/long-term prepared 'Stock Solutions', matrix samples long term and dilution integrity.**

SUGGESTED READINGS

ASTM-Methods,	: Vol. 14.02 E 898-88, June 1990.
ASTM-Methods,	: Vol. 14.03 E 77-89, June 1990.
ASTM-Methods,	: Vol. 14.02 E 542-94, June 1990.
Blanchard *J et al.* S. Karger,	: **Principles and Perspectives in Drug Bioavailability,** New York:1979.
Bourne DWA Dittert LW.	: **Pharmacokinetics,** In:Banker GS, Rhodes CT, Eds. *Modern Pharmaceutics,* 2nd ed. Marcel Dekker, New York, **1996.**
Gibson CG,	: Skett P.**Introduction to Drug Metabolism,** Chapman and Hall, London (UK). 1986.
Hoener BA, Bentet LZ.	: **Factors Influencing Drug Absorption and Drug Availability** In: Banker: [Eds]. *Modern Pharmaceutics.* Marcel Dekker Inc New York GS, Rhodes CT, 1990.
McEnlang IC.	: **Buccal Absorption of Drugs**. In: Swarbrick J *et al.* (Eds). *Encyclopedia of Pharmaceutical Technology, Vol.1.* **Marcel Dekker Inc,** New York: 2007.
Meyer MC.	: **Bioavailability of Drugs and Bioequivalence** In: Swarbrick Swarbrick J *et al.* (Eds). *Encyclopedia of Pharmaceutical Technology, Vol.1.*Marcell Dekker Inc New York: 2007.
Ritschel WA,	: **Handbook of Clinical Pharmacokinetics,** 3rd ed. *In Drug Intelligence* Publication, Inc. Hamillton: 1986.
Rowald M, Tozen TN.	: **Clinical Pharmacokinetics: Concepts and Applications,** 3rd ed. BI Waverly Pvt.Ltd. New York: 1996.
Shargel L *et al.*	: **Applied Biopharmaceutics and Pharmacokinetics,** 5th ed. McGraw Hill, Sydney, Australia. 2005.
Sloan KB. **Prodrugs**	: **Topical and Ocular Drug Delivery**. Marcel Dekker Inc, New York:1992
Stockley IH.	: **Drug Interactions: A Sourcebook of Drug Interactions. their Mechanisms, Clinical Importance and Management,** 2nd ed. Blackwell Scientific Publications (UK) London: 1991.
Synder LR, Stadahus MA.	: **High Performance Liquid Chromatography: Advances and Perspectives,** : Horvath CS, (Ed) Academic Press, New York:1986.

United States Pharmacopedia 27 and NF-22, 2008.

US-FDA Guidelines for Industry-Bioanalytical Method Validation 1992.

Welling PG *et al.*	: **Pharmaceutical Bioequivalence,** Marcell Dekker Inc, New York: 1991.

APPENDIX

Acceptance Criteria	The product specifications and acceptance/rejection criteria, such as acceptable quality level and unaccptable quality level, with an associated sampling plan, that are necessary for making a decision to accept or reject a lot or batch (or any other convenient sub-groups of manufactured units).
Action Levels	Levels or ranges that may be detrimental to end product quality, signaling a drift from normal operating conditions.
Alert Levels	Levels or ranges that signify a drift from normal operating conditions. These ranges are not perceived as being detrimental to end product quality, but corrective action should be taken to ensure that action levels are not obtained.
Audit	An audit is a formal review of a product, manufacturing process, equipment, facility or system for conformance with regulations and quality standards.
Bulk Drug Substance	Any substance that is represented for use in a drug and that, when used in the manufacturing, processing or packaging of a drug, becomes an active ingredient or a finished dosage form of the drug. The term does not include intermediates used in the synthesis of such substances.
Bulk Pharmaceutical Chemical	Any substance that is intended for use as a component in a 'Drug Product', or a substance that is repackaged or relabelLed for drug use. Such chemicals are usually made by chemical synthesis, by processes involving fermentation, or by recovery from natural (animal, mineral or plant) materials.
Calibration	Comparison of a measurement standard or instrument of known accuracy with another standard or instrument to detect, correlate, report or eliminate by adjustment any variation in the accuracy of the item being compared.
Certification	Documented statement by qualified authorities that a validation event has been done appropriately and that the results are acceptable.

Certification is also used to denote the acceptance of the entire manufacturing facility as validated.

Change Control

A formal monitoring system by which qualified representatives of appropriate disciplines review proposed or actual changes that might affect validated status and take preventive or corrective action to ensure that the system retains its validated state of control.

Computer Validation

The validation of computers has been given a particular focus by the US FDA.

Three documents have been published for agency and industry guidance. In February 1983, the agency published the Guide to Inspection of Computerized Systems in Drug Processing; in April 1987, the Technical Reference in Software Development Activities was Published; on 16 April, 1987, the agency published Compliance Policy Guide 7132 in Computerized Drug Processing: Source Codes for Process Control Application Programmes.

In the inspection guide, attention is called to both hardware and software; some key points being the quality of the location of the hardware unit as to extremes of environment, distances between CPU and peripheral devices, and proximity of input devices to the process being controlled; quality of signal conversion, for example, a signal converter may be sending inappropriate signals to a CPU; the need to systematically calibrate and check for accuracy of I/O devices; the inappropriateness and compatibility within the distributed system of command overrides, for example, can an override in one computer controlled process inadvertently alter the cycle of another process within the distributed system? Maintenance procedures are another matter of interest to the agency during an inspection. Other matters of concern are methods by which unauthorized programme changes are prevented, as inadvertent erasures, as well as methods of physical security.

Hardware validation should include verification that the programme matches the assigned operational function. For example, the recording of multiple lot numbers of each component may not be within the programme, thus second or third lot numbers of one component may not be recorded. The hardware validation should also include worse case conditions; for example, the maximum number of alphanumeric code spaces should be long enough to accommodate the longest lot numbering system to be encountered. Software validation must be thoroughly documented-they should include the testing protocol, results, and persons responsible for reviewing and approving the validation. The FDA regards source code, *i.e.*, the human readable form of the programme written in its original programming language, and its supporting documentation for application programs used in any drug process control, to be part of the master production and control records within the meaning of 21CFR parts 210, 211 (Current Good Manufacturing Practice Regulations).

As part of all validation efforts, conditions for revalidations are a requirement.

Concurrent Validation — Establishing documented evidence that the process being implemented can consistently produce a product meeting its predetermined specifications and quality attributes. This phase of validation activities typically involves careful monitoring/recording of the process parameters and extensive sampling/testing of the in-process and finished product during the initial implementation of the process.

Construction Qualification — The documented evaluation of the construction or assembly of a piece of equipment, process or system to assure that construction or assembly agrees with the approved specifications, applicable codes and regulations, and good engineering practices. The conclusion of the evaluation should decidedly state that the equipment, process or system was or was not constructed in conformance with the specifications.

Critical Process Variables — Those process variables that are deemed important to the quality of the product being produced.

Design Review — A 'design review' is performed by a group of specialists (such as an Architect, a Quality Assurance Scientist, a HVAC Engineer, a Process Engineer, a Validation Specialist, a Civil Engineer and a Regulatory Affairs Specialist) to review engineering documents to ensure that the engineering design complies with the cGMPs for the facility. The thoroughness of the design review depends upon whether the engineering project is a feasibility study, a conceptual design, preliminary engineering, or detailed engineering. Minutes of all meetings for design review will be sent to team members and the client to show the compliance of the design to cGMPs.

Drug — Substances recognized in the official USP; substances intended for use in the diagnosis, cure, mitigation or prevention of disease in man or other animals; substances (other than food) intended to affect the structure or any function of the body of man or other animals; substances intended for use as a component of any substances specified above but does not include devices or their components, parts or accessories.

Dynamic Attributes — Dynamic attributes are classified into functional, operational and quality attributes, which are identified, monitored, inspected and controlled during actual operation of the system.

Edge of Failure	A control or operating parameter value that, if exceeded may have adverse effects on the state of control of the process and/or on the quality of the product.
Facilities	Facilities are areas, rooms, spaces, such as receiving/shipping, quarantine, rejected materials, approved materials warehouse, staging areas, process areas, etc.
Functional Attributes	Functional attributes are such criteria as controls, instruments, interlocks, indicators, monitors, etc., that operate properly, are pointing in the correct direction, and values that allow flow in the correct sequence.
Good Manufacturing Practice (GMP)	The minimum requirements by law for the manufacture, processing, packaging, holding or distribution of a material as established in Title 21 of the Code of Federal Regulations.
Installation Qualification Protocol	An installation qualification protocol (IQ) contains the documented plans and details of procedures that are intended to verify/system, or process equipment. Installation qualification (IQ), when executed, is also a documented verification that all key aspects of the installation adhere to the approved design intentions and that the manufacturer's recommendations are suitably considered.
Intermediate (Drug/ Chemical)	Any substance, whether isolated or not, which is produced by chemical, physical, or biological action at some stage in the production of a bulk pharmaceutical chemical and subsequently used at another stage in the production of that chemical.
Life-Cycle	The time-frame from early stages of development until commercial use of the product or process is discontinued.
Master Plan	The purpose of a master plan is to demonstrate a company's intent to comply with cGMPs and itemizes the elements that will be completed between the design of engineering and plant start-up. A typical master plan may contain, but is not limited to, the following elements: approvals, introduction, scope, glossary of terms, preliminary drawings/facility design, process description list of utilities, process equipment list, list of protocols, list of SOPs, equipment matrices, validation schedule, protocol summaries, recommended tests, calibration, training, manpower estimate, key personnel (organization chart and resumes), protocol examples, SOP examples.
Medical Devices	A medical device is defined in the Federal Food Drug and Cosmetic Act Section 201(h) as: *An instrument, apparatus, implement or contrivance intended for use in diagnosis, cure, mitigation, prevention or other treatment of disease in man or other animals, or intended to alter a bodily function or structure of man or other animal.*

	This is the definition used in the code of Federal Regulations 21 parts 800 to 1299. Medical Devices.
Operational Attributes	Operational attributes are such criteria as a utility/system's capability to operate at rated ranges, capacities, intensities, such as: revolutions per minute, Kg per square cm, temperature range, Kg of steam per second, etc.
Operation Qualification Protocol	An operation qualification (OQ) contains the plan and details of procedures to verify specific dynamic attributes of a utility/system or process equipment throughout its operated range, including worse case conditions. Operation qualification (OQ) when executed is documented verification that the system or subsystem performs as intended throughout all anticipated operating ranges.
Operating Range	A range of values for a given process parameter that lie at or below a specified maximum operating value and/or at or above a specified minimum operating value, and are specified on the production worksheet or the standard operating instruction.
OverKill Sterilization Process	A process which is sufficient to provide at least 12 log reduction of microorganisms having a minimum D-Value of 1 minute.
Process Parameters	Process parameters are the properties or features that can be assigned values that are used as control levels or operating limits. Process parameters assure the product meets the desired specifications and quality. Examples might be: pressure at 5.2 psig, temperature at $37°C \pm 0.5C$, flow rate at 10 ± 1.01 min^{-1}, pH at 7.0 ± 0.2.
Process Variables	Process variables are the properties or features of a process which are not controlled or which do not change product specifications or quality.
Process Validation	Establishing documented evidence that provides a high degree of assurance that a specific process will consistently produce a product meeting its predetermined specifications and quality attributes.
Process Validation Protocol	Process validation protocol (PV) is a documented plan, and detailed procedures to verify specific capabilities of a process equipment/ system through the use of simulation material, such as the use of a nutrient broth in the validation of an aseptic filling process.
Product Validation	A product is considered validated after completion of three successive successful lot size attempts. These validation lots are saleable.
Prospective Validation	Validation conducted prior to the distribution of either a new product or a product made under a revised manufacturing process, where the revisions may have affected the product's characteristics, to ensure that the finished product meets all release requirements for functionality and safety.
Protocol	A protocol is defined in this book as a written plan stating how validation will be conducted.

Quality Assurance	The activity of providing evidence that all the information necessary to determine that the product is fit for intended use is gathered, evaluated and approved.
Quality Attributes	Quality attributes refer to those measurable properties of a utility, system, device, process or product such as resistivity, impurities, particulate matter, microbial and endotoxin limits, chemical constituents and moisture content.
Quality Control	The activity of measuring process and product parameters for comparison with specified standards to assure that they are within predetermined limits and, therefore, the product is acceptable for use.
Retrospective Validation	Validation of a process for a product already in distribution based upon establishing documented evidence through review/analysis of historical manufacturing and product testing data, to verify that a specific process can consistently produce a product meeting its predetermined specifications and quality attributes. In some cases a product may have been on the market without sufficient pre-market process validation.
	Retrospective validation can also be useful to augment initial pre-market prospective validation for new products or changed processes.
Revalidation	Repetition of the validation process or a specific portion of it.
Specifications	Document that defines what something is by quantitatively measured values. Specifications are used to define raw materials, in-process materials, products, equipment and systems.
Standards Operating Procedures (SOP)	Written procedures followed by trained operators to perform a step, operation, process, compounding or other discrete function in the manufacture or production of a bulk pharmaceutical chemical, biologic, drug or drug product.
State of Control	A condition in which all process parameters that can affect performance remain within such ranges that the process performs consistently and as intended.
Static Attributes	Static attributes may include conformance to a concept, design, code, practice, material/finish/installation specifications and absence of unauthorized modifications.
Utilities/Systems	Utilities/systems are building mechanical equipment and include such things as heating, ventilation and air conditioning (HVAC) systems, process water, product water (purified water, water for injection), clean steam, process air, vacuum, gases, etc. Utilities/systems include electro-mechanical or computer-assisted instruments, controls, monitors, recorders, alarms, displays, interlocks, etc., which are associated with them.

Validation	Establishing documented evidence to provide a high degree of assurance that a specific process will consistently produce a product meeting its predetermined specifications and quality.
Validation Programme	The collective activities related to validation.
Validation Protocols	Validation protocols are written plans stating how validation will be conducted, including test parameters, product characteristics, production equipment, and decision points on what constitutes acceptable test results. There are protocols for installation qualification, operation qualification, process validation and product validation. When the protocols have been executed it is intended to produce documented evidence that the system has been validated.
Validation Scope	The scope identifies what is to be validated. In the instance of the manufacturing plant, this would include the elements that impact critically on the quality of the product. The elements requiring validation are facilities, utilities/systems, process equipment, process and product.
Worst Case	A set of conditions (encompassing upper and lower processing limits and circumstances including those within standard operating procedures), which pose the greatest chance of process or product failure when compared to ideal conditions. Such conditions do not necessarily induce product or process failure.

Appendix

2

LIST OF SYMBOLS

A	Amount of drug in the body at any time
A_e	Amount of drug excreted unchanged in the urine
AUC	Area under plasma concentration-time curve from zero to infinity
C	Drug concentration in plasma at any time
$C(0)$	Initial (fictive) plasma drug concentration following rapid intravenous infection
C_{max}	Maximum (peak) plasma drug concentration after single dose administration
C^{SS}	Steady-state drug concentration in plasma during constant rate drug delivery
C_{av}^{SS}	Average steady-state drug concentration in plasma during multiple dosing
C_{max}^{SS}	Maximum (peak) steady-state drug concentration in plasma during each multiple dosing interval
C_{min}^{SS}	Minimum steady-state drug concentration in plasma during each multiple dosing interval
CL	Total body clearance of drug from plasma
CL_H	Hepatic clearance of drug from plasma
CL_{int}	Intrinsic hepatic clearance of free (unbound) drug in plasma
CL_{NR}	Nonrenal clearance of drug from plasma
CL_R	Renal clearance of drug from plasma
CL_{CR-}	Creatinine clearance
D	Dose
DL	Loading dose in repetitive dosing or constant-rate infusion
DM	Maintenance dose in repetitive dosing
f	Fraction of administered dose systemically available; the bioavailable fraction
f_e	Fraction bioavailable dose excreted in the urine
k	First-order rate constant
k_a	Apparent first-order absorption rate constant
K_m	Michaelis-Menten constant
k_o	Zero-order rate constant, used to describe constant-rate sustained-release drug delivery

λ_i	Exponent of the ith exponential term of a polyexponential equation
λ_1	Largest apparent first-order rate constant in a polyexponential disposition equation
λ_z	Smallest apparent first-order rate constant in a polyexponential disposition equation. The terminal ln-linear negative slope following intravenous dosing
Q_H	Liver blood flow
Q_R	Renal blood flow
R_0	Constant (zero-order) infusion rate
S_Z	Terminal negative ln-linear slope following extravascular administration and so indicated when the true pharmacokinetic meaning of the slope is not certain (See also $t^*_{1/2}$).
T	Duration of constant-rate infusion or other zero-order drug delivery
t_{max}	Time to reach peak or maximum concentration following extravscular drug administration
t_{pi}	Time elapsed since end of a constant-rate infusion
$t_{1/2}$	Elimination half-life associated with negative terminal slope $(-\lambda_z)$ ln-linear plot following intravenous administration
$t^*_{1/2}$	Apparent half-life associated with a ln-linear terminal pahse following extravscular administration when true meaning of the slope is not known (see also S_z)
τ	Dosing interval in repetitive dosing
V_C	Pharmacokinetic volume of central or plasma compartment
V	Apparent volume of distribution during terminal (λ_z) phase
V	Volume of distribution at steady state
V_{max}	Apparent maximum rate of metabolism in nonlinear pharmacokinetics described by the Michaelis-Menten equation

Appendix

LIST OF ACRONYMS

The following is a list of acronyms used in this book. It is followed by a glossary of the more important validation terms.

ADR	Adverse Drug Reaction
AGMP	Automated Good Manufacturing Practice
AGV	Automated Guided Vehicles
AHU	Air Handling Unit
ALARP	As Low As Reasonably Practicable
ANDA	Abbreviated New Drug Application
ANSI	American National Standards Institute
API	Active Pharmaceutical Ingredient
ASME	American Society of Mechanical Engineers
BATNEEC	Best Available Techniques Not Entailing Excessive Costs
BL1	Biosafety Level 1
BL2	Biosafety Level 2
BL3	Biosafety Level 3
BL4	Biosafety Level 4
BMR	Batch Manufacturing Record
BMS	Building Management System
BOD	Biological Oxygen Demand
BP	British Pharmacopeia
BPC	Bulk Pharmaceutical Chemical
BPEO	Best Practicable Environmental Option
BS	British Standard
BSI	British Standards Institution
cAGMP	Current Automated Good Manufacturing Practice
CAMMS	Computer Aided Maintenance Management System
CCTV	Closed Circuit Television

CDER	Centre for Drug Evaluation and Research
CDM	Construction (Design and Management) Regulations
CFC	Chloroflurocarbons
CFR	Code of Federal Regulations
CFU	Colony Forming Unit
cGCP	Current Good Clinical Practice
cGLP	Current Good Laboratory Practice
cGMP	Current Good Manufacturing Practice
CHAZOP	Computer HAZOP
CHIP	Chemical Hazard Information and Packaging regulations
CIMAH	Control of Industrial Major Accident Hazards regulations
CIP	Clean In Place
CMH	Continuous Motion Horizontal
COD	Chemical Oxygen Demand
COMAH	Control of Major Accident Hazards regulations
COSHH	Control of Substances Hazardous to Health
CPMP	Committee on Proprietary Medicinal Products
CPU	Central Processing Unit
CSS	Continuous Sterilization System
CV	Curriculum Vitae
DAF	Dissolved Air Flotation
DIN	Deutsches Institute Fur Normung
DMF	Drug Master File
DNA	Deoxyribonucleic Acid
DOP	Dioctyl Phthalate
DQ	Design Qualification
EC	European Community
EEC	European Economic Community
EMEA	European Agency for the Evaluation of Medical Products
EPA	Environmental Protection Agency
EPDM	Ethyl Propylene Diene Terapolymer
ERP	Enterprise Resource Planing
EU	European Union
FAT	Facility Acceptance Testing
FDA	Food and Drug Administration
FMEA	Failure Mode Effects Analysis
FS	Functional Specification
GAMP	Good Automated Manufacturing Practice

GC	Gas Chromatograph
GCP	Good Clinical Practice
GLP	Good Laboratory Practice
GLSP	Good Large Scale Practice
GMP	Good Manufacturing Practice
GRP	Glass Reinforced Plastic
GSL	General Sales List
HAZOP	Hazard and Operability Study
HEPA	High Efficiency Particulate Arrestor
HFC	Hydrofluorocarbons
HIC	Hydrophobic Interaction Chromatography
HMAIP	Her Majesty's Inspectorate of Air Pollution (now defunct)
HMSO	Her Majesty's Stationery Office
HPLC	High Pressure Liquid Chromatograph
HS	Hazard Study
HSE	Health and Safety Executive
HSL	HAZOP Study Leader
HVAC	Heating Ventilation and Air Conditioning
IBC	Intermediate Bulk Container
ICH	International Conference on Harmonization
IDF	International Diary Foundation
IEC	Ion Exchange Chromatography
IEEE	Institute of Electrical and Electronics Engineers
IMV	Intermittent Motion Vehicle
IND	Investigational New Drug Application
I/O	Inputs and Outputs
IPA	Iso Propyl Alcohol
IPC	Integrated Pollution Control
IQ	Installation Qualification
ISO	International Standards Organization
ISPE	International Society for Pharmaceutical Engineering
LAPC	Local Authority Air Pollution Control
LAF	Laminar Air Flow
LIMS	Laboratory Information Management System
LTHW	Low Temperature Hot Water
mAb	Monoclonal Antibody
MCA	Medicines Control Agency
MCB	Master Cell Bank

MCC	Motor Control Centre
MEL	Maximum Exposure Limit
MRA	Mutual Recognition Agreement
MRP	Manufacturing Resource Planning
MSDS	Material Safety Data Sheet
NCE	New Chemical Entity
NDA	New Drug Application
NDT	Non-Destructive Testing
NICE	National Institute for Chemical Excellence
NMR	Nuclear Magnetic Resonance
OEL	Occupational Exposure Limits
OES	Occupational Exposure Standards
OQ	Operational Qualification
OSHA	Occupational Safety & Health Administration
OTC	Over The Counter
P	Pharmacy Only
PBTB	Polybutylene Teraphthalate
PC	Programmable Controller
PCB	Printed Circuit Board
PDA	Personal Digital Assistants
PEG	Polyethylene Glycol
PFD	Process Flow Diagram
PHA	Preliminary Hazard Assessment
Ph.Eur	European Pharmacopeia
PHS	Puck Handling Station
P&ID	Piping and Instrumentation Diagram
PLA	Product Licence Application
PMI	Positive Material Identification
POM	Prescriptions Only Medicines
PP	Polypropylene
PPE	Personal Protective Equipment
PQ	Performance Qualification
PSF	Performance Shaping Factors
PTFE	Polytetrafluoroethylene
PV	Process Validation
PVC	Ployvinyl Chloride
PVDF	Ployvinylidene Fluroide
PW	Purified Water

QA	Quality Assurance
QC	Quality Control
QRA	Quantitative Risk Assessment
R&D	Research and Development
RF	Radio Frequency
RH	Relative Humidity
RHS	Rolled Hollow Section
RIDDOR	Reporting of Injuries, Disease and Dangerous Occurrences Regulations
RP-HPLC	Reverse Phase High Performance Liquid Chromatography
SCADA	Supervisory Control And Data Acquisition system
SEC	Size Exclusion Chromatography
SHE	Safety, Health and Environment
SIP	Sterilize In Place/Steam In place
SOP	Standard Operating Procedure
SS	Suspended Solids
THERP	Technique for Human Error Rate Prediction
TOC	Total Organic Carbon
TWA	Time-Weighted Average
UK	United Kingdom
UPVC	Unplasticized Polyvinyl Chloride
URS	User Requirement Specification
USA	United States of America
USP	United States Pharmacopeia
UV	Ultra Violet
VDU	Visual Display Unit
VMP	Validation Master Plan
VOC	Volatile Organic Compound
WCB	Working Cell Bank
WFI	Water for Injection

GUIDING PRINCIPLES FOR HUMAN AND ANIMAL RESEARCH

[A] ETHICAL PRINCIPLES FOR MEDICAL RESEARCH INVOLVING HUMAN SUBJECTS

The *Declaration of Helsinki*, first published in 1964 by the World Medical Association, established recommendations guiding medical doctors in biomedical research involving human subjects (**www.wma.net/e/policy/b3.htm**). The Declaration governs international research ethics and defines rules for "research combined with clinical care" and "non-therapeutic research". The Declaration of Helsinki has been revised periodically and is the basis of Good Clinical Practices used today. A copy of the latest revision is reproduced in this Appendix. The Declaration of Helsinki addressed the following issues:

- "Medical research is subject to ethical standards that promote respect for all human beings and protect their health and rights".
- Research protocols should be clearly formulated into an experimental protocol and reviewed by an independent committee prior to initiation.
- Informed consent from all research participants is necessary.
- Research should be conducted by medically/scientifically qualified individuals.
- Risks should not exceed benefits.

The *Belmont Report*, Ethical Principles and guidelines for the Protection of Human Subjects of Research, was published by the National Commission for the Protection of Human Subjects of Biomedical and Behavioral Research on April 18, 1979 (http://ohsr.od.nih.gov/mpa/belmont.php3). The Belmont Report identifies three principles, or general prescriptive judgments, that are relevant to research involving human subjects.

1. Boundaries between Practice and Research

1. *Practice* refers to interventions that are designated solely to enhance the well-being of an individual patient or client and that have a reasonable expectation of success. The purpose of medical or behavioral practice is to provide diagnosis, preventive treatment, or therapy to particular individuals.
2. *Research* designates an activity designed to test an hypothesis, permit conclusions to be drawn, and thereby to develop or contribute to generalizable knowledge (expressed, for example, in theories, principles, and statements of relationships). Research is usually described in a formal protocol that sets forth an objective and a set of procedures described in a formal protocol that sets forth an objective and a set of procedures designed to reach that objective.
3. *Experimental* is when a clinician departs in a significant way from standard or accepted practice. The fact that a procedure is "experimental", in the sense of new, untested, or different, does not automatically place it in the category of research.

2. Basic Ethical Principles

1. Respect for Persons
2. Beneficence
3. Justice

3. Applications

1. Informed Consent
2. Assessment of Risks and Benefits
3. Selection of Subjects

The United States' *Code of Federal Regulations* (CFR) publishes regulations for the protection of human subjects. Title 45 Code of Federal Regulations Part 46 (45CFR46) contains federal regulations which directly apply to most of human research done in the United States and are intended to protect all human subjects. 45CFR46 does the following:

- Defines activities that are subject to regulation
- Details the composition and function of an Institutional Review Board (IRB)
- Describes expedited review procedures
- Lists the criteria for review of research
- Provides a detailed description of the informed concent process, including waivers
- Describes the process for documenting consent, including waivers.
- There are three subparts of the regulations that include additional protections for vulnerable populations:
  - Pregnant women, fetuses, and neonates
  - Prisoners
  - Children

Various resources concerning ethics involving human subjects research and institutional Review Boards (IRBs) have been collected by the National Institutes of Health (www.nih.gov/sigs/bioethics/IRB.html).

[B] GUIDING PRINCIPLES IN THE CARE AND USE OF ANIMALS

Animal experiments are to be undertaken only with the purpose of advancing knowledge. Consideration should be given to the appropriateness of experimental procedures, species of animals used, and number of animals required.

Only animals that are lawfully acquired shall be used in the Laboratory, and their retention and use shall be in every case in compliance with federal, state, and local laws and regulations and in accordance with the NIH Guide.

Animals in the Laboratory must receive every consideration for their comfort; they must be properly housed, fed, and their surroundings kept in a sanitary condition.

Appropriate anesthetics must be used to eliminate sensibility to pain during all surgical procedures. Where recovery from anesthesia is necessary during the study, acceptable technique to minimize pain must be followed. Muscle relaxants or paralytics are not anesthetics and they should not be used alone for surgical restraint. They may be used for surgery in conjunction with drugs known to produce adequate analgesia. Where use of anesthetics would negate the results of the experiment, such procedures should be carried out in strict accordance with the NIH Guide. If the study requires the death of the animal, the animal must be killed in a humane manner at the conclusion of the observations.

The postoperative care of animals shall be such as to minimize discomfort and pain, and in any case shall be equivalent to accepted practices in schools of veterinary medicine.

When animals are used by students for their education or the advancement of science, such work shall be done under the direct supervision of an experienced teacher or investigator. The rules for the care of such animals must be the same as for animals used for research.

ESTIMATION OF AREA UNDER THE CURVE [AUC]

There are several methods for estimating the area under a drug concentration-time curve. An estimate of area is required to determine bioavailability, clearance, apparent volume of distribution, and other pharmacokinetic parameters. The most common method of estimating area is the use of the *trapezoidal rule*.

A blood level-time curve can be described by a series of trapezoids that are determined by each concentration-time point (Fig. I-1). The area bounded by the trapezoids approximates the the area under the curve; the greater the number of data points, the closer is the approximation.

The area of trapezoid is equal to one half the product of the sum of the heights times the width. The area under a drug concentration in plasma versus time curve is approximated by the following equation:

$$\text{Area} = (1/2)\,(C_1 + C_2)\,(t_2 - t_1)$$
$$+ (1/2)\,(C_2 + C_3)\,(t_3 - t_2)$$
$$+ (1/2)\,(C_{n-1} + C_n)\,(t_n - t_{n-1})$$

where C denotes drug concentration, t denotes time, and the subscript refers to the sample number.

The use of the trapezoidal rule is illustrated in table I-1. By way of example, the areas of the first, fifth, and seventh trapezoids are calculated as follows:

$\text{Area (1)} = (\tfrac{1}{2})\,(0 + 6.6)\,(1\text{-}0) = 3.3$ µg-hr/ml (I-2)

$\text{Area (5)} = (\tfrac{1}{2})\,(9.4 + 8.7)\,(6\text{-}4) = 18.1$ µg-hr/ml (I-3)

$\text{Area (7)} = (\tfrac{1}{2})\,(6.6 + 3.7)\,(12\text{-}8) = 20.6$ µg-hr/ml (I-4)

The area under the curve from $t = 0$ to $t = 12$ hr is the sum of the areas of all trapezoids or 83.3 µg-hr/ml.

Table I.1. Drug Concentration as a Function of Time after Oral Administration			
Sample	**Time (hr)**	**Concentration (µg/ml)**	**Area**
1	0	0.0	3.30
2	1	6.6	7.55
3	2	8.5	9.00
4	3	9.5	9.45

5	4	9.4	18.10
6	6	8.7	15.30
7	8	6.6	20.60
8	12	3.7	–
		Total	83.3
			(µg/ml per hr)

METHOD OF SUPERPOSITION

The method of superposition is a useful non-compartmental approach for predicting drug accumulation and steady-state concentrations on repetitive dosing from data obtained after a single dose. The theoretical basis for superposition is merely that drug concentration is proportional to dose.

The application of superposition to predict the time course of drug concentration under different conditions requires several assumptions. The first is that, irrespective of time of administration, a given single dose administered by a given route will always give rise to the same drug concentration-time curve. A change in dose, but not in route of administration, is reflected by a proportional change in drug concentration at any time after administration. During repetitive administration, blood levels arising from a given dose are simply an additive function of the blood levels resulting from previous doses. This principle is illustrated in Table II-1.

Table II-1 shows how the method of superposition can be used to predict drug concentrations during multiple dosing. In this particular example, drug concentration-time data was obtained after a single dose (see column 2). We wish to predict drug concentration on repetitive administration of the same dose given every 3hr. Each subsequent dose, if given independently, would give rise to the same concentrations as the first dose; this is indicated by the values in parentheses. The net concentration after the second, third, or subsequent doses, however, must also reflect the contribution of previous doses.

If given independently, the second dose would provide a drug concentration of 7 µg/ml 1 hr after administration. When given after the first dose, however, the second dose gives rise to a drug concentration of 9.5 µg/ml 1 hr after dosing; 2.5 µg/ml of drug concentration is contributed by the first dose. One hr after giving the third dose, drug concentration equals 9.7 µg/ml (rather than 7 µg/ml) because of the contributions from the two previous doses.

The data in Table I-1 also indicate that steady state is achieved after the third dose, because drug concentrations following the third, fourth, and subsequent doses are identical.

Table II-1. Drug Concentrations (µg/ml) During 4 Consecutive Doses Given at 3-hr Intervals (See Text Detailed Explanation)

Time	First dose	Second dose	Third done	Fourth dose
0	0			
1	7			
2	10			
4	5	(+0)	5	
	2.5	(+7)	9.5	

5	1.25	(+10)	11.25				
6	0..6	(+5)	5.6	(+0)	5.6		
7	0.2	(+25)	2.7	(+7)	9.7		
8	0	(+1.25)	1.25	(+10)	11.25		
9	–	(+0.6)	0.6	(+5)	5.6	(+0)	5.6
10	–	(+0.2)	0.2	(+2.5)	2.7	(+7)	9.7
11	–	(+0)	0	(+1.25)	1.25	(+10)	11.25
12	–		–	(+0.6)	0.6	(+5)	5.6

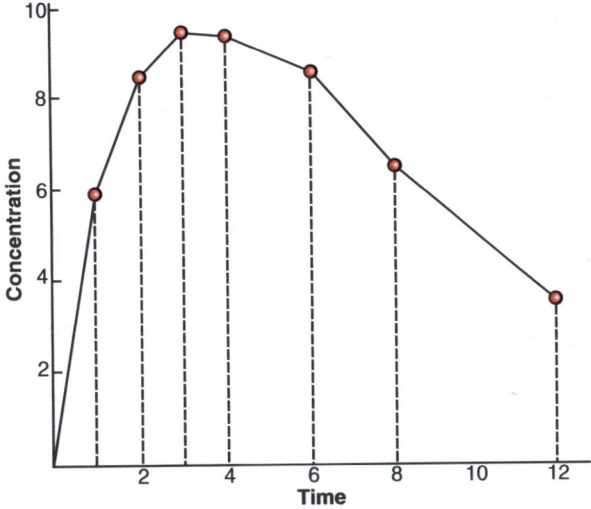

Fig. 4.1. Drug concentration (μg/ml) as a function of time (hr) after oral administration. The data points are connected by straight line segments, rather than a smooth curve, to apply the trapezoidal rule. The area of each trapezoid is delineated.

APPLICATIONS OF COMPUTERS IN PHARMACOKINETICS

PREAMBLE

The availability of computers and improvements in bioanalytical chemistry have greatly accelerated the development of pharmacokinetics. Computer software programs now allow for the rapid solution of complicated pharmacokinetic equations and rapid modeling of pharmacokinetic processes. Computers simplify tedious calculations and allow more time for the development of new approaches to data analysis and pharmacokinetics modeling. In addition, computer software is used for the development of experimental study designs, statistical data treatment, data manipulation, graphical representation of data, pharmacokinetic model simulation, and projection or prediction of drug action. Furthermore, computers are used frequently for written reports, documentation, and archiving.

A variety of computers are now available. Personal computers (PCs) may be used independently or linked together into local networks (LANs) that share many application software packages. Each type of computer has an operating system (OS), which is a collection of programs that allocates resources and enables algorithms (well-defined rules or processes for solving a problem in a finite number of steps) to be processed. UNIX, Windows, and more recently, LINUX, are example of commonly used operating systems. Windows NT is used mostly in network systems that link many PCs. Most PCs today are equipped with a modem to allow access to remote information. Netscape and Microsoft Internet Explorer are browsers that allow PCs to access remote information at various sites on the Internet referred to as Websites.

A program of instructions known as a computer package or software is written in a computer language. This software is needed to run the computer. The computer operating system must support the computer language of the software. In the past, computer users needed to be competent in computer programming and usually had knowledge of at least one computer language such as Pascal, C, or Basic. As a result of the availability of various commercial and noncommercial pharmacokinetic applications and spreadsheets, such as excel, very little computer programming is required for many applications in pharmacokinetics. Some examples are given below.

1. PHARMACOKINETIC SOFTWARE

Pharmacokinetic software consists of computer programs designed for computation and easy solution of pharmacokinetic problems. Not all computer programs satisfy the user's full requirements, but many provide the following:

1. Fitting drug concentration-versus-time data to a series of pharmacokinetic models, and choosing the one that best describes the data statistically.

   Typically, a least-squares program is employed, in which the sum of squared differences between observed data points and theoretic prediction is minimized. Usually, a mathematical procedure is used iteratively (repetitively) to achieve a minimum in the sum of squares (convergence). Some data may allow easier convergence with one procedure rather than another. The mathematical method employed should be reviewed before use.

2. Fitting data into a pharmacokinetic or pharmacodynamics model defined by the user

   This method is by far the most useful, because any list of prepared models is often limited. The flexibility of user-defined models allows continuous refinement of the model as new experimental information becomes available. Some software merely provides a utility program for fitting the data to a series of polynomials. This utility program provides a simple, quantitative way of relating the variables, but offers little insight into the underlying pharmacokinetic processes.

3. Simulation

   Some software programs generate data based on a model with parameter input by the user. When the parameters are varied, new data are generated based on the model chosen. The user is able to observe how the simulated model data matches the experimental observed data. Because pharmacokinetic processes are conveniently described by systems of differential equations, the simulation process involves a numerical solution of the equation with predefined precision.

4. Experimental design

   To estimate the parameters of any model, the experimental design of the study must have points appropriately spaced to allow curve description and modeling. Although statisticians stress the need for proper experimental design, little information is generally available for experimental design in pharmacokinetics when a study is performed for the first time. For the first pharmacokinetic study, an empirical or a statistical experiment design is necessarily based on assumptions that may later prove to be wrong.

5. Clinical pharmacokinetic applications

   Some software programs are available for the clinical monitoring of narrow therapeutic-index drugs (i.e., critical-dose drugs) such as the aminoglycosides, other antibiotics, theophylline, or antiarrythmics. These programs may include calculations for creatinine clearance using the Cockcroft-Gault equation, dosage estimation, pharmacokinetic parameter estimation for the individual patient, and pharmacokinetic simultations.

6. Computer programs for teaching

   Software applications for teaching have been reviewed by Charles and Duffull (2001). These authors taught a course in which students used (download free ware). Pharmacalc and PharmaSim may be used for pharmacokinetic computations. SAAM II or Stella and Model Maker may be used for "system dynamics". The latter takes into account stochastic processes in the simulation and may be more suitable when variability is considered to be an important factor in a clinical situation. Other software reviewed includes ADAPT for use in parameter estimation, simulation, and experimental (sample schedule) design.

2. VALIDATION OF SOFTWARE PACKAGES

Software used for data analysis such as statistical and pharmacokinetic calculations should be validated with respect to the accuracy, quality, integrity, and security of the data. One approach for determining the accuracy of the data analysis is to compare the results obtained from two different software packages using the same set of data (Heatherington et al, 1998). Because software packages may have different functionalities, different results (*e.g*, pharmacokinetic parameter estimates) may be obtained.

3. PHARMACOKINETIC SOFTWARE

Various pharmacokinetic programs (software) are available on the Internet. These programs may not have been validated by the programmer. Thus, the user is responsible for validating the program. Other programs are available from commercial suppliers. Dr. David Bourne of the University of Oklahoma has complied a listing of pharmacokinetic programs, general references in pharmacokinetics, pharmacodynamics, and other information, available at www.boomer.org. The Website www.cpb.uokhsc.edu/pkin/soft.html lists numerous pharmacokinetic software packages with user comments. Students should consult the site for updated information.

(a) Popular Programs

Some popular commercially available computer software programs are listed below. The descriptions may not represent the latest versions. New features are often added or old features improved. The user should contact the program vendor directly for more information. See below for information about Internet resources, including user evaluations of software packages.

(b) PCNonlin

PCNonlin is a powerful least-squares program for parameter estimation. Both a user-defined model and a library of over 20 compartmental models are available. The program accepts both differential and regular (analytical) equations. Users may select the Hartley-modified or Levenberg-type Gauss-Newton algorithm or the (Nelder and Mead) simplex algorithm for minimizing the sum of squared residuals. Some training is needed. Until its commercial release. Nonlin was installed mostly on mainframe computers. PCNonlin includes additional features and was designed to run on PCs. PCGRAPH (Version 4) was bundled to improve the quality of the plots from previous versions of Nonlin. Compartmental models, curve fitting, and simulations are specially designed for pharmacokinetics.

(c) WinNonlin

Pharsight Corporation Main
800 W.El Camino Real, Suite 200
Mountain View, CA 94040
(650) 314-3800
www.pharsight.com/products/winnonlin

WinNonlin is Windows-based software for pharmacokinetic, pharmacodynamic, and noncompartmental analysis. It is designed for easy interfacing and secure data management with PkS Suite. WinNonlin can calculate individual bioequivalences for all of the common replicated crossover designs. WinNonMix is associated software for population pharmacokinetic analysis. WinNonlin has an improved user interface that makes it easier to use and to interface with other Windows applications. WinNonlin is relatively easy to use for modeling with other Windows applications. WinNonlin is relatively easy to use for modeling or noncompartmental analysis of data files and handles large numbers of subjects or profiles. WinNonlin's input and output data may be managed via Excel (Microsoft)-compatible spreadsheet files. The Noncompartmental Analysis module computes derived pharmacokinetic parameters ($AUC_{t\to0}$, $AUC0_{\to}$", C_{max}, cumulative excretion, etc). PCNonlin's extensive library of models for nonlinear regression and parameter estimation are included in this software. Standard descriptive statistics and confidence intervals are determined from datasets.

(d) SAS

SAS Institute, Inc.

Cary, NC 27511

(919) 677-8000

www.sas.com

An al-purpose data analysis with a flexible application-development languages, SAS Graph allows for multidimension plots, for bar, pie, and contour charts, and for all sorts of other graphs. Over 5000 SAS products are reported to be available. Various "procs" (subroutines) are available for statistics as well as general linear and nonlinear regression models. There are over 80 procedures for univariate descriptive statistics; t-test, chi-square, correlation, autoregression, multidimensional scaling, nonparametric test, chi-square, correlation, autoregression, multidimensional scaling, nonparametric test, factor analysis, and discriminant and stepwise analysis. SAS runs in many user environments, including PCSAS for personal computers. A special startup interface, ASSIST, facilitates beginners who are unfamiliar with the default batch data entry.

The U.S. Code of federal Regulations, 21CFR Part 11, requires all datasets to be provided in special format for review and inspection. SAS Institute published the SASXPORT format (Version 5) for electron data submission for regulatory purposes. Details about SAS EXPORT can be found at www.sas.com/fda-esub. *Guidance for industry: Providing regulatory submissions in electronic format-General considerations 1999.*

(e) RSTRIP

Micro Math Research

1710 South Brentwood Blvd.

Saint Louis, MO 63144

www.micromath.com

RSTRIP is menu-driven and very suitable for student use; it fits data to models, mono-, bi-, and tri-exponentials based on model selection criteria (Akaike Information Criteria). A good statistics menu is available for AUC, C_{max}, T_{max}, and mean residence time. The program gives initial parameter estimates and final parameters after iteration. However, the program does not handle differential equations or user-defined models. Plot outputs are available, as are pharmacokinetic curve stripping, and least-squares parameter optimization. The original software was written for PCDOS but has now been replaced by a Windows version with additional features.

(f) Scientist for Windows

Scientist for Windows V2.01 is a general mathematical modeling application from MicroMath, www.micromath.com. It can perform nonlinear least-squares minimization and simulation. Models can consist of both analytic and differential equations. The software has many functions with pharmacokinetic applications.

(g) PKAnalyst for Windows

MicroMath Scientific Software

PO Box 21550

Salt Lake City, UT 84121

PKAnalyst is a bundled pharmacokinetic software incorporating many features of RSTRIP but with more statistics and mathematical functions. The program operates under Windows and is generally easy to use. It is very user-friendly for routine data analysis in pharmacokinetics.

(h) DIFFEQ and DIFFEQ Pharmacokinetics Library

MicroMath Scientific Software

PO Box 2121550

Salt Lake City, UT 84121

DIFFEQ is a nonlinear least-squares program for PCs. Model entry uses a generic languages with syntax similar to Basic; it may be used with DIFFEQ Pharmacokinetic Library, which includes many models used in Pharmacokinetics. The original version was updated under a different name.

(i) P-STAT

P-Stat Inc.

Princeton, NJ 08540

(609) 924-9100

This program supplies statistical data handling for mainframe computers.

(j) STELLA

High Performance Systems

Lyme, NH 03755

(603) 643-9636

STELLA is a structural thinking experimental learning laboratory with animation, available for Windows-based PCs. The program was developed on the MAC. STELLA solves differential equations and simulates pharmacokinetic models and other physiologic systems. The software is particularly suitable for teaching because of its animation and learning simulation by drawing the model.

(k) NONMEN

NONMEN Project Group, C255

University of California

San Francisco, CA 94143

NONMEN (Nonlinear Mixed Effects Model), developed by S.L. Beal and L.B. Sheiner, is a statistical program used for fitting parameters in population pharmacokinetics. The NONMEN program first appeared in 1979. It is useful in evaluating relationship between pharmacokinetic parameters and demographic data such as age, weight, and disease state. Average population parameters and inter-subject variance are estimated. The program fits the data of all the subjects simultaneously and estimates the parameters and their variances. The parameters are useful in estimating doses for individuals based on population pharmacokinetics with calculated risks. A regression program is written in ANSI (American National Standards Institute) Fortran 77 for mainframe computers.

The current version of NONMEN (Version IV) consists of several parts. The NONMEN program itself is a general (noninteractive) regression program which can be used to fit many different types of data. PREDPP consists of subroutines that can be used to fit many different types of data. PREDPP consists of subroutines that can be used by NONMEN to compute predictions for population pharmacokinetics. NM-TRAN is a preprocessor, allowing control and other needed inputs and error messages to NONMEN/PREDPP.

(l) MKMODEL

Biosoft

PO Box 10398

Ferguson, MO

MKMODEL, by N. Holford, is a pharmacokinetic program from the National Institutes of Health-supported PROPHET system. The program, available for the PC, performs nonlinear least-squares regression and includes both pharmacokinetic and pharmacodynamic models (effect compartment).

(m) ADAPT II

D.Z. D'Argenio and A.Schumizky

Biomedical Simulation Resource

University of Southern California

Los Angeles, CA

Supplied as Fortran code for various operating systems, this program performs simulations, nonlinear regression, and optimal sampling, and includes extended least-squares and Bayesian optimization. Models can be expressed as integrated or differential equations (D'Argenio and Schumitzky, 1992).

(n) USC PACK PC PROGRAMS

USC Laboratory of Applied Pharmacokinetics

2250 Alcazar St, CSC 134B

Los Angeles, CA 90033

www.usc.edu/hsc/lab_apk

This software package consist of various Pharmacokinetic programs bundled for clinical Pharmacokinetic applications and model parameter estimation. The program NPEM2 (Version 3) is an improved version of the nonparametric expectation maximization algorithm that is well adapted for population Pharmacokinetics. The program is now available for a three-compartment model with various route of dosing. Lahey Fortran F77EM32 and its associated package is used in this program.

Clinical programs include related routines in which past therapy data for individual patients are entered into files along with parameter and dose-prediction programs for various drugs (*e.g,* aminoglycosides, other antibiotics, and drugs of special interest). Bayesian fitting procedures are included to fit a selected drug population model to a patient's data of doses and serum concentrations and to adaptive control of the individual dose regimen. Some program selections include:

- Amikacin (Amik)
- Gentamicin (Gent)
- Netilmicin (Net)
- Tobramycin (Tob)
- Bayesian General Modeling (MB)
- Least-Squares General Modeling (MLS)

Many patient-oriented programs for adaptive dosing based on pharmacokinetics and pharmacodynamic are featured in the package. Maximum Aposteriori Probability (MAP) Bayesian fitting is useful in individual dosing; an example is shown in Figure B-1 for gentamicin dose prediction. This method yields better prediction than conventional clinical methods even in patients with unstable renal function.

(o) S-Plus

S-plus is a versatile package that can be used for analyzing data using the included software, and also includes its own programming language, which can be used to write your own routines. S is a statistical package developed at AT & AS Bell Laborataries. S-Plus is an extension of this statistical language produced by the StatSci Division of MathSoft in Seattle. The software is used extensively by many pharmacokinetics and statisticians for model analysis.

(p) MathCAD

www.mathcad.com

MathCAD 11 has many general mathematical and statistical functions which can be easily adaptable for data analysis or fitting data to probability distribution models. Differential equation solvers support ordinary differential equations, systems of differential equations, and boundary-value problems both at the command line and in Solve blocks that use natural notation to specify the differential equations and constraints.

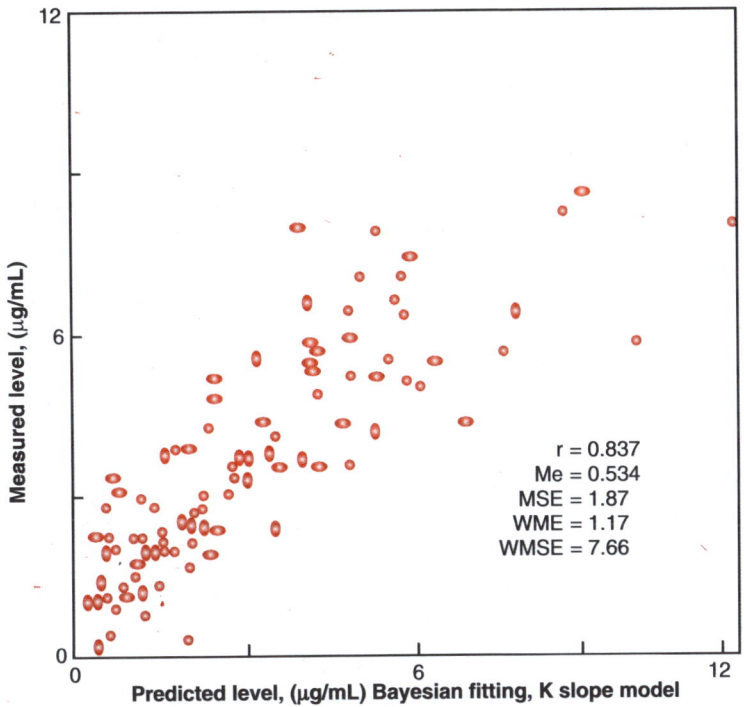

Fig. B-1. An example of gentamicin dosing prediction in patients using MAP Bayesian fitting and K slope method (one compartment): Predicted versus measured serum gentamicin. (r=correlation coefficient, ME = mean error, MSE = mean squared error, WME=mean weighted error. WMSE= weighed mean squared error). (From Jelliffe et al. 1995, with permission).

(q) Cyber Patient

Cyber Patient is a Windows-based multimedia pharmacokinetic simulation program that can be used for development and presentation of problem-solving case studies from Michael B. Bloger, USC School of Pharmacy. This program is suitable for simulations in pharmacy courses and research in development of pharmacokinetic drug models.

(r) GastroPLUS

GastroPlus is a computer simulation program that predicts the rate and extent of drug absorption from the gastrointestinal tract. This innovative program was developed by a team of scientist-programmers under the direction of Dr. Michael B. Bolger at Simulations Plus, Inc., in collaboration with Dr. Gordon L. Amidon.

(s) Instructional Programs

The **Modern Biopharmaceutics Version 6** Computer Based Training Software provides a complete information base for both university biopharmaceutics courses and continuing education courses. The program teaches both basic principles and important applications. Course material is available in modules on CD for individualized learning. For more information see www.tsrlic.com/mbindex.htm or www.simulations-plus.com.

4. OTHER PHARMACOKINETIC PROGRAMS

- **ACSL. BioMed:** Software based on the ACSL language that is used to simulate clinical trials of drugs. Pharsight Corporation, www.pharsight.com
- **BIOPAK:** A pharmacokinetic program for bioavailability/bioequivalence studies, available from SCI Software.
- **BOOMER/MULTI-FORTE:** A simulation program by D.W.A. Bourne, College of Pharmacy, University of Oklahoma.
- **PCDCON:** A convolution/deconvolution program by W.R. Gillespie (see Karol et al, 1991).
- **FUNFIT:** A parameter estimation regression program.
- **Kinetica 4.0:** A pharmacokinetic/pharmacodynamic analysis and simulation program that supports nonlinear mixed-effect model fitting. Available at www.innaphase.com.
- **LAGRAN:** A parameter estimation regression program.
- **MATLAB:** A powerful program that handles complex models, mostly in chemical engineering but found useful in pharmacokinetics.
- **NCOMP:** An Excel-based program for noncompartmental analysis of pharmacokinetic data, by Paul B. Laub. For integration of AUC and other uses, with choice of splines obtained from Lagrange polynomials or the hybrid method recommended by Purves (1996). J Pharm Sci 85:393-395, 1996.
- **NPEM:** A nonparametric expectation maximization program by A. Schumitzky (1991). It is part of the USC*PACK collection (see above).
- **Pharsight Trial Simulator**: A comprehensive computer-assisted trial simulation software system by Pharsight Corporation, www.pharsight.com/products/trial_simulator.
- **PDx-Pop:** Integrates with NONMEM and other software to expedite population modeling and analysis. UNIX version published by GloboMax LLC.
- **SAAM:** A program for pharmacokinetics and other biological models that was developed at the National Institute of Health (NIH).
- **SAAM/CONSAM:** Performs nonlinear regression in batch (SAAM) or conversational mode (CONSAM). The SAAM/CONSAM programs are provided by the NIH. Available from L.A. Zech and P.C. Grief, Laboratory of Mathematical Biology, NIH, **zech@ncifcrf.gov.**
- **P-PHARM:** A population pharmacokinetic-dynamic data modeling program from InnaPhase, science@innaphase.com.
- **PK-Sim:** A whole-body physiology-based pharmacokinetic (PBPK) simulation software by Bayer Technology Services GmbH, www.pk-sim.com.

- **PopKinetics:** A population pharmacokinetics analysis program. It is a companion application to SAAM II that uses parametric algorithms, Standard Two-Stage and Iterated Two-Stage, to compute population parameters. Available from the SAAM Institute, info@saam.com.
- **TOPFIT:** A PC-based pharmacokinetic program with both data fitting and clinical application, available from Gustav Fischer (VCH Publishers, Transwell and Koup, 1993).
- **WinNonMix:** A program for nonlinear mixed-effects modeling provided in an interactive and easy-to-use Windows application. By Pharsight Corporation, www.pharsight.com.
- **Win SAAM:** A Windows version of the original interactive biological modeling program. CONSAAM, developed in 1980 at the NH. WinSAAM Windows features and enhances application environment and is maintained by Peter C. Grief.

5. ELECTRONIC SPREADSHEETS

For general computation, many programs, such as electronic spreadsheets, are very adaptable to calculation and pharmacokinetic curve plotting. Spreadsheet software programs such as Quattro and Microsoft Excel are easy to use. Data are entered in columns (referred to alphabetically as A,B,C,....) and rows (referred to numerically as 1,2,3,....). Manuals are generally displayed on screen and can be selected by moving the arrow keys followed by pressing the return or Enter key. An example of a Microsoft Excel worksheet used to generate time-versus-concentration data after n doses of a drug given orally according to a one-compartment model is given in Figure B-2. The parameter inputs are in column B, time is in column D, and concentration is in column E.

EXAMPLE [1]

From a series of time-concentration data (Fig. B-3, rows A and B), determine the elimination rate constant using the regression feature of MS Excel.

Solution

(a) Type in the time and concentration data shown in columns A and B (Fig. B-3).

(b) Convert in column C all concentration data to ln concentration. Data point #1 may be omitted because ln of zero cannot be determined.

(c) From the main menu, select Insert:

Select function

SLOPE

Y data range (select last 4 value)

X data range (select last 4 value)

The slope, given in Fig. B-3 is -0.1. in this case, the ln concentration is plotted versus time, and the slope is simply the elimination rate constant.

| NOTE | To check this result, students may be interested in simulating the data with dose $= 10,000 \ \mu g/kg$, $V_D = 1000 \ mL/Kg$, $k_a = 0.8 \ hr^{-1}$, and $k = 0.1 \ hr^{-1}$. |

	A	B	C	D	E	F
1	D	100000		0	0.00	
2	KA	2		0.1	1.78	
3	K	0.4		0.2	3.16	
4	V	10000		0.3	4.23	
5	TAU	4		0.4	5.04	
6	F	1		0.5	5.64	
7	N	1		0.6	6.07	
8	EXP(-KA*TAU)	0.00033546		0.7	6.36	
9	EXP(-KT*AU)	0.20189652		0.8	6.55	
10	FKAD	200000		0.9	6.65	
11	V(K-KA)	-16000		1	6.69	
12	AA	1		1.1	6.67	
13	BB	1		1.2	6.60	
14				1.3	6.50	
15	FD/VK	25	AUC	1.4	6.38	
16				1.5	6.24	
17	FD/V...	8.86435343	C_{max}-ss	1.6	6.08	
18				1.7	5.92	
19				1.8	5.74	
20	TMAX	1.0058987	t_{max}-1	1.9	5.57	
21				2	5.39	
22				2.1	5.21	
23	TMAX-SS	0.86516026	t_{max}-ss	2.2	5.03	
24				2.3	4.86	
25				2.4	4.68	
26				2.5	4.51	
27				2.6	4.35	
28				2.7	4.19	
29				2.8	4.03	
30				2.9	3.88	
31				3	3.73	
32				3.1	3.59	
33				3.2	3.45	
34				3.3	3.32	
35				3.4	3.19	
36				3.5	3.07	
37				3.6	2.95	
38				3.7	2.84	
39				3.8	2.73	
40				3.9	2.62	
41				4	2.52	C_{min}
42			t_{min}			
43						
44						
45						
46						
47	Parameter	Param. val	Pharm-Term	Time (hrs)	Conc (mcg/ml)	

Fig. B-2. Example of a Microsoft Excel spreadsheet used to calculate time-concentration data according to an oral one-compartment model after *n* doses.

S. No.	A	B	C	
1	Time	Conc	Ln	
2	(hr)		(conc)	
3	0	0.00		
4	2	7049.53	8.86	
5	4	7194.95	8.88	
6	6	6178.08	8.73	
7	8	5116.20	8.54	
8	10	4200.50	8.34	
9	12	3441.45	8.14	Slope -0.1
10	14	2818.09	7.94	
11	16	2307.36	7.74	

Fig. B-3. A sample spreadsheet showing a set of time-concentration data (Time and Conc) being analyzed to obtain the slope or the elimination constant. Note: Only four points from the terminal part of the curve were regressed [t versus ln (conc)].

Example [2]

Generate some data for a two-compartment model using two differential equations. Initial conditions are dose = 1, $V = 1$, and $k_{12} = 0$, $k_{21} = 1$, and $k = 3$.

Solution

The data may be generated with MathCAD (Fig. B-4). Note that k_{12} is abbreviated as k_1, k_{21} is abbreviated as k_2, and k is abbreviated at k_3 in the program for simplicity. Also, $dC_p/dt = F(t, x, y)$; $x = C_p$; $y = C_i$; t = time; and $dCt/dt = G(t, x, y)$.

Model Fitting

An example of a set of oral plasma data was fitted to a one-compartment model by RSTRIP (Fig B-5). The software makes an initial estimate as well as a final parameter after several iterations. An example of some oral plasma data was generated with PCNonlin (Figs. B-6A, B, C).

SOLVING A SYSTEM OF DIFFERENTIAL EQUATIONS $k_1 = 0.2$ $k_2 = 1$ $k_3 = 3$

x and y are functions of the time variable t, and F and G are the

$$F (t,x,y) = k_2.Y-[k_3 + k_1].x$$

derivatives dx/dt and dy/dt.

$$G(t,x,y) = k_1.x-k_2.y$$

Start $t = 0$ end $t + 4$ $n = 100$ intervals   init $x = 1$ init $y = 0$

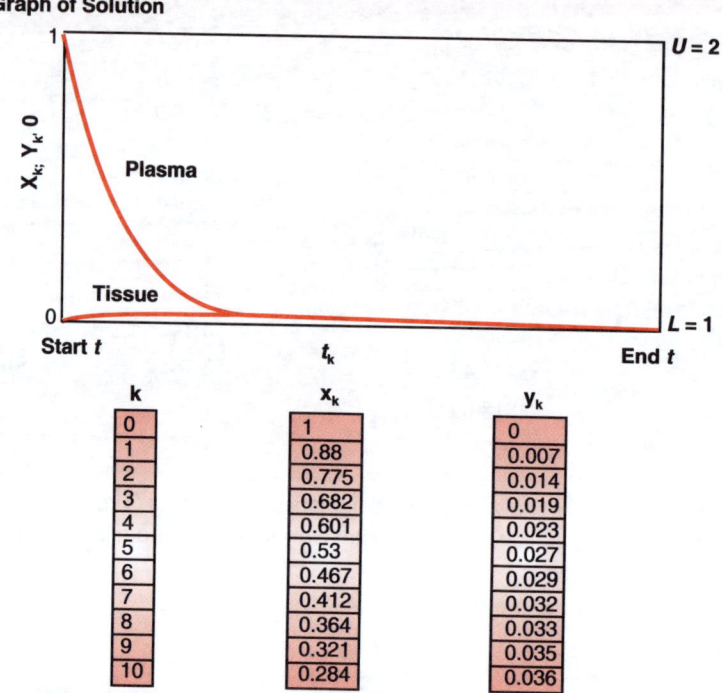

Graph of Solution

k	x_k	y_k
0	1	0
1	0.88	0.007
2	0.775	0.014
3	0.682	0.019
4	0.601	0.023
5	0.53	0.027
6	0.467	0.029
7	0.412	0.032
8	0.364	0.033
9	0.321	0.035
10	0.284	0.036

Fig. 5.1. A sample of the MathCAD application program used to solve the two-differential equation for a two-compartment model after IV bolus dose. (The first 10 data points are shown).

Summary of Least squares for dataset oral absorption

Computation time : 1.04 secs	$A[1] = 12.801$	$k[1] = 0.40724$
calculated lag time : 0.00000	$k[2] = -12.800$	$k[2] = 1.9428$

Sum of squared residuals : 0.0048572

Model Selection Criterion : 8.1157

Weighting Factor: 0.00000

time	y-obs	y-calc	resid	wt*res-sq
0.00000	0.00000	0.00051906	-0.00051906	2.694E-007
0.40000	5.0000	4.9919	0.0080675	6.509E-005
0.80000	6.5000	6.5363	-0.036276	0.0013160
1.2000	6.6600	6.6087	0.051306	0.0026323
2.0000	5.3900	5.4062	-0.016228	0.00026334
2.4000	4.6800	4.6961	-0.016060	0.00025791
2.8000	4.0300	4.0373	-0.0072648	5.278E-005
3.2000	3.4500	3.4520	-0.0020411	4.166E-006
3.6000	2.9500	2.9431	0.0069157	4.783E-005
4.0000	2.5200	2.5053	0.014746	0.00021745

Press any key to continue

Fig. B-5: Sample output from RSTRIP pharmacokinetic software showing a good fit of the theoretical data to actual data (column 2 and 3). The parameters estimated are given in top right-hand corner.

Example: 3

After a drug is administered orally, a series of plasma drug concentration-time data may be fitted to a one-compartment model, to estimate the absorption rate constant, elimination rate constant, and volume of distribution. Other pharmacokinetic parameters of interest may also be calculated using the NONLIN program, as shown in Figure B-6. Three parameters were estimated- V, k_{01}, and k_{10}-representing volume of distribution, k_a, and k (see model). Initial estimates were derived from either curve stripping or feathering. Dose is CON (1). In this case, NOBS = 9, showing that there are 9 data points. There is only function that describes the model FUNC 1. S(1) represents the calculation of AUC, S(2) the calculation of absorption, and S(3) the calculation of elimination half-life.

LISTING OF INPUT COMANDS

```
MODEL 3, 'ONE'
MODEL 3
REMARK ONE COMPARTMENT MODEL- FIRST ORDER INPUT AND OUTPUT
REMA
REMA      NO.    PARAMETER    CONSTANT      SECONDARY PARM.
REMA
REMA      ────    ──────────    ────────      ──────────────
REMA      1      VOLUME        DOSE          AUC
REMA      2      K01                         K01 HALF LIFE
REMA      3      K10                         K10 HALF LIFE
REMA      4                                  TMAX
REMA      5                                  CMAX
REMA*******************************************************
REMA              I──────────────────────────I
REMA              I                           I
REMA      K01     I       compartment         I---------K10
REMA              I──────────────────────────I
REMA*******************************************************
COMM
NPARM 3
NCON 1
MSEC 5
PNAMES 'VOLUME', 'K01', 'K10'
SNAMES 'AUC', 'K01-HL, K10-HL', 'TMAX', 'CMAX'
END
TEMP
D = CON (1)
V = P(1)
K01 = P(2)
K10 = P(3)
```

```
T = X
END
FUNC1
COEF=D*K01/(V*(K01-K10))
F=COEF*(DEXP (-K10*T)-DEXP (-K01*T))
END
SECO
S(1) = D/V/K01
S(2) = DLOG (.5)/K01
S(3) = DLOG (.5)/K10
TMAX = (DLOG (K01/K10)/(K01-K10))
S(4) = TMAX
S(5) = (D/V)* DEXP (-K10* TMAX)
END
EOM
CONS 250
INIT 100.7, 1.03, .13
NOBS 9
DATA
BEGIN
```

PCNONLIN NONLINEAR ESTIMATION PROGRAM

ITERATION	WEIGHTED		SS	VOLUME		K01		K10
0	1.34180			100.7		1.030		.1300
		TAU =		.1583E–04		RANK = 3	COND =	1049.
1	.136818			100.7		.5689		.1706
		TAU =		.1108E–04		RANK = 3	COND =	1701.
2	.358976E–01			100.7		.4396		.1788
		TAU =		.1008E–04		RANK = 3	COND =	2489.
3	.357194E–01			100.7		.4439		.1795
		TAU =		.1005E–04		RANK = 3	COND =	2451.
4	.357049E–01			100.7		.4442	.	.1791
		TAU =		.1008E–04		RANK = 3	COND =	2447.
5	.356635E–01			99.63		.4392		.1816
		TAU =		.9998E–05		RANK = 3	COND =	2473.
6	.356553E–01			99.63		.4383		.1815
		TAU =		.1000E–04		RANK = 3	COND =	2481.
CONVERGENCE ACHIEVED								
RELATIVE CHANGE IN WEIGHTED SUM OF SQUARES LESS THAN								.000100
6	.356533E–01			99.57	.	4377		.1817

Fig B-6A. Sample output from PCNONLIN showing data fitted to Model 3, a one-compartment model with First-Order Absorption and First-Order Elimination.

PARAMETER	ESTIMATE	STANDARD ERROR	95% CONFIDENCE LIMITS	
VOLUME	99.568030	19.182331	52.630524	146.505537 UNIVARIATE
			24.795837	174.340224 PLANAR
K01	.437738	.117793	.149508	.725969 UNIVARIATE
			.021417	.896894 PLANAR
K10	.181749	.043746	.074706	.288792 UNIVARIATE
			.011228	.352271 PLANAR

SUMMARY OF NONLINEAR ESTIMATION

FUNCTION 1

X	OBSERVED Y	CALCULATED Y	RESIDUAL	WEIGHT	SD-YHAT	STANDARDIZED RESIDUAL
1.000	.7000	.8085	-.1085	1.000	4987E-01	-1.847
2.000	1.200	1.196	.3927E-02	1.000	.4740E-01	.6460E-01
3.000	1.400	1.334	.6581E-01	1.000	.4034E-01	1.002
4.000	1.400	1.330	.7008E-01	1.000	.4253E-01	1.090
6.000	1.100	1.132	-.3226E-01	1.000	.4620E-01	-5.228
8.000	.8000	.8737	-.7371E-01	1.000	.4000E-01	-1.119
10.00	.6000	.6435	-.4349E-01	1.000	.3919E-01	-.6552
12.00	.5000	.4624	.3760E-01	1.000	.4469E-01	.5986
16.00	.3000	.2305	.6954E-01	1.000	.4888E-01	1.167

CORRECTED SUM OF SQUARED OBSERVATIONS = 1.28889
  WEIGHTED CORRECTED SUM OF SQUARED OBSERVATIONS = 1.28889
  SUM OF SQUARED RESIDUALS = .356533E-01
  SUM OF WEIGHTESD SQUARED RESIDUALS = .356533E–01
  S = .770857E-01 WITH   6 DEGREES OF FREEDOM

SUMMARY OF ESTIMATED SECONDARY PARAMETERS

PARAMETER	ESTIMATE	STANDARD ERROR
AUC	13.814898	.847009
K01-HL	1.583474	.425680
K10-HL	3.813757	.917038
TMAX	3.433715	.217994
CMAX	1.345203	.040455

Fig B-6B Sample output from PCNONLIN.

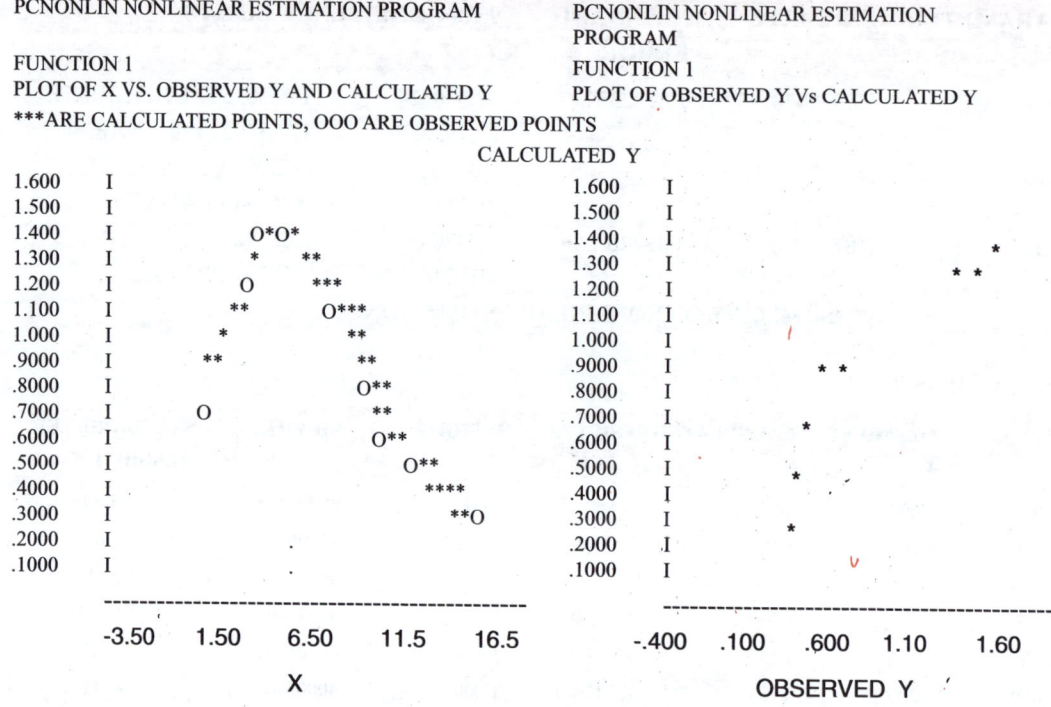

PCNONLIN NONLINEAR ESTIMATION PROGRAM

FUNCTION 1
PLOT OF X VS. OBSERVED Y AND CALCULATED Y
***ARE CALCULATED POINTS, OOO ARE OBSERVED POINTS

PCNONLIN NONLINEAR ESTIMATION PROGRAM

FUNCTION 1
PLOT OF OBSERVED Y Vs CALCULATED Y

Fig. B-6C. Sample Output From PCNONLIN.

REFRENCES

Charles BG, Duffull SB: **Pharmacokinetic Software for the Health Sciences: Choosing the Right Package for Teaching Purposes**. *Clin Pharmacokinet* 40(6): 395-403, 2001

D'Argenio DZ, Schumitzky A: *ADAPT II User's Guide, Los Angeles,* Biomedical Simulation Resorce, University of Southern California, 1992

Heatherington AC, Vicini P, Golde H: **A Pharmacokinetic/Pharmacodynamic Comparison of SAAM II and PC/WIN Nonlin Modelling Software.** *J Pharm Sci* **87**: 1255-1263, 1998

Jelliffe RW, Schumitzky A, Van Guilder M, Jiang F: User Manual for Version 10.7 *USC*PACK Collection of PC Programs*. **USC Laboratory of Applied Pharmacokinetics**, University of Southern California, 1995

Karol M, Gillespie WR, Veng-Pederson P: *AAPS Short Course: Convolution Deconvolution and Linear Systems,* Washington, DC, AAPS (1991)

Schumitzky A: **Nonparametric EM Algorithms for Estimating Prior Distributions.** Appl Math Comput **45**: 143-157, 19911

Tanswell P, Koup J: *Int J Clin Pharmacol Ther Toxicol* **31**(10): 514-420, 1993

BIBILOGRAPHY

Boune DWA: **Mathematical Modeling of Pharmaceutical Data.** In Swarbrick J, Boylan JC (Eds), *Encyclopedia of Pharmaceutical Technology*, Vol 9. Marcel Dekker, New York, 1994

Gabrielsson J, Wiener D: ***Pharmacokinetics and Pharmacodynamic Data Analysis:* Concepts and Applications,** 2nd ed. Swedish Pharmaceutical Press, 1998

Gex-Fabry M, Balant LP: **Consideration on Data Analysis Using Computer Methods and Currently Available Software for Personal Computers.** In Welling PG, Balant LP (Eds), *Handbook of Experimental Pharmacology,* Vol. 110, Pharmacokinetics of Drugs, Springer-Verlag Berlin, 1994.

Maronda R (Ed): **Clinical Applications of Pharmacokinetics and Control Theory: Planning, Monitoring, and Adjusting Dosage Regiments of Aminoglycosides, Lidocaine, Digoxitin, and Digoxin.** In Jelliffe RW (ed), Selected Topics in clinical Pharmacology. Springer-Verlag, New York, 1986.

The NONMEN Project Group: *NONMEN User Manuals I-VI.* University of California San Fransico, www.micromath.com/http://www.micromath.com,1995

Appendix

6

STATISTICS

[A] PROBABILITY

Probability is widely applied to measure risk associated with disease and drug therapy. *Risk factor* is a condition or behavior that increases the chance of developing disease in a healthy subject over a period of time. An example could be the risk of developing lung cancer over time with tobacco smoking. Another example of risk factor is the possibility of developing hearing loss after receiving an aminoglycoside antibiotic for a period of time.

The term *relative risk* (RR) or risk ratio is the most frequently used probability term to measure association of risk with exposure (to a drug or a behavior). Risk factors may be genetic, environmental, or behavioral. They have important implications in both pharmacokinetics and drug therapy (see Chapter 12). Risk factors may be casual or merely a marker that increases the probability of a disease.

$$RR = \frac{risk_{(exposed)}}{risk_{(unexposed)}}$$

$$RR = relative\ risk = \frac{disease\ probability\ of\ exposed}{disease\ probability\ of\ unexposed}$$

Often risk information is collected in a controlled manner over a period of time by survey, either from the past or forward in time. In a *prospective cohort study* (also known as a cohort *study, prospective, follow-up,* or *longitudinal study*), a cohort of healthy subjects exposed to different levels of a suspected risk is followed forward in time to determine the incidence of risk in each group. For example, in a hypothetical study, the risk of thrombophlebitis was studied in a group of randomly selected women: 500 women taking and 500 matched women not taking a birth control pill for 10 years. The RR of 10 for thrombophlebitis was calculated from a risk of thrombophlebitis in women exposed to the birth control pill versus women not exposed to the drug using a dichotomous 2×2 table as shown in Table A.1, where A and b are the number of subjects who developed thrombophlebitis. The probability of exposed in this case is $A/(A + B)$ and that of not exposed is $C/(C + D)$. In this case, assume the exposed risk is 0.025 and the not exposed risk is 0.0025. Then $RR = 0.025/0.0025 = 10$. Thus, the relative risk of thrombophlebitis in women on the birth control pill for 10 years is 10 for this group of women studied.

A second method of studying risk is the historical or retrospective cohort study, which looks backward in time to determine the present risk. The cohort of exposed and unexposed subjects is retrieved from past records to determine risk outcome. In the next section relative risks are described in terms of odds, a similar concept that is also widely applied.

TABLE A.1 Tabulation from a Hypothetical Cohort Study of Female Subjects on the Pill with and without Developing Thrombophlebitis for 10 Years.

	POSITIVE OUTCOME (+THROMBOPHLEBITIS)	NEGATIVE OUTCOME (-THROMBOPHLEBITIS)	SUBTOTAL
Risk factor present (*e.g.* Taking the pill-exposed)	A	B	A + B
Risk factor absent (*e.g.* Not taking the pill-not exposed)	C	D	C + D
Subtotal	A + C	B + D	

[B] ODDS

The probability of drawing an ace from a deck of cards is 4/52, or 1/13 for a deck of cards containing 4 aces in 52 cards. The odds of drawing an ace is the number of times an ace will be drawn divided by the number of times it will not be drawn. The odds are:

$$\textbf{ODDS} = \frac{4/52}{48/52} = \frac{4}{48} = \frac{1}{12}$$

This can be read as a 1:12 odds of drawing an ace. The absence of four aces in the denominator makes the difference in the odds outcome. Odds are numerically not equal to probability as defined.

The point may be illustrated by considering the opening of a standard deck of cards, one card at a time. For example, we may encounter 4 aces after 40 cards are opened, before the entire deck is open. We can see that the number of cards opened (we stopped at 40 cards) becomes a factor in the odds obtained. In this case, after opening the first 40 cards, 4 cards were aces and 36 cards were not aces. The odds are 4/36 = 1/9 instead of 1/12 as calculated for 52 cards. Using this analogy, it is inappropriate to pick sample sizes that do not reflect the natural risk course of the disease or drug treatment involved. If we decide to sample only 40 cards, stop sampling, and then calculate the odds (or RR in observing a disease), the results will be in error. In statistics, the sample size and how samples represent the population at large are important considerations for accurate determination of the RR of a disease or drug treatment.

A common approach to studying risk outcome is the *case-control study* (also known as the *retrospective study*). In the case-control study, the exposure histories of two groups of subjects are selected on the basis of whether or not they develop a particular disease (*e.g.* Thrombophlebitis), in order to evaluate disease frequently resulting from drug (*e.g,* the pill) exposure. The investigator selects the size of the subject population that has the disease or is disease free to determine exposure to the risk factor. The number of subjects who do and do not have the disease may not necessarily reflect the natural frequency of the disease. It is therefore improper to compute a "relative risk (RR)" from the odds ratio (OR) for a case-control study, because the investigator can manipulate the size of the relative risk.

$$OR = \frac{\text{odds of case exposure}}{\text{odds of case unexposed}}$$

If the disease is rate, then ORH≈RR. When the sample size is large, the differences between OR and RR diminishes.

In statistical analysis, it is important to guard against selection error or bias. Investigators may look harder for cancer, for example, in smokers than in a control group of healthy subjects. The resultant disparity is often called *surveillance bias*. In a case-control group there may also be *recall bias*; for example, medical history taken on surgical lung cancer (case) may be more likely to contain information on smoking than other type of surgical controls (Knapp and Miller, 1992).

[C] EXPERIMENTAL DESIGN AND COLLECTION OF DATA

Statistics have important applications in scientific studies, whether in studies involving hypothesis testing or finding ways to improve a product. Statistical design is widely used at the experimental planning stage. Later, when data are collected, statistical methods are applied for data analysis and to help draw conclusions from the studies.

Experimental design may be simple or may involve an elaborate model. The method may be applied to optimize a drug product based on a set of criteria (Deming and Morgan, 1987). Experimental design may be used to optimize an analytical method to separate drug from impurities, such as HPLC method. In pharmacokinetics, experimental design is used to design better sampling time for drawing blood samples for drug analysis in pharmacokinetic parameter estimation. A common approach to optimizing a drug product is the *factorial design*. For example, we may be interested in determining whether 0, 0.25, 0.5, 0.75 or 1% of magnesium stearate should be formulated into a tablet granulation to allow adequate flow of the tablet granulation mixture during manufacturing. This problem may be viewed as a simple one-factorial-design experiment to determine the amount of lubricant needed to provide best powder flow (1 factor 5 lubricant levels). The object of the experimental design is to try to pick the tablet lubricant level that will result in the optimal powder flow from the hopper to the die cavity during tablet compression.

In practice, tablet granulation flow is more complex. Moisture level, particle size, and tackiness (of the drug substance) are other factors that influence flow. We may decide to reduce the increment level and select the lubricant levels to 0, 0.5, and 1% only. This provides three lubricant levels-high, medium, and low-for each factor. We then can apply a factorial design of 4 factors at 3 levels, which involves $4^3 = 64$ trials in the above case to generate a geometric response space that represents all the factors involved. The full factorial design is tedious, so a reduced design, the fractional factorial design, is often used. How to reach the optimal point efficiently when several factors are involved is a problem for many optimization experiments.

The identical concept for optimizing flow can be applied to optimizing the media composition supporting antibiotic production by fermentation using Streptomyces or a new microbe engineered by recombinant DNA. The factorial design may be employed to find the optimum composition for the growth medium. Factorial design yields knowledge about the system but is tedious. An alternative approach to carry out the optimization is the sequential simplex method, which optimizes the factors through sequentially planned experiments. This method is often applied in parameter estimation from data using computerized iteration algorithms. In designing experiments, it is important to know the factors involved and the range of each factor. How much change in drug concentration can the analytical method detect? Good design requires some knowledge of the system and a strategy to obtain data for analysis that saves time and resources.

The same principle applies to human clinical studies. In clinical trials, studies are often done with a limited number of subjects, due to either cost or the availability of subjects who meet the study requirements. Based on good clinical practices, the study subjects are selected according to exclusion and inclusion criteria that are written into the protocol. All subjects must give informed consent to be in the study. Since most studies are done over a period of time, it is important to ensure that both the treatment and control groups are balanced and to avoid any temporal influence. For example, in bioequivalency trials, adequate time (wash-out time) between study dosing periods is allowed for the drug to be eliminated from the subject and to avoid residual effects due to carryover of the drug from the first dosing period to the next dosing period.

All scientific studies must be designed properly to obtain valid conclusions that may be applied to the population intended. The experimental design of a study includes the following:

1. **A clearly stated hypothesis for the study**
2. **Assurance that the samples have been randomly selected**
3. **Control of all experimental variables**
4. **Collection of adequate data to allow experimental testing of the hypothesis**

Example: We may wish to test the hypothesis that the average weight of young males is greater than the average weight of females in the United States. First, we may decide that young male and female subjects aged 18 to 24 will be selected and other ages excluded. The subjects are randomly selected from a pool opf subjects who are not interrelated in a way that might affect their body weights. We may want to exclude subjects with certain diseases (exclusion criteria). A sufficient number of subjects must be selected (sampled) randomly so that the total number of subjects (sample size) represents the general population in the United States. The need for randomization is easily understood but often poorly met because of the difficulties in recruiting subjects, or in the methods used for recruiting. For example, if all the subjects in this example are randomly recruited from one health club in a given city, the samples will not be typical of the population intended even though the subjects are randomly selected. Are we too ambitious to include the population of the entire United States? Second, many of the subjects exercise at the health club to lose weight, and this may not be representative of the general population. A true sample is one selected randomly from the population of the entire country without connection by any variable that affects their weights.

The identification of all covariates in a study is generally difficult and requires through consideration. The subject of sample size, inclusion criteria, and exclusion criteria are major considerations in experimental design that will affect the statistical outcome. After careful consideration, we may realize that there are many variables to be considered and may wish to modify the scope to tailor the study objectives more efficiently.

Age, gender, genetic background, and health of the subjects are important variables in clinical drug testing. The statistical design of a study is based on the study objectives. Each study should have clearly stated objectives and an appropriate study design indicating how the study is to be performed. Often, the population may be subdivided according to the objectives of the study. For example, a new drug for the treatment of Alzheimer's disease in the elderly may initially be tested in male subjects aged 55 and above. Later, clinical studies might test the drug in other patient populations. May different statistical designs are possible. Some of these designs control experimental variables better than others. Specific statistical designs are given in other chapters are in standard statistical texts.

The quality of the data is very important and may be controlled by the researcher and the method of measurement. For example, if the weights of the young males and females in the example above are obtained using different scales, the investigator must ascertain that each scale weighs the subject accurately. Accuracy refers to the closeness of the observation (*i.e.*, observed weight) to the actual or true value. Reproducibility or precision refers to the closeness of repeated measurements.

[D] ANALYSIS AND INTERPRETATION OF DATA

The objective of data analysis is to obtain as much information about the population as possible based on the sample data collected. A common method for analyzing data of a sample population is to classify the data and then plot the frequency of occurrence of all samples. For example, the frequency of weight distribution of a class of students may be plotted in the form of a histogram that relates frequency to weight (Fig A-1).

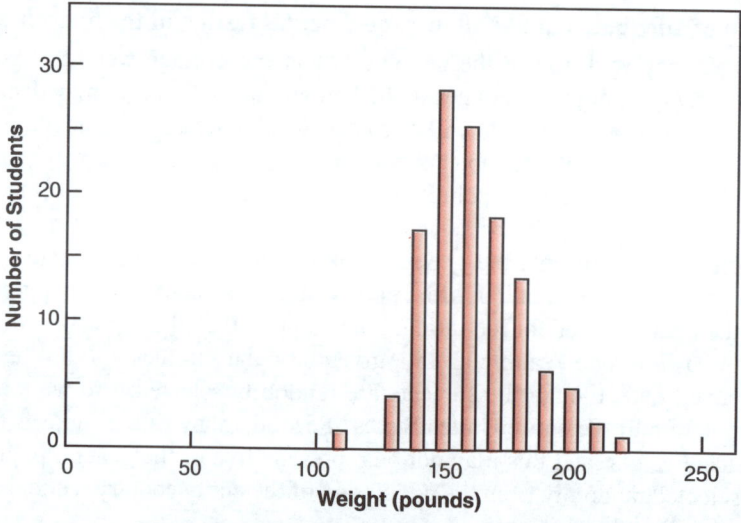

Fig. A-1. Weight distribution of 120 students.

An important observation in this example is that the weight of most students lies in the middle of the weight distribution. There is a common tendency for most sample values to occur around the mean. This is described in the central limit theorem, which states that the frequency of the values of measurements drawn randomly from a population tends to approximate a bell-shaped curve or normal distribution. Extensive data collection is needed to determine the distributional nature of a sample population. Once the parameters of a distribution are determined, the probability of a given sample's occurrence in the population may be calculated.

[E] DESCRIPTIVE TERMS

Descriptive terms are used in statistics to generalize the nature of the data and provide a measure of central tendency. The mean or average is the sum of the observations divided by the numbers, n, of observations (Table A.2). The median is the middle value of the observation between the highest and lowest value. The mode is the most frequently occurring value. The term range is used to describe the dispersion of the observations and is the difference between the highest and lowest values. For data that are distributed as a normal distribution (discussed below), the mean, median, and mode have the same value.

[F] THE NORMAL DISTRIBUTION

If data are plotted according to the frequency of occurrence, a pattern for the distribution of the data is observed. Most data approximate a normal or *Gaussian distribution*. The *normal distribution* is a bell-shaped curve that is symmetric on both sides of the mean. Statistical tests that assumes the data follow normal distribution patterns are known as *parametric tests. Nonparametric tests* do not make any assumption about the central tendency of the data and may be used to analyze data without assuming normal distribution. Nonparametric tests require no assumption of normality and are less powerful. Examples are the Wilcoxan test and the side test.

Table A.2 Descriptive Statistics for a Set of Data[a]

DATA		DESCRIPTIVE TERMS
21	63	Sum = 1274
25	67	Mean = 57.9
29	67	Mode = 67
35	67	Median = 62
37	67	$n = 22$
42	67	Range = 21-91
45	72	SD = 20.3
49	73	RSD = 35.1%
56	75	
57	88	
61	91	

[a]The data represent a set of measurements (observations) in study. The descriptive terms are often used to describe the data. Each term is defined in the text.

SD, standard deviation; RSD, relative standard deviation.

The shape of the normal distribution is determined by only two parameters, the population mean and the variance, both of which may be estimated from the samples. The variance is a measure of the spread or variability of the sample. Many biological and physical random variables are described by the normal distribution (or may be transformed to a normal distribution). These may include the weight and height of humans and animal species, the elimination half-lives of many drugs in a population of patients, the duration of a telephone call, and other variables. In statistics, the item investigated is termed the random variable. For convenience, the standardized normal distribution is introduced to allow easy probability calculation when the standard deviation is known (Fig. A-2). The probability of a sample value occurring from 1 standard deviation (SD) above to 1 SD below the mean is 68% (z of –1 to +1). This value is calculated by finding the probability corresponding to z = –1 and z = 1 from curve B in figure A-2 as follows:

- Probability between z of –4 to –1 is 0.16.
- Probability between z of –4 to +1 is 0.84.
- Therefore, the probability between z of – 1 to + 1 is 0.84 – 0.16 = 0.68 or 68%.

The area representing probability between any two points on the normal distribution is calculated from this graph. In practice, a cumulative standardized normal distribution table is used top allow better accuracy.

Standard deviation measures the variability of a group of data. SD for n number of measurement is calculated according to the following equation:

$$SD = \sqrt{\frac{\sum_{i}^{n}(x_i - x)^2}{n-1}}$$

Where x is the mean, x_i is the observed value, and n is the number of observations (data). The standard deviation is often calculated by computer or calculator and gives an indication of the spread of data (Fig A-2). A larger standard deviation indicates that the spread of data about the mean is larger compared to data with the same mean but with a smaller standard deviation.

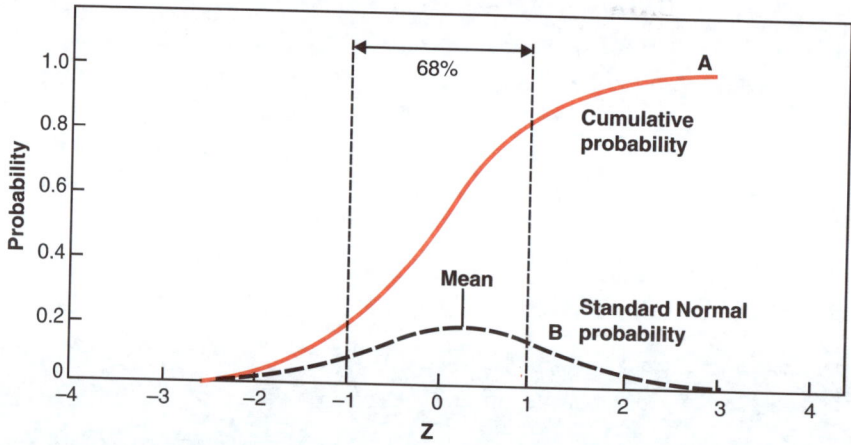

Fig. A-2. Probability of a normal distribution. (A = cumulative probability, B = standard normal probability).

Relative standard deviation or coefficient of variation allows comparison of the variance of measurements. The standard deviation is divided by the mean to give the relative standard deviation (RSD) or coefficient of variation (CV).

$$SD = \frac{SD}{\bar{x}}$$

The RSD may be expressed as a percent or %CV by multiplying the RSD by 100. This is commonly known as percent standard deviation or *percent standard deviation or percent variation.*

The difference between the mean, $\bar{x}$, and each observed datum, x_i, is the deviation from the mean. Because the deviation from the mean can be either negative or positive, the deviations are squared and summed to give an estimation of the total spread, or deviation of the data from the mean. The term is the sum of squares. This term $\Sigma_i^n (x_i - \bar{x})^2$ incorporates measurement error as well as inherent variance of the samples. If a single sample is measured several times, the sum of the squares should be very small if the method of measurement is reproducible. The concept of least squares for miunimizing error due to model fitting is fundamental in many statistical methods.

[G] CONFIDENCE LIMIT

If normal distribution of the data is assumed, the probability of a random variable in the population can be calculated. For example, data that falls within 1 SD above and below the mean ($\bar{x} \pm 1$ SD) represents approximately 68% of the data, whereas data that falls within 2 SD above and below the mean ($\bar{x} \pm 2$ SD1) represents approximately 95% of the data. In the examples below, the random variable in which we are interested is the diameters of drug particles of drug measured from a powdered drug sample lot.

Examples

The particle size of a powdered drug sample was measured. The average (mean) particle size was 130 μm with a standard deviation of 20 μm.

Q1. Determine the range of particle sizes that represents the middle 68% of the powdered drug.

Solution

From a normal distribution table or Figure A-2, 68% of the middle particles represent 34% above and below the mean, corresponding to the mean ±1 SD.

Small particle size = mean − SD = 130 − 20 = 110 μm

Large particle size = mean + SD + 130 + 20 = 150 μm

Therefore, 68% of the particles will have a particle size ranging from 110 to 150 μm.

Q2. **Determine the range of particle sizes that represents the middle 95% of the powdered drug.**

Solution

95% or 47.5% on each side of the mean, corresponding to ±2 SD (Fig. A-2)

Smallest particle size = 130 − (2 × 20) = 90 μm

Largest particle size = 130 + (2 × 20) = 170 μm

Therefore, 95% of the particles will have a particle size ranging from 90 to 170 μm.

Explanation

- In the above example, the calculation shows that most of the particles lie around the mean. To be 95% certain, simply extend from the mean ±2 SD. This approach estimates the 95% confidence limit. A 95% confidence limit implies that if an experiment is performed 100 times, 95% of the data will be in this range above and below the mean.

❑ This example shows how to reconstruct a population based on the two parameters, mean and variance (approximated by the SD). A more common application is the estimation of experimental data such as assay measurements. Such 95% confidence limits are often calculated from the standard deviation to estimate the reliability of the assay measurement.

❑ In the example above, the mean for the particle size was 130 μm and the SD was 20 mm. Therefore, from equation A.2, the RSD = 20/130 or 0.15. the RSD may be expressed as a percent or % CV by multiplying the RSD by 100.

Accuracy: As mentioned, accuracy refers-to 'the agreement with the observed value or measurement in a group of data and the actual or true value of the population'. Unfortunately, the true value is unknown in many studies. The term precision refers to the reproducibility of the data or the variation within a set of measurements. Data that are less precise will demonstrate a larger variance or a larger relative standard deviation, whereas more precise data will have a similar variance.

Example

Q.1. A lot of 10-mg tablets was assayed five times by three students (Fig. A-3). Which student assayed the tablets most accurately?

Solution

The mean and SD of assays by each student were determined. Because the same lot was assayed, the difference in SD among the students is attributed to assay variations. Student A is closest to the target-that is, the labeled claimed dose (LCD) of 10 mg. Student C is most precise (with the smallest %SD), but is consistently off target.

The data obtained by Student C is considered biased because all the observed data are above 10 mg. data are also considered biased if all the observed data are below the true value of 10 mg.

[H] BIAS

Bias refers to-'**a systematic error when the measurement is consistently not on target**'. Repeated measurements may be very reproducible (precise) but miss the target. In the example above, Student C was most precise, but Student A was most accurate. **In determining accuracy and precision, a standard (known sample) is usually prepared and assayed several times to determine the variation due to assay errors**. In the example above, we assumed that the students used known 10-mg standard tablets. If the tablets were unknown samples, it would not be possible to conclude which students was more accurate, because the true value would be unknown. In practice, assay methods are validated for precision and accuracy based on known standards before unknown samples (*e.g.* Plasma Samples) are assayed.

In the analysis and interpretation of data, statistics makes inferences about a population using experimental data gathered in a sample. After analysis of data, the statistician calculates the likelihood or probability that a given result would happen. Probability (P) is the fraction of the population indicating that a given result or event would occur by random sampling or chance. For example, if P<0.05%, then the likelihood that a result occurs by random sampling is 5/100, 1/20, or 5%. By convention, if the statistical inference produces a P value of 0.05 or less, it is considered atypical or uncommon of the population. As shown in Figure A-1, the probability of finding a student weighing above 250 Ib is small (P<0.05), and we may conclude (somewhat erroneously) that a student who weighs 250 Ib is significantly different from the rest. This concept for determining the probability of how typical a given sample value occurs in a population may be extended to hypothesis testing. Hypothesis testing estimates the probability of whether a given value is typical of the control group or of the treated group.

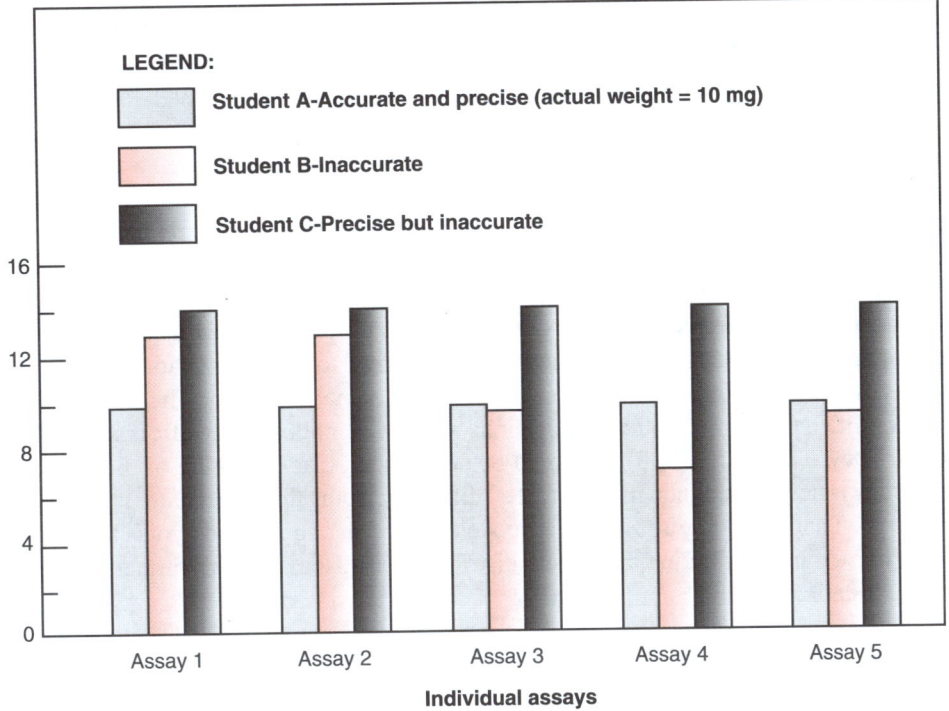

Fig. A-3. Comparison of assays (5 each) of 10-mg tablet by three students.

[I] STATISTICAL DISTRIBUTIONS AND APPLICATION

The frequency distribution of some data does not appear to be symmetrically shaped. The term skewness relates to the asymmetry of the data. The data distribution may be skewed to the left or right of the mean. In many pharmacologic studies, the sample size in the study is small, and the investigator cannot always be certain that the data obtained from the study are normally distributed. An incorrect assumption of a normal distribution may lead to a biased conclusion. In such cases, a nonparametric test may be used, because it does not make any assumption about the underlying test except that it may be continuous.

During data analysis, a value or observation may be observed that is several standard deviation above or below the mean; such a value is called an *outlier.* A value that is an outlier is difficult to use statistically. An observed value that deviates far from the majority of the data may indicate non-normal distribution, an error in measurement, or an error in data entry. If an error is found during checking, it should be corrected. In general, outlier values should not be excluded from the statistical analysis. Some investigators use log transformation of the data to make the distribution of the data appear to be more normally distributed. A geometric mean is obtained after log transformation of the data to make the distribution of the data appear to be more normally distributed. A geometric mean is obtained after log transformation of the data. In some cases, with sufficient data collection, a bimodal distribution may be observed. For example the acetylation of isoniazid in humans follows a bimodal distribution, indicating two populations consisting of fast acetylators and slow acetylators. In this study, if the data were obtained from subjects of whom all but one were fast acetylators, then the single datum for the slow acetlator might be considered an outlier (and possibly be discarded from the data analysis).

When a specific distribution is not known, it may be possible to use the bootstrap/jackknife method. A **bootstrap** is a paradoxical means of getting started on something when you need some of that something in order to get started. The concept derives from the phrase "**to pull oneself up by one's bootstrap**s". Rather than attributing an assumption to the distribution, the actual data collected will be used to extrapolate further about the larger population it represents. Instead of collecting more samples by actual experiment, one simply puts all the data into a "**virtual bag**" and randomly samples (not actually taking the original data out) from the bag until the desired number of samples is collected to yields a glimpse of what the population will be like. The method was a great innovation by Bradley Efron and is easily adapted to many applications with computer technology. The basic bootstrap method is essentially the same. The method has worked well and has been modified for many practical applications where assumption of specific distribution failed (Efron, Bradley, Tibshirani, 1993). It should be appreciated that the nature of the data from an original study is new and unknown. The greatest difficulty facing the investigator is characterizing the distribution and applying it to a proper model. The bootstrap method avoids the problem of assuming the wrong distribution. Statistical distribution is discussed with further application to **Pharmacokinetics**.

The normal, binomial, Poisson, chi-square distributions are frequently applied in statistics and engineering. Some distributions are related mathematically. References for further information are listed at the end of this appendix.

Statistical Analysis is referred to-'as a statistical test when the data are formulated for hypothesis testing'. The most common test involves the *Student's t-test*, which is a test of means of two groups assuming the same variance. If the variances are different, the Student's *t-test* will be a *t-test* with unequal variance. When the sample size increases to very large, the t-distribution approaches the normal distribution. The *t-test* becomes more powerful if the subjects meet the criteria for a paired *t-test*. The *F-test* is a simple test of variance of two groups. When more groups are involved, analysis of variance may be applied.

Statistics are broadly applied in pharmacokinetics. Special statistical methods have been developed to provide a platform for rational argument or decision making in accepting or rejecting a theory. The information generated in many controlled clinical studies is often sparse due to limited sample size (*e.g,* few subjects) and limited sampling (*e.g,* **few blood samples**). For this reason, all drugs under development in clinical studies are monitored for side effects and rare events. After **FDA approval** and **marketing, pharmacovigilance** is needed to assure safety in the larger population of patients who will be using the drug.

In testing the effect of a drug across different groups, the term interaction is often heard. An effect is a difference in treatment response, and an interaction is a difference in differences. Examples might be **treatment-by-centre interactions**, or treatment-by-gender interactions. When large interactions are noted, it is not appropriate to combine groups and make an overall assessment of the treatment effect statistically. **Clinical trials** often involve pivotal and supporting studies. An analysis that combines multiple studies to obtain an overall result, such as an overall estimate of the size of the treatment effect of a drug, is termed meta-analysis.

[J] HYPOTHESIS TESTING

Hypothesis testing is an objective way of analyzing data and determining whether the data support or reject the hypothesis postulated. For example, we might want to test the hypothesis that a given steroid causes a weight increase. We want to test this hypothesis using two groups of healthy volunteers, one group (treated) that took the given steroid and another (control) that took no drug. The two hypotheses generated are as follows:

H_0: **There is no difference in weight between the treated and control groups (null hypothesis).**

H_1: **There is a difference in weight between the treated and control groups (alternative hypothesis).**

The **Null Hypothesis** H_0, states that-'**there is no difference between the treatments**'. The **experimental data** will either reject or fail to reject (accept) the **Null Hypothesis**. If the **Null Hypothesis** is rejected, then the alternative hypothesis is accepted, since there are only two possibilities. A **simple hypothesis** testing data from two groups is the two-sample Student's t-test involving a control group and a treated group (the *t*-distribution approximates the normal distribution and is commonly used).

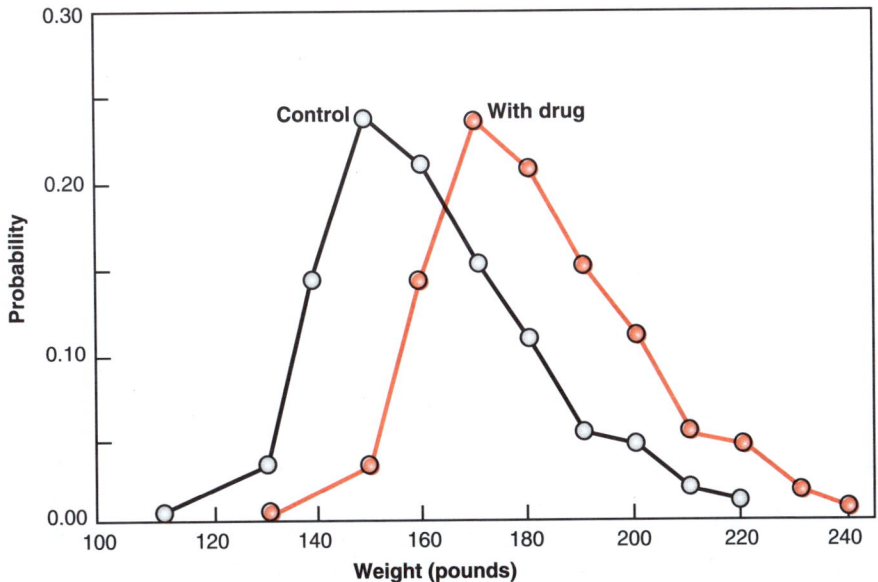

Fig. A-4 Hyothesis Testing Example

The data for the study (simulated) is shown in Figure A-4 using 120 students in the control and treated groups. The mean weight of the treated group is about 175 Ib, whereas the mean weight for the control group is about 155 lb. There is a shift to the right in the weight distribution of the treated group. However, a considerable overlapping (**shaded area**) in weights is observed, making it difficult to reject the null hypothesis. In practice, H_0 is rejected at a known level of uncertainty called the **level of significance**. A level of 5% ($\alpha = 0.01$) is considered statistically significant, and a level of 1% ($\alpha = 0.01$) is considered highly significant. Commonly, this level of significance is reported as P<0.05 or P<0.01, respectively, to indicate the different levels of significance. Because uncertainty is involved, whenever the null hypothesis is rejected or accepted, the level of significance is stated. A significance level of 25% (P<0.25) in the above example suggests that there is a 25% probability that the weight change is not due to drug treatment. A 25% probability is a level far too large to reject the H_0 with certainty. The level of significance is therefore related to the probability of incorrectly rejecting H_0 when it should have been accepted. This level of error is called Type I error. Whenever a decision is made, there is the possibility of making the wrong decision. Four possible decisions for a statistical test may be made (Table A.3). A type II error is committed when H_0 is rejected when it should have been accepted.

The probability of committing a Type I error is defined as the significance level of the statistical test, and is denoted as P or α (alpha). The probability of a Type II error, denoted as β (beta), can also be computed.

The **Power Test** determines the probability that the statistical test results in the rejection of the null hypothesis if H_0 is really false. The larger the power, the more sensitive are the tests. Because power is defined as $1-\alpha$ the larger the β-error (**Type II error**), the weaker is the power. The power of the test would equal $1-\beta$ for a particular power.

Table A.3. Decisions Based on a Statistical Test		
	ACCEPT NULL HYPOTHESIS (H_0)	**REJECT NULL HYPOTHESIS (H_0)**
H_0 true	Correct decision	Type I error
H_1 true	Type II error	Correct decision

To reduce Type I or Type II errors, the sample sizes need to be increased or the assay method improved. Because time, expense, and ethical concerns for performing a study are important issues, the investigator generally tries to keep the sample size (usually the number of subjects in a clinical study) to a minimum. The variability within the samples, number of samples (sample size), and desired level of significance will affect the power of the statistical test. Usually, the greater the variability within the samples, the larger will be the sample size needed to obtain sufficient power.

[K] ANALYSIS OF VARIANCE (ONE-WAY)

When more than two data sets are compared, **Analysis of Variance (ANOVA)** is used to determine the probability of the data sets being identical or different among groups. One-way analysis of variance is a method for testing the differences between the population means of k treatment groups, where each group i ($i =1,2,……k$) consists of n_i **observations** X_{ij} ($j =1,2,…..n_i$). for example, we may want to test whether there is a difference in the peak plasma level of a drug resulting from the administration of three different dosage forms- solution, capsule, and tablet. If we decide to have three groups of 20 patients per group $i=1,2,3, j=1,2,\ldots\ldots,20$, and decide to have three group will be X_{ij}. The formulas for calculation are as follows:

$$\text{Sum of observation in group} = \sum_{i}^{n_j} x_{ij}$$

$$\text{Total sum of squares SS} = \sum_{i}^{k} \sum_{j}^{n_j} x_{ij}^2 - \frac{\left(\sum_{i}^{k} \sum_{j}^{n} x_{ij}^2\right)}{\sum_{i} n_i}$$

$$\text{Total sum of squares TSS} = \sum_{i}^{k} \sum_{j}^{n_j} x_{ij}^2 - \frac{\left(\sum_{i}^{k} \sum_{j}^{n_j} x_{ij}^2\right)}{\sum_{i} n_i}$$

Error sum squares (ESS) = SS-TSS = total sum of squares – treatment sum of squares
The value of the F-statistic is Found to be:

$$F = \frac{DF_2 \times TSS}{DF_1 \times ESS} = \frac{TSS/DF_1}{ESS/DF_2}$$

Alternatively, F is expressed as the ratio of **Treatment Mean Squares (TMS)/Error Mean Squares (EMS).**

$$F = \frac{TSS/DF_1}{ESS/DF_2} = \frac{TMS}{EMS}$$

Error degrees of freedom $DF_1 = k-1$

Error degrees of freedom $DF_2 = \sum_{j=1}^{k} n_i - k$

The **ANOVA** employed depends on the objectives and design of the study. ANOVA methods can estimate the variance among different subjects (inter subject variability), groups, or treatments. Using ANOVA, the statistician determines whether to accept or reject the null hypothesis (H_0), deciding whether there is no significant difference (**accept H_0**) or there is a significant difference (reject H_0) between the data groups.

ANOVA is-'**a test for a difference in means between two or more groups**'. It is very similar to the *t-test*, which tests for a difference between two groups. It is applicable when several groups are involved. An ANOVA on two groups is analogous to as a *two*-**sample t-test. ANOVA** assumes that the groups have equal sample sizes for each group (as with t-test). If one rejects the null hypothesis in the ANOVA, one can conclude that the groups are not all equal, but the test does not yield any information on each pair of comparisons.

After completion of the study and statistical analysis of the data, the investigator must decide whether any statistically significant differences in the data groups have clinical relevance. For example, it may be possible to demonstrate that a new antihypertensive agent lowers the systolic blood pressure in patients by 10 mm Hg and that this effect is statistically significant (P<0.05) using the appropriate statistical test. From these results and statistical treatment of the data, the principal investigator must decide whether the study is clinically relevant and whether the drug will be efficacious for its intended use.

In clinical tests involving a comparison of a drug to a control, it is important to establish some criteria in advance with the clinicians. What is the size of the **difference (Δ)** that is considered clinically meaningful? How large should the sample size be in order to have adequate statistical power? If the variance is large, a large sample may be needed. On the other hand, "Over-powering" may occur if the study sample size is so large that an extremely small treatment effect could be found statistically significant but not clinically useful. When two similar studies testing the treatment effect of a drug found different results and conclusions, as is sometimes reported in the literature, it is important to look for study flaws and biases. If an estimate is biased, it means that it is not accurately estimating the true value (true mean, true median, true standard deviation, etc). It may be due to a flaw in the study design, conduct, or analysis. Any of these can shift the results in favor of either the new drug or the control. Is the drug tested in one of the studies using an old standard of care? A new drug believed by most physicians to be superior can influence the result. **Bias includes not blinding the study or having many dropouts, especially if the dropouts are due to the study drug**. The consequence of the study bias may lead to a drug that may be found statistically better than the control but not clinically important. **Clinical judgment** should be used to evaluate the magnitude of the treatment and eliminate over-powering. This is especially important for superiority trials of new drugs. **Most clinical trials** for regulatory purposes are quality checked or audited to assure accuracy. On the other hand, the literature or information published, although useful, may not be adequately reviewed or does not always meet statistical design requirements. It is important for the pharmacist to check the source of information and determine whether test methods are validated.

[L] POWER TEST

A type I error may be observed when the result of an ANOVA rejects the null hypothesis when it should have been accepted. The power of a statistical hypothesis test provides a high level of certainty that the correct decision was made-that is, to reject the null hypothesis when it is actually false. The power of a hypothesis test is the probability of not committing a Type II error. It is calculated by subtracting the probability of a Type II error from 1, usually expressed as

$$\text{Power} = 1 - P \text{ (Type II error)} = 1 - \beta$$

The values for the power test range from 0 to 1. Ideally, the values for the power test should have a high power or value close to 1. To calculate the power of a given test, it is necessary to specify a (the probability that the test will lead to the rejection of the hypothesis is true) and to specify a specific alternative hypothesis. Usually, a is set at 0.05. the power test is influenced by sample size and by intrasubject variability. For drugs whose bioavailability demonstrates high intrasubject variability (> 30% CV), a larger number of subjects (larger sample size) is required to obtain a high power (> 0.95).

[M] BIOEQUIVALENCE STUDIES

Statistics have wide application in bioequivalence studies for the comparison of drug bioavailability for two or more drug products. The FDA has published two Guidance for Industry for the **Statistical Determination of Bioequivalence (2001, 1992) that describes the comparison between a test (T) and reference (R) drug product. These trials are needed for approval of New or Generic Drugs, several investigational formulations may be used at various stages, or one formulation with several strengths must show equivalency by extent and rate** (*e.g.*, 2250-mg tablet versus 1 500- mg tablet, suspension versus capsule, immediate-release versus extended-release product). The blood levels of the drug are measured for both the new and the reference formulation. The derived pharmacokinetic parameters, such as **Maximum Concentration (C_{max})** and area under the curve (**AUC**) must meet accepted statistical criteria for the two drugs to be considered bioequivalent. **In Bioequivalence Trials, a 90% confidence interval of the ratio of the mean of the New Formulation to the Mean of the Old Formulation (test/Reference) is calculated**. That **Confidence Interval** critically needs to be completely within 0.80 to 1.25 for the drugs to be considered **Bioequivalent.** Adequate power should be built into the design and validated methods used for analysis of the samples. Typically, both the rate (reflected by C_{max}) and extent (**AUC**) are tested. The **ANOVA** may also reveal any sequence effects, period effects, treatment effects, or inter- and intrasubject variability. Because of the small subject population usually employed in bioequivalence studies, the **ANOVA** uses log-transformed data to make an inference about the difference of the two groups.

[N] PHARMACOKINETIC MODELS

In data analysis involving a model, the number of data points should exceed the number of parameters in the model with a sufficient degree of freedom. Otherwise, the model is unconstrained and the parameters estimated are not valid.

REFERENCES

Deming SN, Morgan SL: *Experimental Design: A Chemometric Approach*, **Elsevier,** London (UK), 1987

Efron, Bradely, Tibshirani RJ: *An Introduction to the Bootstrap*, **Chapman & Hall** New York, London 1993

FDA Guidance for Industry-*Statistical Approaches to Establishing Bioequivalence* [*www.fda.gov/cder/guidance, 2001*]

FDA Guidance for Industry-Statistical Procedures for Bioequivalence Studies Using a Standard Two-Treatment Crossover Design [*www.fda.gov/cder/guidance, 1992*]

Knapp RG, Miller MC III: *Clinical Epidermiology and Biostatistics.* Lippincott Williams & Wilkins, New York, 1992.

POPULAR DRUG AND PHARMACOKINETIC PARAMETERS

DRUG	ORAL AVAILABILITY (%)	URINARY EXCRETION (%)	BOUND IN PLASMA (%)	CLEARANCE[2] (mL/min)	VOLUME OF DISTRIBUTION (L)	HALF-LIFE (hr)	EFFECTIVE[3] CONCENTRATIONS	TOXIC CONCENTRATIONS
Acetaminophen	88±15	3±1	0	350±100	67±8	2.0±0.4	10-20µg/mL	>300µg/mL
Acyclovir	15-30	75±10	15±4	330±80	48±13	2.4±0.7		
Alendrenate	0.59 (0.58-0.98)						very long (related to bone turnover)	
Alprazolam	88±16	20	71±3	0.74±0.14 ml/min/kg	0.72±0.12 L/Kg	12±2	20-40 ng/mL	
Alteplase (TPA)	-	LOW	-	10±4 ml/min/kg	0.1±0.01 L/kg	0.08±0.04		
Amikacin		98	4	91±42	19±4	2.3±0.4		
Amoxicillin	93±10	86±8	18	180±28	15±2	1.7±0.3		
Amphotericin B		2-5	>90	32±14	53±36	18±7		
Ampicillin	62±17	82±10	18±2	270±50	20±5	1.3±0.2		
Aspirin[4]	68±3	1.4±1.2	49	650±80	11±2	0.25±0.3	See Salicyclic acid	
Atenolol	56±30	94±8	<5	170±14	67±11	6.1±2.0	1µg/mL	
Atropine	50	57±8	14-22	410±250	120±49	4.3±1.7		
Captopril	65	38±11	30±6	840±100	57±13	2.2±0.5	50 ng/mL	
Carbamazepine	>70	<1	74±3	89±37	98±26	15±5	6.5± 3 µg/mL	>9 µg/mL
Cephalexin	90±9	91±18	14±3	300±80	18±2	0.90±0.18		
Cephalothin		52	71±3	470±120	18±8	0.57±0.3		
Chloramphenicol	75-90	25±15	53±5	170±14	66±4	2.7±0.8	07 µg/mL	
Chlordiazepoxide[4]	100	<1	96.5±18	38±34	21±2	10±3		0.25 µg/mL
Chloroquine[4]	89±16	61±4	61±9	750±120	13,000±4600	8.9±3.1 days	15-30 ng/mL	
Chlorpropamide	>90	20±18	96±1	2.1±0.4	6.8±0.8	33±6		
Cimetidine	62±6	62±20	19	540±130	70±14	1.9±0.3	0.8 µg/mL	
Ciprofloxacin	60±12	65±12	40	420±84	130±28	4.1±0.9	0.2-2 ng/mL	
Clonidine	95	62±11	20	210±84	150±30	12±7	100-400 ng/mL	>400 ng/mL
Cyclosporine	23.7	<1	93±2	410±70	85±15	5.6±2	300-400 ng/mL	
Diazepam[4]	100	<1	98.7±0.2	27±4	77±20	43±13	>10 ng/mL	>35 ng/mL
Digitoxin	>90	32±15	97±1	3.9±1.3	38±10	6.7±1.7	>0.8 ng/mL	>2 ng/mL
Digoxin	70±13	60±11	25±5	130±67	440±150	39±13		
Diltiazem[4]	44±10	<4	78±3	840±280	220±85	3.7±1.2		
Diflunisal	90	6±3	99.9±0.01	0.1±0.02 mL/min/kg	0.1±0.02 L/kg	11±2		
Disopyramide	83±11	55±6	Dose-dependent	84±28	41±11	6.0±1.0	3 ± 1 µg/mL	>8 µg/mL

Drug								
Erythromycin	35±25	12±7	84±3	640±290	55±31	1.6±0.7		
Erythropoietein				7.88 mL/min	3.70 Per 1.73 m²	4.92		
Ethambutol	77±8	79±3	<5	600±60	110±14	3.1±0.4		>10 µg/mL
Ethosuximide	–	25±15	0	0.19±0.04 mL/min/kg	0.72±0.16 L/kg	45±8	40-100 µg/mL	
Famciclovir	77±8	74±9	<20	8.0±1.5	0.98±0.13	2.3±0.4		
Famotidine	45±14	67±15	17±7	7.1±1.7 mL/min/Kg	1.3±0.2 L/kg	2.6±1.0	13 ng/ml	
Fluoxetine	>60	<2.5	94	9.6±6.9	35±21	53±41		
Furosemide	61±17	66±7	98.8±0.2	140±30	7.7±1.4	1.5±0.1	<500 ng/mL	
Ganciclovir	3	73±31	1-2	4.6±1.8 mL/min/kg	1.1±0.3 L/kg	4.3±1.6		<25 µg/mL
Gentamicin	20-60	>90	<10	90±25	18±6	2-3		
Hydralazine		1-15	87	3900±900	105±70	1.0±0.3	100 ng/mL	
Imipramine[4]	40±12	<2	90.1±1.4	1050±280	1600±600	18±7	100-300 ng/mL	>1 µg/mL
Indinavir	98							
Indomethacin	18±5	15±8	90	140±30	18±5	2.4±0.4	0.3-3 µg/mL	>5 µg/mL
Labetalol	35±11	<5	50	1750±700	660±240	4.9±2.0	0.13 µg/mL	
Lidocaine	100	2±1	70±5	640±170	77±28	1.8±0.4	1.5-6 µg/mL	>6 µg/mL
Lithium	97±2	95±15	0	25±8	55±24	22±8	0.5-1.25 meq/L	>2 meq/L
Lomefloxacin	<5	65±9	10	3.3±0.5 mL/min/kg	2.3±0.3 L/kg	8.0±1.4		
Lovastatin		negligible	95	4-18 mL/min/kg	-	1.1-1.7 hr		
Meperidine	52±3	1-25	58±9	1200±350	310±60	3.2±0.8	0.4-0.7 µg/mL	10 µM
Methotrexate	70±27	48±18	34±8	150±60	39±13	7.2±2.1		
Metoprolol	38±14	10±3	11±1	1050±210	290±50	3.2±0.2	25 ng/mL	
Metronidazole[4]	99±8	10±2	10	90±20	52±7	8.5±2.9	3-6 µg/mL	
Mexiletine	87±13	4-15	63±3	6.3±2.7 mL/min/kg	4.9±0.5 L/kg	9.2±2.1 hr	0.5-2.0 µg/mL	>2.0 µg/mL
Midazolam	44±17	56±26	95±2	460±130	77±42	1.9±0.6		
Morphine	24±12	6-10	35±2	1600±700	230±60	1.9±0.5	65 ng/mL	
Moxalactam	–	76±12	50	120±30	19±6	2.1±0.7		
Notilmicin	–	80-90	<10	1.3±0.2 ml/min/kg	0.2±0.02 L/kg	2.3±0.7 hr		
Nifedipine	50±13	0	96±1	490±130	55±15	1.8±0.4	47 ± 20 ng/m	
Nortriptyline[4]	51±5	2±1	92±2	500±130	1300±300	31±13	50-140 ng/mL	>500 ng/mL
Phenobarbital	10±11	24±5	51±5	4.3±0.9	38±2	4.1±0.8 days	10-25 µg/mL	>30 µg/mL
Phenytoin	90±3	2	89±23	Dose-Dependent	45±3	Dose-Dependent	>10 µg/mL	>20 µg/mL

Drug								
Pravastain	18±8	47±7	43-48	3.5±2.4 ml/min/kg	0.46±0.04 L/kg	1.8±0.8 hr		
Prazosin	68±17	<1	95±1	210±20	42±9	2.9±0.8		
Procainamide[4]	83±16	67±8	16±5	350-840	130±20	3.0±0.6	3-14 µg/mL	>14 µg/mL
Ptopranolol[4]	26±10	<0.5	87±6	840±210	270±40	3.9±0.4	20 ng/mL	
Pyridostogmine	14±3	80-90		600±120	77±21	1.9±0.2	50-100 ng/mL	
Quinidine[4]	80±15	18±5	87±3	330±130	190±80	6.2±1.8	2-6 µg/mL	>8 µg/mL
Ranitidine	52±11	69±6	15±3	730±80	91±28	2.1±0.2	100 ng/mL	
Ribavirin	45±5	35±8	0	5±1.0 ml/min/kg	9.3±1.5 L/kg	28±7 hr		
Rifampin	<5	7±3	89±1	240±110	68±25	3.5±0.8~3 hr		
Ritonavir	<5		high (AAG)	*<988 L/hr	*<1503 L	7-12 hr (beta) (1.38 hr)		
Saquinavir			high (AAG					
Salicylic acid	100	2-30	80-90[5]	14[5]	12±2	10-15[5]	150-300 µg/mL	>200 µg/mL
Simvastatin	<5	negligible	94	7.6 ml/min/kg	–	1.9 hr		
Sotalol	90-100	>75	0	2.6±0.5 ml/min/kg	2.0±0.4 L/kg	12±3 hr		
Sulfamethoxazole	100	14±2	62±5	22±3	15±1.4	10±5		
Sulfisoxazole	9.6±14	49±8	91±1	23±3.5	10.5±1.4	6.6±0.7		
Sumatriptan	14±5 (oral) 97±16 (SQ)	22±4	14-21	16±2 ml/min/kg	0.65±0.1 L/kg	1.9±0.3 hr		
Tamoxifen	–	<1	>98	1.4 ml/min/kg	50-60 L/kg	4-11 days		
Terbutaline	14±2	56±4	20	240±40	125±15	14±2	23±1.8 ng/mL	
Tetracycline	77	58±8	65±3	120±20	105±6	11±1.5		
Theophylline	96±8	18±3	56±4	48±21	35±11	8.1±2.4	10-20 µg/mL	>20 µg/mL
Tobramycin	90	<10		77	18±6	2.2±0.1		
Tocainide	89±5	38±7	10±15	180±35	210±15	14±2	6-15 µg/m	
Tolbutamide	93±10	0	96±1	17±3	7±1	5.9±1.4	80-240 µg/mL	
Trimethoprim	100	69±17	44	150±40	130±15	11±1.4		
Tubocurarine		63±35	50±8	135±42	27±8	2.0±1.1	0.6 ± 0.2 µg/mL	
Valproic acid	100±10	1.8±2.4	93±1	7.7±1.4	9.1±2.8	14±3	30-100 µg/mL	>150 µg/mL
Vancomycin		79±11	30±10	98±7	27±4	5.6±1.8		
Verapamil	22±8 (oral) 35±13 (Sublingual)	<3	90±2	15±6 ml/min/kg	5.0±2.1 L/kg	4.0±1.5 hr	120 ± 20 ng/mL	
Warfarin	93±8	<2	99±1	3.2±1.7	9.8±4.2	37±15	2.2 ± 0.4 µg/mL	
Zidovudine	63±13	18±5	<25	26±6 Ml/min/kg	1.4±0.4 L/kg	1.1±0.2hr		
Zalcitabine	88±17	65±17	<4	4.1±1.2 Ml/min/kg	0.53±0.13 L/kg	2.0 ±0.8 hr		

The values in the table represent the parameters determined when the drug is administered to healthy volunteers ot to patients who are generally free from disease except for the condition for which the drug is being prescribed. The values presented here are adapted, with permission, from Hardman JG: Design and optimization of dosage regimens: Pharmacokinetic data In: Goodman and Gliman's The Pharmacological Basis of Therapeutics. 9th ed. Gilman AG et al (editors). McGraw-Hill, 1995. This source must be consulted for the effects of disease states on the pertinent pharmacokinetic parameters.

[2] For a standard 70-kg person

[3] No pharmacodynamic values are given for antibiotics since these vary depending upon the infecting organism.

[4]One or more metabolites are active. Clearance given for aspirin is for conversion to the active metabolite, salicylic acid; see that compound for further clearance data.

[5]The values are within the therapeutic range for drugs exhibiting dose-dependent pharmacokinetics.

[6]Volume of distribution and clearance determined orally (when F is unknown, CI/F, or VD/F) are listed as less than actual since F may be less than I.

[7]Effective levels for antibiotics are variable depending on the susceptibility of the microorganisms.

[8]Generally, the beta half-life is listed, but it may be essential to consult the alpha half-life if the effective concentration is high or the distributive phase is long.

[9]The percent of urinary drug excretion is 100 fe, fe is the fraction of drug excreted unchanged, "100-100 fe" yields the percent of drug eliminated by other routes, often assumed to be metabolism. It is worth noting that in some cases the mass balance may be off, and sometimes biliary excretion is significant.

[10]For simplicity, most PK parameters are listed without consideration of the curvilinear phase which is present for most drugs.

[11]Some parameters are listed on a per kilogram basis, whereas others are parameters based on average BW or body surface reported in the study.

From Katzung BG: Basic & Clinical Pharmacology. 7th ed. Norwalk, CT, Appleton & Lange, 1998.

Physician's Desk Reference, 1997

Dirithromycin:

Sides GD et al, Anti Micr. Chem. 31; Supp C: P65-75, 1993

Erythropoietin:

Jensen-JD et al; J-Am-Soc-Nephrol. 1994 Aug; 5(2); 177-85

Indinavir:

Lin JH et al: Drug Metab Dispos 1996 Oct; 24(10): 1111-1120

Alendronate:

Gertz BJ, Holland SD, Kine WF, Matuszewski BK, Freeman A, Quan H, Lasseter KC, Mucklow JC, Porras: Clin Pharmacol Ther, 1995 Sep (3): 288-298

Protease inhibitors:

Barry M, Gibbons S, Back D, Mulcahy F; Clin Pharmacokinet 1997 Mar; 32(3): 194-209

Zidovudine, zalcitabine, and saquinavir:

Vanhove GF, Kastrissios H, Gries JM, Verotta D, Park K, Collier AC, Squires K, Sheiner LB, Blaschke; Antimicrob Agents Chemother 1997 Nov; 2428-2432

Appendix

8

HELSINKI DECLARATION [WORLD MEDICAL ASSOCIATION OF HELSINKI]

ETHICAL PRINCIPLES FOR MEDICAL RESEARCH INVOLVING HUMAN SUBJECTS

- Adopted by the 18th WMA General Assembly, Helsinki, Finland, June 1964; amended by the 29th WMA General Assembly, Tokyo,
- Japan, October 1975; 35th WMA General Assembly, Venice, Italy, October 1983; 41st WMA General Assembly, Hong Kong,
- September 1989; 48th WMA General Assembly, Somerset West, Republic of South Africa, October 1996, and the 52nd WMA
- General Assembly, Edinburgh, Scotland, October 2000

A. Introduction

1. The World Medical Association has developed the Declaration of Helsinki as a statement of ethical principles to provide guidance to physicians and other participants in medical research involving human subjects. Medical research involving human subjects includes research on identifiable human material or identifiable data.

2. It is the duty of the physician to promote and safeguard the health of the people. The physician's knowledge and conscience are dedicated to the fulfillment of this duty.

3. The Declaration of Geneva of the World Medical Association binds the physician with the words, "The health of my patient will be my first consideration," and the International Code of Medical Ethics declares that, "A physician shall act only in the patient's interest when providing medical care which might have the effect of weakening the physical and mental condition of the patient."

4. Medical progress is based on research which ultimately must rest in part on experimentation involving human subjects.

5. In medical research on human subjects, considerations related to the well-being of the human subject should take precedence over the interests of science and society.

6. The primary purpose of medical research involving human subjects is to improve prophylactic, diagnostic and therapeutic procedures and the understanding of the aetiology and pathogenesis of disease. Even the best proven prophylactic, diagnostic, and therapeutic methods must

continuously be challenged through research for their effectiveness, efficiency, accessibility and quality.

7. In current medical practice and in medical research, most prophylactic, diagnostic and therapeutic procedures involve risks and burdens.

8. Medical research is subject to ethical standards that promote respect for all human beings and protect their health and rights. Some research populations are vulnerable and need special protection. The particular needs of the economically and medically disadvantaged must be recognized. Special attention is also required for those who cannot give or refuse consent for themselves, for those who may be subject to giving consent under duress, for those who will not benefit personally from the research and for those for whom the research is combined with care.

9. Research Investigators should be aware of the ethical, legal and regulatory requirements for research on human subjects in their own countries as well as applicable international requirements. No national ethical, legal or regulatory requirement should be allowed to reduce or eliminate any of the protections for human subjects set forth in this Declaration.

B. Basic principles for all medical research

10. It is the duty of the physician in medical research to protect the life, health, privacy, and dignity of the human subject.

11. Medical research involving human subjects must conform to generally accepted scientific principles, be based on a thorough knowledge of the scientific literature, other relevant sources of information, and on adequate laboratory and, where appropriate, animal experimentation.

12. Appropriate caution must be exercised in the conduct of research which may affect the environment, and the welfare of animals used for research must be respected.

13. The design and performance of each experimental procedure involving human subjects should be clearly formulated in an experimental protocol. This protocol should be submitted for consideration, comment, guidance, and where appropriate, approval to a specially appointed ethical review committee, which must be independent of the investigator, the sponsor or any other kind of undue influence. This independent committee should be in conformity with the laws and regulations of the country in which the research experiment is performed. The committee has the right to monitor ongoing trials. The researcher has the obligation to provide monitoring information to the committee, especially any serious adverse events. The researcher should also submit to the committee, for review, information regarding funding, sponsors, institutional affiliations, other potential conflicts of interest and incentives for subjects.

14. The research protocol should always contain a statement of the ethical considerations involved and should indicate that there is compliance with the principles enunciated in this Declaration.

15. Medical research involving human subjects should be conducted only by scientifically qualified persons and under the supervision of a clinically competent medical person. The responsibility for the human subject must always rest with a medically qualified person and never rest on the subject of the research, even though the subject has given consent.

16. Every medical research project involving human subjects should be preceded by careful assessment of predictable risks and burdens in comparison with foreseeable benefits to the

subject or to others. This does not preclude the participation of healthy volunteers in medical research. The design of all studies should be publicly available.

17. Physicians should abstain from engaging in research projects involving human subjects unless they are confident that the risks involved have been adequately assessed and can be satisfactorily managed. Physicians should cease any investigation if the risks are found to outweigh the potential benefits or if there is conclusive proof of positive and beneficial results.

18. Medical research involving human subjects should only be conducted if the importance of the objective outweighs the inherent risks and burdens to the subject. This is especially important when the human subjects are healthy volunteers.

19. Medical research is only justified if there is a reasonable likelihood that the populations in which the research is carried out stand to benefit from the results of the research.

20. The subjects must be volunteers and informed participants in the research project.

21. The right of research subjects to safeguard their integrity must always be respected. Every precaution should be taken to respect the privacy of the subject, the confidentiality of the patient's information and to minimize the impact of the study on the subject's physical and mental integrity and on the personality of the subject.

22. In any research on human beings, each potential subject must be adequately informed of the aims, methods, sources of funding, any possible conflicts of interest, institutional affiliations of the researcher, the anticipated benefits and potential risks of the study and the discomfort it may entail. The subject should be informed of the right to abstain from participation in the study or to withdraw consent to participate at any time without reprisal. After ensuring that the subject has understood the information, the physician should then obtain the subject's freely-given informed consent, preferably in writing. If the consent cannot be obtained in writing, the non-written consent must be formally documented and witnessed.

23. When obtaining informed consent for the research project the physician should be particularly cautious if the subject is in a dependent relationship with the physician or may consent under duress. In that case the informed consent should be obtained by a well-informed physician who is not engaged in the investigation and who is completely independent of this relationship.

24. For a research subject who is legally incompetent, physically or mentally incapable of giving consent or is a legally incompetent minor, the investigator must obtain informed consent from the legally authorized representative in accordance with applicable law. These groups should not be included in research unless the research is necessary to promote the health of the population represented and this research cannot instead be performed on legally competent persons.

25. When a subject deemed legally incompetent, such as a minor child, is able to give assent to decisions about participation in research, the investigator must obtain that assent in addition to the consent of the legally authorized representative.

26. Research on individuals from whom it is not possible to obtain consent, including proxy or advance consent, should be done only if the physical/mental condition that prevents obtaining informed consent is a necessary characteristic of the research population. The specific reasons for involving research subjects with a condition that renders them unable to give informed consent should be stated in the experimental protocol for consideration and approval of the

review committee. The protocol should state that consent to remain in the research should be obtained as soon as possible from the individual or a legally authorized surrogate.

27. Both authors and publishers have ethical obligations. In publication of the results of research, the investigators are obliged to preserve the accuracy of the results. Negative as well as positive results should be published or otherwise publicly available. Sources of funding, institutional affiliations and any possible conflicts of interest should be declared in the publication. Reports of experimentation not in accordance with the principles laid down in this Declaration should not be accepted for publication.

C. Additional principles for medical research combined with medical care

28. The physician may combine medical research with medical care, only to the extent that the research is justified by its potential prophylactic, diagnostic or therapeutic value. When medical research is combined with medical care, additional standards apply to protect the patients who are research subjects.

29. The benefits, risks, burdens and effectiveness of a new method should be tested against those of the best current prophylactic, diagnostic, and therapeutic methods. This does not exclude the use of placebo, or no treatment, in studies where no proven prophylactic, diagnostic or therapeutic method exists.

30. At the conclusion of the study, every patient entered into the study should be assured of access to the best proven prophylactic, diagnostic and therapeutic methods identified by the study.

31. The physician should fully inform the patient which aspects of the care are related to the research. The refusal of a patient to participate in a study must never interfere with the patient–physician relationship.

32. In the treatment of a patient, where proven prophylactic, diagnostic and therapeutic methods do not exist or have been ineffective, the physician, with informed consent from the patient, must be free to use unproven or new prophylactic, diagnostic and therapeutic measures, if in the physician's judgement it offers hope of saving life, reestablishing health or alleviating suffering. Where possible, these measures should be made the object of research, designed to evaluate their safety and efficacy. In all cases, new information should be recorded and, where appropriate, published. The other relevant guidelines of this Declaration should be followed.

INDEX